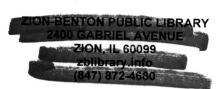

D1266093

"The story Rosner and Markowitz tell of generations of children gravely damaged by promiscuous dispersal of lead, and the persistent attempts made to evade responsibility for the harms caused, is both true and shocking. This book will not just educate future environmental and health leaders, it should outrage them."

RICHARD J. JACKSON, MD, MPH, Professor and Chair, Environmental Health Sciences, UCLA Fielding School of Public Health

"Can being poor justify differing standards for research or a focus merely on harm reduction and the politically feasible? Markowitz and Rosner make the compelling case that in public health the practical and possible may in the end be immoral and dangerous, and a consequence of the war on science. A necessary read for anyone who cares about public health, the role of government, children, medical experimentation and environmental justice."

SUSAN M. REVERBY, McLean Professor in the History of Ideas and Professor of Women's and Gender Studies, Wellesley College

"Lead poisoning remains a tragedy (and scandal) of immense proportions, and the authors utilize new sources—including previously unexamined court records—to tell a story that is as gripping as it is important."

ROBERT N. PROCTOR, Professor of the History of Science at Stanford University and author of *Cancer Wars*

"Markowitz and Rosner have majestically woven the key characters and elements of the history of lead poisoning into a captivating narrative that exposes a tremendous and terrifying truth; unless it serves the needs of private enterprise, public health is incapable of controlling the causes of chronic disease and disability. In place of prevention, we have settled for partial solutions. Everyone who has an interest in public health, health policy or history should read this book."

BRUCE LANPHEAR, MD, MPH, Clinician Scientist, Child & Family Research Institute BC Children's Hospital and Professor of Health Sciences, Simon Fraser University, Vancouver, BC

Lead Wars

Lead Wars

The Politics of Science and the Fate of America's Children

GERALD MARKOWITZ AND DAVID ROSNER

University of California Press

BERKELEY   LOS ANGELES   LONDON

Milbank Memorial Fund

NEW YORK

University of California Press, one of the most distinguished university presses in the United States, enriches lives around the world by advancing scholarship in the humanities, social sciences, and natural sciences. Its activities are supported by the UC Press Foundation and by philanthropic contributions from individuals and institutions. For more information, visit www.ucpress.edu.

The Milbank Memorial Fund is an endowed operating foundation that engages in nonpartisan analysis, study, research, and communication on significant issues in health policy. In the Fund's own publications, in reports, films, or books it publishes with other organizations, and in articles it commissions for publication by other organizations, the Fund endeavors to maintain the highest standards for accuracy and fairness. Statements by individual authors, however, do not necessarily reflect opinions or factual determinations of the Fund. For more information, visit www.milbank.org.

University of California Press
Berkeley and Los Angeles, California

University of California Press, Ltd.
London, England

Library of Congress Cataloging-in-Publication Data
Markowitz, Gerald E.
Lead wars : the politics of science and the fate of
    America's children / Gerald Markowitz and David Rosner.
        p. cm.   (California/Milbank books on health and the public ; 24)
    Includes bibliographical references and index.
    ISBN 978-0-520-27325-2 (cloth : alk. paper) :
        1. Lead Poisoning—history—United States. 2. Child—United States.
3. Environmental Exposure—United States.   4. History, 20th
Century—United States.   5. Politics—United States.   6. Public
Health—history—United States.
    QV 11 AA1   2013
    363.738/492— dc23

                                                    2012042916

Manufactured in the United States of America
22   21   20   19   18   17   16   15   14   13
10   9   8   7   6   5   4   3   2   1

For Andrea and Kathy

And

*In memory of John Rosen, MD, whose life was
dedicated to protecting children and their families
from the scourge of lead poisoning.*

Contents

Foreword

The Milbank Memorial Fund is an endowed operating foundation that works to improve health by helping decision makers in the public and private sectors acquire and use the best available evidence to inform policy for health care and population health. The Fund has engaged in nonpartisan analysis, study, research, and communication since its inception in 1905.

Lead Wars: The Politics of Science and the Fate of America's Children, by Gerald Markowitz and David Rosner, is the twenty-fourth book in the series California/Milbank Books on Health and the Public. The publishing partnership between the Fund and the University of California Press encourages the synthesis and communication of findings from research and experience that could contribute to more effective health policy.

Markowitz and Rosner's first book published in the California/Milbank series, *Deceit and Denial: The Deadly Politics of Industrial Pollution,* provided the early history of the lead industry's efforts to sell its product while knowing the devastating health effects it had on those exposed to it, particularly factory workers employed in lead-based industries and children living in homes decorated with lead paint. In *Lead Wars,* the authors reveal how this preventable, century-long public health scourge continues to plague children because partial removal of lead from homes—a process that proponents claim yields safe levels of lead—has been the chosen policy over complete abatement. While children rarely die of lead poisoning today, their exposure to "safe" levels of lead, instead of being protective, has caused them irreparable damage in the form of neurological, physiological, and behavioral problems.

Lead Wars underscores the present-day challenge of public health, with the field's shift of focus from prevention to harm reduction in the face of declining resources, lack of political mandate, and questionable professional will. As a result of the authors' thorough research and analysis, this book will provide compelling reading for historians, sociologists, public health officials, ethicists, environmentalists, and anyone else interested in the effects that public policies have on people's health and the environment.

Carmen Hooker Odom
President, Milbank Memorial Fund
Samuel L. Milbank
Chairman, Milbank Memorial Fund

Preface

In 1996 the City of New York Law Department asked us if we would evaluate a huge cache of documents they had received on lead poisoning and the lead industry. Several families whose children had been injured by lead paint used in some of the city's public housing had sued the City; the City, in turn, had filed a suit against the lead industry, claiming that the industry bore some responsibility for injuries to these children. Through the discovery process the City had now amassed a roomful of documents that were drawn largely from the Lead Industries Association, the trade association for manufacturers of lead paint and other lead-bearing products. What, the City wanted to know, was in these voluminous papers it had accumulated? Could we help them figure out what these records showed about the history of lead, lead pigment, lead poisoning, and what the industry knew of lead's dangers? Thus began a journey into the world of childhood lead poisoning that led ultimately to the writing of this book.

What we found in that roomful of material and the further investigations it spurred became the basis for part of our earlier book, *Deceit and Denial: The Deadly Politics of Industrial Pollution.* That account of industry's role in the development of a public-health tragedy would not have been possible without litigation, which brought to light literally hundreds of thousands of pages of company documents. In fact, without the cases, historians would never have seen internal memos and minutes of meetings in which company representatives from the National Lead or Sherwin-Williams companies, among others, discussed among themselves the dangers that lead paint posed to children as early as the 1920s. Nor would we have been able to learn of marketing campaigns aimed at counteracting public concerns over the dangers of lead—ads claiming lead paint was safe, sanitary, and useful on children's walls, furniture, and the like.

The documents gave us a new perspective on the history of lead poisoning, especially childhood lead poisoning, and its effects. The immediate fruit of our efforts was a lengthy affidavit that became part of the New York City case and then was quickly incorporated in other legal actions that, by the end of 2002, were under way in Chicago, New York, Buffalo, San Francisco, St. Louis, Milwaukee, and other cities around the country. Some of these cases were quickly dismissed by judges, but others were allowed to go forward. We were contacted and agreed to serve as expert witnesses in a number of these suits and, subsequently, other ones.

As we were preparing *Deceit and Denial*, the Attorney General's Office of Rhode Island asked if we would serve as historical consultants and, possibly, expert witnesses, in what would prove to be a groundbreaking lawsuit against the lead pigment industry.[1] After years of document review and preparation, we were each deposed for many days and then appeared on the stand as experts for six days each. The jury verdict in favor of the State was exhilarating for us: history, we saw, had played an important role in addressing one of public health's oldest and most frustrating epidemics—childhood lead poisoning. Two years later, however, Rhode Island's Supreme Court overturned the jury verdict, reasoning that the case had been brought to court under the wrong law.[2] Controlling the lead poisoning disaster, like resolving so many other environmental problems that currently plague the nation, would require more than history and good science.

In 2006 we were asked to testify about the history of lead poisoning in Maryland's House of Delegates in conjunction with a hearing on proposed legislation. Lead poisoning had a special resonance in Maryland at the time because of the continuing epidemic that affected Baltimore's children in particular and because of a highly controversial court case that had attracted national attention and was still fresh in the minds of community advocates, researchers, and legislators. This case, which revolved around research conducted at Johns Hopkins University involving more than a hundred African American children, is a leitmotif that runs through this book. As we looked into the case (in which we had played no role) and the circumstances behind it, we realized that it offered a window into the broader arguments about lead poisoning, society, and the emerging scientific evidence on the harmful health effects of relatively low-level exposure to various pollutants, lead among them.

If the history of lead poisoning has taught us anything, it is that the worlds we as a society construct, or at least allow to be built in our name, to a large extent determine how we live and how we die. The social, economic, political, and physical environments humans create bring about specific diseases that are emblematic of these conditions. If poverty, for example, and great disparities of wealth result in those on the bottom of the social scale living in crowded conditions without access to pure water, adequate sanitation, or pure air, we can expect infectious and communicable diseases to predominate as they did in nineteenth-century American cities. If we systematically pollute our water and air, we can expect chronic diseases emblematic of the late twentieth century to predominate.

Lead poisoning is a classic example of what happens when we take a material that was once buried deep underground and with which humans rarely had contact and introduce it widely into humans' ecology. In the 1920s, the additive for gasoline, tetraethyl lead, was called a "gift of God" by an industry intent on profiting from it. Despite warnings at the time that this industrial toxin might pollute the planet, more than a half century passed before it was finally removed from gasoline. In the 1920s and 1930s, asbestos was touted as a "miracle mineral" despite its identification as a cause of fibrosis and cancers among industrial workers. Yet it too was broadly introduced into our homes, schools, and workplaces with little or no controls. From the depths of the Depression through the Cold War years, the tobacco industry used physicians themselves to sell cigarettes, promoting smoking as a means to reduce stress and enhance one's personal appeal. In the 1940s and 1950s, DDT (marketed as "Doomsday for Pests" and even sold to consumers in a Sherwin-Williams paint called "Pestroy"),[3] PCBs, and a variety of other poisonous chlorinated hydrocarbons were poured over our farmlands and began appearing in the tissue and blood of virtually all animals, people included, the world over. Today, bisphenol A, a proven endocrine disruptor, has been used in a wide variety of consumer products, including baby bottles, superglue, and water bottles, leading to the discovery that, like PCBs, it is in virtually all of us. Few of the synthetic materials that have been introduced into our environment and therefore into our bodies have been tested for their long-term health effects. Even more troubling, we are often not sure how to go about doing the appropriate testing or evaluating whatever data we accumulate.

This book is about an ongoing grand human experiment in which we as a society are unwitting subjects. It is about a test that is taking place on all of us, a test of thousands of existing materials and chemicals, like mercury and PCBs, and new chemicals and materials whose safety is largely unproven and whose effects are unknown. None of the industries that are introducing these new chemicals and materials have told us that they are unsure of the potential harm these products may cause, nor have we consented to be part of this "study."

We tell of this grand experiment through the modern history of the oldest and perhaps most widely dispersed environmental toxin, lead, a material that has ofttimes been marketed as an essential ingredient in industrial society. For the past hundred years mining concerns, pigment manufacturers, the auto and chemical industries, and a host of other companies have based their profits on this material. But for the past hundred years it has also been known that lead was killing workers in the factories that used it and children in the homes that were painted with it. Now scientists are learning that even those adults who thought they had escaped its immediate effects are at higher risk of heart disease, kidney damage, and even dementia. In *Deceit and Denial*, we detailed the early history of the industry's knowledge of lead's dangers, showing how lead was sold to the American public through advertisements and marketing campaigns that "catered to the children" and portrayed lead products as essential to American life.

This new book takes a wider view. It attempts to show how, in the case of lead, growing scientific understanding of the effects of the grand experiment has led to the "Lead Wars" of the title—sharp contests among advocates for children's well-being, the lead industry and other interests that have played out in federal, state, and local government; the media; the courts; and the university. These contests have involved everything from the meaning of disease, primary prevention, and abatement to who should bear responsibility for risk and poisoning in the nation. For a century, children, poisoned primarily by leaded gasoline fumes and lead paint in their homes, have borne the overwhelming burden of this grand experiment in the form of permanent brain damage, school failure, loss of intelligence, and even death.

In these contests over lead exposure the public health profession has played a critical role, and it accordingly has a prominent position in this book; the struggles within it offer a microcosm of the contending forces as they have played out in the larger society over how best to regulate our environment and how to protect our children. As we showed in our earlier work, the lead industry ensured that children would be forced, as one physician put it, "to live in a lead world."[4] But the task of protecting children was left to a public health profession divided within itself that, despite some remarkable successes, has neither the resources nor the authority to do what's needed on its own. The remedies that do exist have so far proven to be politically unfeasible. In the meantime, the nation continues to sacrifice thousands of children yearly, deeming them not worthy of our protection.

Acknowledgments

The journey we have taken over the past decade writing about the lead wars has given us the opportunity to meet and work with an extraordinary group of dedicated people. We have gotten to know and to learn from public health scientists who, at various times, have been invaluable guides through the maze of the science and politics as well as the moral and ethical dimensions of our story. We are indebted to the people we have interviewed and who provided us with primary documents, including minutes of meetings at the National Institutes of Health (NIH), the U.S. Environmental Protection Agency (EPA), and other government agencies and public forums.

Paul Mushak was particularly helpful, forwarding boxes of documents from his personal files as well as providing us with extremely useful interviews. He generously and quickly responded to our numerous requests for information and clarification as we drafted portions of our book. Bruce Lanphear has also been an invaluable source of information and critical comment. He twice read the entire manuscript and provided detailed and thoughtful criticisms that have proved enormously important to us. Dave Jacobs, whose work with the U.S. Department of Housing and Urban Development (HUD) was a critical part of lead's history but largely lies outside of this account, was another extremely generous source. We spent days in his home sorting through the files he had accumulated from his years at HUD as well as other boxes of material of his wife, Kathryn R. Mahaffey, whose work on the dangers of mercury, lead, and other heavy metals while at various government agencies (including the National Institute for Occupational Safety and Health, the National Institute of Environmental Health Sciences, the U.S. Food and Drug Administration, and the EPA), deserves its own special attention. We will never forget

Dave's generosity, despite his still-recent loss. Don Ryan, founding executive director of the Alliance to End Childhood Lead Poisoning, and whose career we briefly outline, was another important source and generous colleague. He too gave unstintingly of his time, documents, and insights. One of the special pleasures we had was visiting Jane Lin-Fu at her home in suburban Washington, D.C. The day we spent with her provided us with invaluable information and perspectives on her efforts to awaken the federal government to the lead-poisoning epidemic. Herbert Needleman, of course, is a hero for public health practitioners, both for his pioneering research as well as his willingness to confront powerful forces that sought to undermine his work. We are forever grateful for his advice over the years. Two of the early pioneers, then young researchers, Philip Landrigan and Ellen Silbergeld, were always supportive and enthusiastic about our efforts, helping us understand how important it was to get the science right and always explaining how their scientific work was part of a broader effort to improve the lives of Americans.

Over the years, chance encounters played a role that could not possibly be predicted. New York's subway system, always a source of amusements and interactions among the city's citizens, led us to strike up morning conversations with Robert Mellins, a professor of pediatrics at Columbia. Through these discussions we learned that he began his career with the U.S. Public Health Service in Chicago, documenting and treating lead-poisoned children. We had referred to his work, but only through the happy accident of meeting him on the 7:30 AM Broadway local did we put two and two together. He soon sent us his personal files from the early 1950s, which again gave us insight into the importance of lead in the lives of pediatricians and public health workers during that decade and beyond.

It is not uncommon to hear plaintiffs' attorneys be denigrated as "ambulance chasers" solely interested in exploiting the legal system and their clients. But over the years we have developed a very different view of plaintiffs' lawyers, many of whom decided to represent workers, children, and consumers, people who otherwise would never have had a voice in the courts or the history books. In fact, many of the lawyers we met are truly public health advocates dedicated to their clients, particularly the children. Neil Leifer, Jack McConnell (who has since been appointed by President Obama as a federal district court judge for the District of Rhode Island), Fidelma Fitzpatrick, Robert McConnell, and Jonathan Orent not only played central roles in the historic Rhode Island lawsuit but also were critical in providing poisoned children and their parents a public voice in what all too easily could have been a closed discussion among professionals, politicians, and industry lawyers. We are so grateful for their willingness to provide documents and oral histories of their experiences. It was a special pleasure to meet with Sheldon Whitehouse, then attorney general of Rhode Island and now U.S. senator from that state. Laura Holcolm, the senior paralegal for Motley Rice, deserves special mention. Her vast knowledge of the lead industry's archive is itself truly irreplaceable. Her memory, generosity, friendship, humor, and good will were critical to our research.

We asked attorneys for the lead industry for interviews but they politely declined. Suzanne Shapiro and Saul Kerpelman, the attorneys who first brought suit against Johns Hopkins, were forthcoming and generous with their time and documents. Gerson Smoger, the main attorney in a historic lawsuit by citizens of Herculaneum, Missouri, against Fluor Corporation, which owned the lead smelter that polluted the town, provided us with unfettered access to important documents regarding the history of the Lead Industries Association, the International Lead Zinc Research Organization, and the smelter industry.

This is the third book we have published with the University of California Press and the Milbank Memorial Fund Series on Health and the Public. The series began under the leadership of Dr. Dan Fox, then president of Milbank, and Lynne Withey, editor and, later, director of the University of California Press. It continued under the leadership of Carmen Hooker Odom, president of Milbank, and Hannah Love, associate editor for health at UC Press. What makes this series attractive to us is its unusually rigorous and fruitful review process. Initially, the press went through its traditional anonymous review procedure, and we are grateful to the external reviewers. We are particularly grateful for the second part of the review process, in which Milbank sent this manuscript to thirteen scholars, legislators, and lead experts; they provided written reviews, and most then spent a full day with us in New York City going over their comments in detail. All of us who participated in this session came out of it recognizing how special this process was. The participants were Heidi Bresnahan, director of publications at Milbank; Jonathan Cobb, editor; Daniel M. Fox, president emeritus of Milbank; Nicholas Freudenberg, distinguished professor, Hunter College School of Health Sciences, City University of New York (CUNY); Richard N. Gottfried, chair, Health Committee, New York State Assembly; Pete Grannis, first deputy comptroller, Office of the New York State Comptroller; Sheldon Krimsky, now Zicklin Professor, Brooklyn College, CUNY; Bruce P. Lanphear, professor of public health, Simon Fraser University; Susan E. Lederer, Robert Turell Professor of Medical History and Bioethics, University of Wisconsin–Madison; Jane Lin-Fu, now retired from the U.S. Children's Bureau and the U.S. Public

Health Service; John J. McConnell Jr., judge, U.S. District Court for the district of Rhode Island; Carmen Hooker Odom, president of Milbank; Samuel K. Roberts, associate professor of history, Columbia University; Charles K. Scott, chair, Labor Health and Social Services Committee, Wyoming Senate; Tara Strome, publications associate at Milbank; and Christian S. Warren, associate professor of history, Brooklyn College, CUNY. In addition, Ilene Abala, Kathleen Bachynski, Elisa Gonzalez, Alison Bateman-House, Marian Moser Jones, Sarah Vogel, and Laura Bothwell, at Columbia, and Faye Haun, at CUNY—our brilliant, enthusiastic, and always helpful past and present doctoral students—provided us needed help at many stages of this project.

Two colleagues who spent many years at Johns Hopkins University provided us with essential background information regarding the history of Johns Hopkins and its relationship to the surrounding community. Cynthia Connolly, now associate professor at the University of Pennsylvania, and Constance Nathanson, now professor of sociomedical sciences at Columbia University's Mailman School of Public Health, have been wonderful resources and friends. Early on in our project we approached numerous faculty and administrators at Johns Hopkins itself and, in fact, had appointments with three senior professors who had been at the university for decades. We made clear that we understood they might not feel able to speak freely about the recent lawsuits and controversies surrounding the Kennedy Krieger Institute (KKI) study but that we were interested in more general information about the history of Johns Hopkins and its relationship to the broader community of Baltimore. We were surprised when each of our appointments was cancelled and we were directed to contact the administration of the schools of public health and medicine. We were advised by administrators to speak with the medical center's head attorney, who kindly forwarded us an article she had written on the KKI controversy (whose first citation was to an article we wrote). However, two professors at Johns Hopkins's Bloomberg School of Public Health, Ellen Silbergeld and Nancy Kass, were both helpful. J. Julian Chisolm and Mark Farfel, the two head researchers in the KKI study, could not be interviewed. Chisolm passed away long before we began this project, and Farfel, understandably, was reluctant to be interviewed.

Our colleagues at Columbia University, John Jay College, and the Graduate Center of the City University of New York were always generous and supportive of our work. We presented various portions of this story during the long process of research and writing. At Columbia, we thank Ron Bayer, Betsy Blackmar, James Colgrove, Sally Conover, Matt Connelly, Tom D'Aunno, Yasmin Davis, Amy Fairchild, Eric Foner, Linda Fried, Tomás

Guilarte, Barron Lerner, Mark Mazower, Lisa Metsch, Gerry Oppenheimer, Kavita Sivaramakrishnan, Pamela Smith, Toya Smith, and Ezra Susser. Samuel Roberts was especially generous with his vast knowledge of Baltimore's history and of the racial and health politics of the city. Nitanya Nedd was always good natured and expert, particularly in addressing the worlds of Columbia and the National Science Foundation bureaucracies. At John Jay and the Graduate Center, we thank Priscilla Acuna, Andrea Balis, Michael Blitz, Jane Bowers, Steve Brier, Josh Brown, Blanche Wiesen Cook, Josh Freeman, Nick Freudenberg, Mary Gibson, Betsy Gitter, Amy Green, Carol Groneman, Richard Haw, Allison Kavey, Susan Klitzman, Sondra Leftoff, David Nasaw, Jordan Pascoe, Bertha Peralta, Shirley Sarna, Dennis Sherman, Abby Stein, and Jeremy Travis. We are especially grateful to Fritz Umbach for providing us with his knowledge of the history of housing. Sheila King of the Columbia Health Sciences Library cheerfully handled our numerous interlibrary loan requests. Also, the support of the National Library of Medicine was invaluable.

The National Science Foundation (NSF) and the Milbank Memorial Fund have been generous supporters of our work. The NSF provided us with the time and resources to research and interview the numerous actors in this recent history, and the Milbank Memorial Fund supported the review process, which has been critical in making this a stronger historical work. We particularly thank Carmen Hooker Odom, president of Milbank, for her enthusiastic support.

Our two primary editors, Hannah Love at the University of California Press and Jonathan Cobb, one of the premier scientific editors in the country, deserve special thanks. Hannah was an unflagging supporter of this project from its inception and navigated the review process with thoughtful expertise. We cannot praise Jonathan enough for his extraordinary skill as a knowledgeable and thoughtful reader, critic, and editor. It was clear to us at many moments that he "knew" this book as well as we did and was able to bring out our work in a broader context of science politics because of his vast reading and commitment over the decades to science, environmentalism, and social justice. He read and commented on too many drafts to even count and improved this manuscript immeasurably. Recently, Naomi Schneider at the University of California Press has enthusiastically assumed editorial responsibility for our book, and Julie Van Pelt has expertly copyedited the manuscript with grace and warmth.

Finally, we want to thank various family friends who have lived through our obsession with lead, poisons, and our endless stories about the children and families whose lives were changed by lead: Jane Bond, Blanche Wiesen

Cook, Clare Coss, Steve Curry, Julie List, Annie Meeropol, Elli Meeropol, Michael Meeropol, Robby Meeropol, Michael Penland, Pennee Bender, Steve Safyer, Paula Marcus, Josh Freeman, Debbie Bell, Maddy deLone, Bobby Cohen, Dennis Sherman, Pat Sherman, Dinitia Smith, Beverly Lewis, Bill Lewis, Lisandro Perez, and Liza Carbajo.

Of course, our families were, as always, patient and loving. Adrienne Markowitz and Ruth Heifetz have devoted their professional lives to improving the health of the society. Our children and grandchildren fill us with pride: Billy and Toby Markowitz, Elena and Steve Kennedy, Anton and Isa Vasquez, Zachary and Molly Rosner, Emilie FitzMaurice, and Mason and Ceci Kennedy.

Finally, we want to thank Kathy Conway and Andrea Vasquez. They both know how much we love them for their warmth, intelligence, and patience with these two old guys.

1 Introduction

A Legacy of Neglect

In August 2001, the Court of Appeals of Maryland, that state's highest court, handed down a strongly worded, even shocking opinion in what has become one of the most contentious battles in the history of public health, a battle that goes to the heart of beliefs about what constitutes public health and what our responsibility to others should be. The court had been asked to decide whether or not researchers at Johns Hopkins University, among the nation's most prestigious academic institutions, had engaged in unethical research on children. The case pitted two African American children and their families against the Kennedy Krieger Institute (KKI), Johns Hopkins's premier children's clinic and research center, which in the 1990s had conducted a six-year study of children who were exposed by the researchers to differing amounts of lead in their homes.

Organized by two of the nation's top lead researchers and children's advocates, J. Julian Chisolm and Mark Farfel, the KKI project was designed to find a relatively inexpensive, effective method for reducing—though not eliminating—the amount of lead in children's homes and thereby reducing the devastating effect of lead exposure on children's brains and, ultimately, on their life chances. For the study, the Johns Hopkins researchers had recruited 108 families of single mothers with young children to live in houses with differing levels of lead exposure, ranging from none to levels just within Baltimore's existing legal limit, and then measured the extent of lead in the children's blood at periodic intervals. By matching the expense of varying levels of lead paint abatement with changing levels of lead found in the blood, the researchers hoped to find the most cost-effective means of reducing childhood exposure to the toxin. Completely removing lead paint from the homes, Chisolm and Farfel recognized, would be ideal for children's health; but they believed, with some justification, that a legal

1

requirement to do so would be considered far too costly in such politically conservative times and would likely result in landlord abandonment of housing in the city's more poverty-stricken districts.

Despite the intentions of KKI researchers to benefit children, the court of appeals found that KKI had engaged in highly suspect research that had direct parallels with some of the most infamous incidents of abuse of vulnerable populations in the twentieth century. The KKI project, the court argued, differed from but presented "similar problems as those in the Tuskegee Syphilis Study, . . . the intentional exposure of soldiers to radiation in the 1940s and 50s, the test involving the exposure of Navajo miners to radiation . . . and the secret administration of LSD to soldiers by the CIA and the army in the 1950s and 60s." The research defied many aspects of the Nuremberg Code, the court said, and included aspects that were similar to Nazi experimentation on humans in the concentration camps and the "notorious use of 'plague bombs' by the Japanese military in World War II where entire villages were infected in order for the results to be 'studied.'"[1] More specifically, the court was appalled that many of the children selected for the study were recruited to live in homes where the researchers knew they would be exposed to lead and thus knowingly placed in harm's way. Children, the court argued, "are not in our society the equivalent of rats, hamsters, monkeys and the like."[2] The court was deeply troubled that a major university would conduct research that might permanently damage children, given what was already known about the effects of lead.

How could two public health researchers who had devoted their scientific lives to alleviating one of the oldest and most devastating neurological conditions affecting children be likened to Nazis? Was this just a "rogue court," an out-of-control panel of judges, as many in the public health community would argue? These were the questions that initially drew our attention. We soon became aware, however, of the much more complex and troubling story underlying the case, about not just the KKI research but also the public health profession, the nation's dedication to the health of its citizens in the new millennium, and the conundrum that we as a society face when confronting revelations about a host of new environmental threats in the midst of a conservative political culture. In its ubiquity and harm, lead is an exemplary instance of these threats. Yet there are many others we encounter in everyday life that entail similar issues, from mercury in fish and emitted by power plants to cadmium, certain flame retardants, and bisphenol A, the widely distributed plastics additive that has been identified as a threat to children.[3]

For much of its history, the public health field provided the vision and technical expertise for remedying the conditions—both biological and social—that created environments conducive to harm and within which disease could spread. And throughout much of the profession's history, public health leaders have joined with reformers, radicals, and other social activists to finds ways within the existing political and economic structures to prevent diseases. Although the medical profession has often been given credit for the vast improvements in Americans' health and life span, the nineteenth- and early-twentieth century public health reformers who pushed for housing reforms, mass vaccination campaigns, clean water and sewage systems, and pure food laws in fact played a major role in improving children's health, lowering infant mortality, and limiting the impact of viral and bacterial diseases such as cholera, typhoid, diphtheria, smallpox, tuberculosis, measles, and whooping cough. In the opening years of the twentieth century, for example, Chicago's public health department joined with Jane Addams and social reformers at Hull House to successfully advocate for new housing codes that, by reducing overcrowding and assuring fresh air in every room, led to reduced rates of tuberculosis. And New York's Commissioner of Health Hermann Biggs worked with Lillian Wald and other settlement house leaders to initiate nursing services for the poor, pure milk campaigns, vaccination programs, and well-baby clinics that dramatically reduced childhood mortality. Biggs, Addams, and other Progressives worked from a firm conviction that as citizens we have a collective responsibility to maintain conditions conducive to every person's health and well-being.

These broad public health campaigns to control infectious diseases yielded great victories from the 1890s through the 1930s. But with the first decades of the twentieth century, a different view of the profession began to gain ascendancy, redefining the mission of public health in ways that belied its role as an agent of social reform. In 1916 Hibbert Hill, a leading advocate of this new direction, put it this way: "The old public health was concerned with the environment; the new is concerned with the individual. The old sought the sources of infectious disease in the surroundings of man; the new finds them in man himself. The old public health ... failed because it sought [the sources] ... in every place and in every thing *where they were not*."[4] In this view, the idea was for the fast-growing science of biological medicine to concentrate on treating disease person by person rather than on eradicating conditions that facilitated disease and its spread, in some cases encouraging reforms in behavior to reduce individual exposure to harm. Hence, like numerous other fields in the early decades of the century, public health became professionalized, imbuing itself with the aura of science and setting itself off as possessing special expertise.

By the middle decades of the twentieth century, public health officials thus typically conceived of their field mainly as a laboratory-based scientific enterprise, and many public health professionals saw their work as a technocratic and scientific effort to control the agents that imperiled the public's health individual by individual.[5] We can see this shift in perspective in treating tuberculosis, for example. An infectious disease that terrified the American public in the eighteenth and nineteenth centuries, tuberculosis had begun to decline as a serious threat by the early twentieth century, mainly because of housing reforms, improvements in nutritional standards, and general environmental sanitation. By midcentury, public health officials tended to downplay such environmental conditions and came to rely instead on the armamentarium of new antibiotic therapies to address the relatively small number of tuberculosis victims. The history of responding to industrial accidents and disease offers another example. In the early years of the twentieth century, reformers such as Crystal Eastman addressed the plague of industrial accidents and disease in the steel and coal towns of Pennsylvania by advocating for higher wages, shorter hours, and better working conditions through unionization. By the 1950s, industrial disease and accidents had largely faded from public health view—ironically, in part because the earlier reform efforts had led to protective legislation—and it was left to company physicians to treat individual workers. This turn toward technological and individualistic solutions to problems that had once been defined as societal was by midcentury part of a general shift in American culture away from divisive class politics and toward a faith in ostensibly class-neutral science, technology, and industrial prowess as the best way to address social or public-health-related problems.

Since the early twentieth century, a tension has existed within the public health field—which mirrors a societal one—between, on the one hand, those who set their sights on prevention of disease and conditions dangerous to health through society-wide efforts and, on the other, those who believe in the more modest and pragmatic goal of ameliorating conditions through piecemeal reforms, personal education, and individual treatments. Despite the tremendous successes of environmental and political efforts to stem epidemics and lower mortality from infectious diseases, the credit for these improvements went to physicians (and the potent drugs they sometimes had at hand), whose role was to treat individuals. This shift also coincidentally, or not so coincidentally, undermined a public health logic that was potentially disruptive to existing social and power relationships between landlord and tenant, worker and industrialist, and poor immigrants and political leaders.

At elite universities around the country—from Harvard, Yale, and Columbia to Johns Hopkins and Tulane—new schools of public health were established in the first two decades of the twentieth century with funds from the Rockefeller and Carnegie Foundations. Educators at these new schools had faith that science and technology could ameliorate the public health threats that fed broader social conflicts. They envisioned a politically neutral technological and scientific field removed from the politics of reform. The Johns Hopkins School of Hygiene and Public Health was at the center of this movement. William Welch, the school's founder and first director (as well as the first dean of the university's medical school), argued persuasively that bacteriology and the laboratory sciences held the key to the future of the field.[6] By the mid-twentieth century, municipal public health officials in most cities had adopted this approach. If early in the century public health workers in alliance with social reformers succeeded in getting legislation passed to control child labor and the dangers to health that accompanied it, and to protect women from having to work with such dangerous chemicals as phosphorus and lead, by midcentury departments of health worked more often to reduce exposures of workers to "acceptable" levels that would limit damage rather than eliminate it. Similarly, by the 1970s departments of health had established clinics aimed at treating the person with tuberculosis but displayed little interest in joining with reformers to tear down slums and build better houses for at-risk low-income people.[7]

By the 1950s and 1960s, when childhood lead poisoning emerged as a major national issue, public health practitioners were divided between those who defined their roles as identifying victims and treating symptoms and those who in addition sought alliances with social activists to prevent poisoning through housing reforms that would require lead removal. Drawing on the social movements of the 1960s, health professionals joined with antipoverty groups, civil rights organizations, environmentalists, and antiwar activists to struggle for access to health facilities for African Americans in the South and in underserved urban areas, for Chicanos active in the United Farm Workers' strikes in the grape-growing areas of California and the West, for Native Americans on reservations throughout the country, and for soldiers returning from Vietnam suffering from post-traumatic stress disorders, among others. By the end of the twentieth century, though, the effort to eliminate childhood lead poisoning through improving urban infrastructure had largely been abandoned in favor of reducing exposures.

CHILDHOOD LEAD POISONING: PUBLIC HEALTH TRIUMPH OR TRAGEDY?

The campaign to halt childhood lead poisoning is often told as one of the great public health victories, like the efforts to eliminate diphtheria, polio, and other childhood scourges. After all, with the removal of lead from gasoline, blood lead levels of American children between the ages of one and five years declined precipitously from 15 micrograms per deciliter (µg/dl) in 1976–80 to 2.7 µg/dl by 1991–94,[8] and levels have continued to drop. Today, the median blood lead level among children aged one–five years is 1.4 µg/dl, and 95 percent of children in this age group have levels below 4.1 µg/dl. Viewed from a broader perspective, however, the story is more complicated, and disturbing, and may constitute what Bruce Lanphear, a leading lead researcher, calls "a pyrrhic victory."[9] If 95 percent of American children have below what is today considered the danger level for lead, then 5 percent—a half million children—still have dangerous amounts of lead in their bodies. A century of knowledge about the harmful effects of lead in the environ-

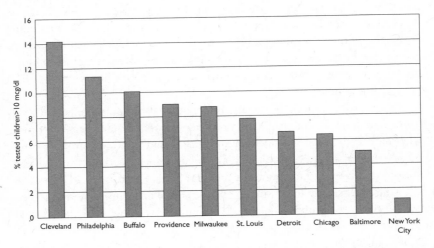

FIGURE 1.   Rates of lead poisoning, 2003. These rates are based on the CDC's 2003 level of concern (10 µg/dl). In 2012, the CDC lowered that to 5 µg/dl, increasing the number of at-risk children from approximately 250,000 to nearly half a million. Source: Environmental Health Watch, available at www.gcbl.org/system/files/images/lead_rates_national.jpg.

ment and the success of efforts to eliminate some of its sources have not staunched the flood of this toxic material that is polluting our children, our local environments, and our planet.

Today, despite broad understanding of the toxicity of this material, the world mines more lead and uses it in a wider variety of products than ever before. Our handheld electronic devices, the sheathing in our computers, and the batteries in our motor vehicles, even in new "green" cars such as the Prius, depend on it. While in the United States the new uses of lead are to a certain degree circumscribed, the disposal of all our electronic devices and the production of lead-bearing materials through mining, smelting, and manufacture in many countries continue to poison communities around the world. Industrial societies in the West may have significantly reduced the levels of new lead contamination, but the horror of lead poisoning here is hardly behind us, exposure coming from lead paint in hundreds of thousands of homes, in airborne particles from smelters and other sources and from contaminated soil, lead solder and pipes in city water systems, and some imported toys and trinkets. Over time, millions of children have been poisoned.

In the past, untold numbers of children suffered noticeably from irritability, loss of appetite, awkward gait, abdominal pain, and vomiting; many went into convulsions and comas, often leading to death. The level of exposure that results in such symptoms still occurs in some places. But today new concerns have arisen as researchers have found repeatedly that what a decade earlier was thought to be a "safe" level of lead in children's bodies turned out to itself result in life-altering neurological and physiological damage. Even by the federal standard in place at the beginning of 2012 (10 µg/dl), more than a quarter of a million American children were victims of lead poisoning, a condition that almost a century ago was already considered with some accuracy as totally preventable. Later in 2012, the Centers for Disease Control (CDC) lowered the level of concern to 5 µg/dl, nearly doubling estimates of the number of possible victims.

The ongoing tragedy of lead poisoning rarely provokes the outrage one might expect, however. If this were meningitis, or even an outbreak of measles, lead poisoning would be the focus of concerted national action. In the 1950s, fewer than sixty thousand new cases of polio per year created a near panic among American parents and a national mobilization of vaccination campaigns that virtually wiped out the disease within a decade. At no point in the past hundred years has there been a similar national mobilization over lead despite its ubiquity and the havoc it can wreak.

For much of the twentieth century we have no systematic records telling us the number of children whose lives have been destroyed by lead. What we have known, as one researcher put it in the 1920s, is that "a child lives in a lead world."[10] By the 1920s, virtually every item a toddler touched had some amount of lead in or on it. Leaded toy soldiers and dolls, painted toys, beanbags, baseballs, fishing lures, and other equipment that were part of the new consumer economy of the time; the porcelain, pipes, and joints in the sparkling new kitchens and bathrooms of the expanding housing stock—all were made of or contained large amounts of lead. But more ominously and disastrously, lead became part of the air Americans breathed when, in 1923, lead was introduced into gasoline to give cars more power. With the dramatic growth of this vast industry, every American child, parent, and neighbor began to systematically incorporate into their bodies a toxic heavy metal that was already known to be poisoning workers in the United States and elsewhere.

For centuries, and particularly with the Industrial Revolution, lead had been causing workers in foundries, smelters, paint factories, and other industries to suffer severe, sometimes fatal neurological damage. By the 1920s, children as well were facing a special threat from the very rooms they lived in every day. Paint, the seemingly innocuous wall covering that replaced wallpaper as the most desirable room decoration in the early twentieth century, contained huge amounts of this deadly material. Up to 70 percent of a can of paint in the first half of the century was composed of lead pigments. Such paint was aggressively marketed as the covering of choice to millions of young families through jingles, advertisements, and even paint books for children, who were told, for example, "This famous Dutch Boy Lead of mine can make this playroom fairly shine."[11]

The vast expansion of America's cities fueled growing use of lead paint as a convenience of modern American life, which also fostered competition among various paint manufacturers eager to gain new sales and capitalize on potential profits. The paint companies could have manufactured their products without lead—zinc-based paints (promoted as safe and nontoxic because they were "lead free") had been on the market as early as 1900, and by the 1930s titanium pigments were available as well. Instead, the lead industry chose to run massive marketing and promotion campaigns all through the first half of the twentieth century despite their knowledge that lead paint was causing children to go into comas, suffer convulsions, and die.[12] The result was a major public health disaster. By the middle decades of the century, millions of children were suffering the effects of acute or chronic lead exposure, and tens of thousands of children had died.[13] Lead was by then certainly among the most prevalent, if not the most well-known, of the threats to children.

The Kennedy Krieger Institute had been identifying such lead-poisoned children and treating them for over a half century when researchers there embarked in 1991 on what became its controversial study.[14] Baltimore, and Johns Hopkins University in particular, had been at the center of work on childhood lead poisoning even longer, for almost a century.[15] Over this period, the city had made some of the more innovative attempts to address what has proven to be one of the nation's most intractable environmental problems. In the 1930s Baltimore's health commissioner identified lead paint as a major source of injury to children, and since the 1950s Johns Hopkins had numbered among its faculty the foremost lead researchers in the nation, including Julian Chisolm, perhaps the preeminent university lead researcher of the middle decades of the twentieth century—and the co-principal investigator for the KKI study. The irony of this history is unmistakable. Here was the premier center for the study of lead poisoning, located in the virtual heart of the country's lead poisoning epidemic, at the eye of a storm over whether or not children were being used, as the Maryland Court of Appeals ultimately opined, as "canaries in the mines"[16] and "guinea pigs."[17]

Fairly typical of the thousands of children that Johns Hopkins had sought to help before the 1960s, when children living in poorly maintained slum housing suffered from convulsions after ingesting lead paint, was John T., aged nine months, who was brought by his distraught parents to the Harriet Lane Home of the Johns Hopkins Hospital in February 1940.[18] John was a well-nourished, playful, and cooperative child, with no history of developmental problems, according to the admitting nurse. John's father was well educated, having spent three years at a theological seminary. He had also trained as an entertainer, but a back injury had incapacitated him and he had gone on relief, receiving fifty-six dollars a month to support his family. Despite their meager income, their home was well maintained and "quite attractively furnished," the visiting social service worker reported.[19]

John was admitted to the hospital because he had developed an ear infection, but that was easily treated; his appetite was good and he slept well. The medical record indicated that John had been breast-fed for six of his first nine months. He was soon eating cereals; started on spinach, string beans, and other vegetables; and given soft-boiled eggs. In his short life he had never suffered from nausea or vomiting. The record reported a happy, healthy infant from a good home who "held up his head at three months; sat up at six months; had first teeth at seven months," and at month nine was able to walk around holding on to objects and walls. "This baby behaves well," said the record. "No problem. Keeps himself entertained all day." He had suffered an attack of chicken pox but had recovered well. In a matter of two days his ear infection seemed to clear up and he was sent back home to 1023 North Caroline Street, a three-story row house just north of the medical center, to rejoin his four other siblings, who ranged in age from two to six years. This healthy child had everything to look forward to.

In the ensuing months John returned periodically to the clinic for treatment of his chronic earaches, but by the time he was two years old he had developed symptoms that were not at all routine. In May 1941 his parents rushed him to the hospital. A few hours earlier, he had "bent over to the left and couldn't straighten up," they told the admitting nurse, and since that time he had "been acting 'crazy-like.'" John had been "eating plaster," they said, and the previous day he had eaten "some paint." The nurse summed up what she had observed: "This is a fairly well-nourished and developed two year old colored boy who is crying and is excitable." At the hospital he "fell to the left side when he tried to walk, and he reeled around to the left. He didn't respond to his name or questions." The hospital raised the possibility that John suffered from lead poisoning, encephalitis, and secondary anemia. He had apparently been eating plaster for the past six months, and his mother reported that "he has been eating paint that peels off from window sills." The blood work showed 390 micrograms of lead per deciliter of blood—almost eighty times the level considered by the CDC to be dangerous for children seventy years later[20] and at the time clearly a cause of acute poisoning. The social worker in charge of the case noted that "because the landlord refused to make any repairs in this home, the family pooled their money and bought some paint which they have used all over the home." When told that paint from the windowsills was dangerous, his mother said she had not realized its danger and had "caught him on frequent occasions with a mouth full of paint chips." She promised that in the future "she would make every effort to keep the child away from the paint." She had "a large play pen and from now on the child [would] be kept there. It gives him adequate room to move about and have a good time," the social worker wrote, "and will make it impossible to get to the window sill and eat more paint."

In mid-June 1941, after more than a month in the hospital, John's symptoms subsided and he was sent back home. But two months later the mother was back at the social service department. In the words of the social worker, the family had "contacted the real estate agency several times about repair work but with no success"; there continued to be problems of "loose plaster throughout the home in spite of their efforts at repair." The social worker contacted the health department, which promised to investigate the home conditions, but we know neither the results nor what befell John in subsequent years.

What did and did not occur in response to the plight of John's family is telling. At the time, Johns Hopkins was the lone institution and Baltimore the lone city in the country that was systematically trying to identify and treat large numbers of children affected by the increasing tonnage of lead polluting the nation's housing. Baltimore and Hopkins had been the epicenter of this issue ever since the area's rapid growth at the turn of the century had created a huge housing boom and, with it, the use of lead-based paint throughout the central city. The first American case of poisoning due to lead paint ingestion was also documented here, in 1914, by Henry Thomas and Kenneth Blackfan at the very same Harriet Lane Home where John was treated. And Baltimore's Department of Health was the first local health agency to mount a campaign to protect a city's children from the effects of lead. In fact, in the 1930s it used the new medium of radio to broadcast public service announcements warning its residents about lead's dangers: "Every year there are admitted to the hospitals of Baltimore a number of children with lead poisoning caused by eating paint. Most of these children die," listeners were told, "but those who live are almost equally unfortunate because lead poisoning leaves behind it a trail of eyes dimmed by blindness, legs and arms made useless by paralysis, and minds destroyed even to complete idiocy."[21]

The response of Johns Hopkins to the epidemic was, however, fraught with practical and institutional problems emblematic of a larger crisis over lead poisoning and other ubiquitous toxic pollutants that continue to plague us today. Lead poisoning was both a medical and a social problem of inordinate proportions. Hopkins could treat the problem by allowing children who came to its attention a brief respite from the environmental assault on their bodies and brains, but such respites were typically just that, and not adequate to stop these assaults. John was returned to his home following the acute episode of lead poisoning that had nearly paralyzed him. But Hopkins, in no position either to compel the landlord to repair the home or to provide the family with a lead-free house, had no answer to the problem of how to protect John from further lead dosings other than to have his desperate mother promise to keep him pent up in a playpen, away from what was assumed to be the major sources of lead.

We may look back on John's treatment and the "discharge protocol" as inadequate (although in many ways it is similar to what occurs in numerous localities today). And we may assume that John would have likely returned to the hospital with a fresh, and possibly fatal, episode of lead ingestion: despite the well-intentioned advice to his parents, no well-functioning toddler could remain for long in a four-by-four pen. But we would be wrong to write off the John Hopkins's effort as an anomaly or proof of special inadequacy of the medical and social service system of the time. True, unlike the Harriet Lane Home, which generally saw its responsibility as treating the acute symptoms of lead poisoning as best it could, the Kennedy Krieger Institute, facing similar problems in serving Baltimore's children a half century later, took as its responsibility finding the means to protect children from lead exposure, treating them when evident symptoms began to appear and planning for their return to a safe environment. But, in the end, despite this wider purview, KKI, like its predecessor, could not overcome the huge social and economic issues that frame the long, troubling, and desperate history of lead poisoning in Baltimore, and in the nation.

The story of John and the public health response to cases such as his are indicative of the entire history of lead poisoning in particular and the crisis of environmental and industrial pollution in general. The root of John's disease lay in the physical conditions in which he and his family lived—poor housing whose walls were covered with a poison. But the only response was from the public health and medical professions, and they could only provide medical care to the individual child. That was important, of course, but the broad social problems that affected huge numbers of children living in similar conditions were left unaddressed, virtually guaranteeing that there would be many more children like John in urgent need of help. John was suffering from more than an environmental exposure to a known neurotoxin, caused by shoddy landlords and peeling paint. He suffered from a social and economic system that condemned his family to poverty and racial discrimination, as well as to the urban decay that put him in harm's way. John's parents could hardly be blamed for the constraints he and his entire family were forced to endure in, for example, the limited choices in housing they would have had. And even vague attempts to "explain away" John's situation by pointing to his color and poverty could not counter the observations that his mother was a hard-working, sincere, and dedicated parent who, according to the social worker at Harriet Lane, was "genuinely interested and concerned about the children" and, using the racist language of the period, "more intelligent than the average negro." Nor could John's well-educated and industrious father be blamed for the family's economic plight and thereby somehow explain away the disease as a family failing. Public health agencies, without such traditional explanations for the diseases of poverty to fall back on—and with no ability to confront the socioeconomic relationships among lead producers, paint manufacturers, housing officials, and landlords that had produced the epidemic of lead poisoning—lacked the tools and the will to control the epidemic effectively as well as the clout to effect much change.

The good doctors of the Harriet Lane Home faced an impossible situation. On the one hand their responsibility was to treat disease and they did so to the best of their abilities. But, in the context of such a glaring threat—children being poisoned by a toxin in their home—one would hope they would have gone beyond that role to advocate more forcefully for housing reforms and rehabilitation as a means of prevention. Public health administrators, advocates, and policy-oriented academics, though, faced a classic dilemma: how does one prevent disease and premature or unnecessary death when the means of effecting such prevention are controlled by a political and economic system over which one has limited influence and that profits from the existing social relationships that produce disease? In this respect, the public health problems of the 1940s are no different than what we face today, though the political climate is quite different. In fact, given the growing attention to the impact of chronic illnesses and low-level environmental exposures to a host of toxic chemicals and industrial products whose chemistry, much less whose health effects, is largely not understood, the problem is only magnified.[22]

Acute lead poisoning, the kind of poisoning John suffered, perhaps the oldest and best understood environmental disease, has been for the most part successfully contained in the United States over the past half century through judicial, legislative, and regulatory decisions as well as scientific discoveries and medical interventions. Removing some of the most obvious sources of lead from the world of children and adults—from gasoline, paint, canned foods, and other widely available consumer products—was an outstanding public health achievement, which in aggregate lowered the average exposure to lead by orders of magnitude. During the 1960s and 1970s, public health authorities joined with various social movements and thereby were instrumental in shaping these regulatory actions and bringing to the nation's attention the huge number of childhood poisonings. Through coalitions with social reformers, public health authorities were able to press national, state, and/or local authorities to enact legislation and authorize agencies to achieve reforms. Because of reduced exposure consequent to those reforms, children in the United States today rarely go into convulsions or suffer massive brain damage from lead poisoning, although this is still a major problem in many areas of the developing world. Similarly, because of other regulatory action, Americans rarely suffer from the most acute symptoms of mercury poisoning, arsenic poisoning, or radiation exposure.

Concern over acute lead poisoning has given way to recognition of the subtler but often still devastating problems induced by lead ingestion, problems only vaguely considered a generation or two ago. Indeed, researchers in the past few decades have changed our understanding of the effects that comparatively low levels of lead exposure have on the brain of the developing child, and with that our understanding of the potential low-dose dangers of other toxins. Mercury, chromium, and other heavy metals still cause damage to children (and adults) even if exposure is rarely fatal; the level of arsenic in some of our water supply is with good reason a cause of concern to the U.S. Environmental Protection Agency and state health officials.

Low-dose effects of such toxins are not new problems; they occurred in the acute age as well. But they typically went unrecognized as toxic because of the glaring damage that accompanied acute poisonings and the limited technological tools available for identifying very low levels of exposure. Today, though, we need only read the newspaper headlines to see the growing alarm over the potential harmful health effects of, for example, bisphenol A, a chemical additive that mimics estrogen and other human hormones and that is found in a myriad of children's toys, baby bottles, plastic containers, adhesives, computer-generated taxi and credit card receipts, and a host of other consumer products.[23] Or we may point to the emerging controversies over the use of nanoparticles in skin creams and cosmetics, or the chemicals used in flame retardants in children's clothing and other consumer items. In these and many other instances, it will require broad population-based public health actions to prevent damage, not just direct individual treatment to deal with these substances' effects.

The decline of the various social movements in the 1970s and 1980s had a telling effect on the public health profession, as it was deprived of the power and energy of political and social allies that could influence legislators and bureaucrats in local, state, and federal agencies. Following the election of Ronald Reagan, even federal agencies whose mission coincided with public health activists were under attack and stymied in their attempts to regulate the environment, identify and remedy unhealthy working conditions, and provide services to the poor. New publicly built housing virtually ceased in these years. In the face of this broad assault, largely at the behest of conservative critics of the Great Society programs of the 1960s, public health activism waned.[24]

A strategy of avoiding confrontation with the political and economic institutions that impede the solutions for public health problems—and indeed may have given rise to them—has led to avoiding confrontation with the structural impediments to improving public health. This is the dilemma of public health today: For generations, many in the public health field have depended on the laboratory, on the development of the next magic bullet, on new technologies and diagnostic and therapeutic interventions to deal with public health problems. But, like lead, other ubiquitous environmental poisons now raise fundamental problems that cannot easily be addressed by these methods. If detection of endocrine disruption is truly a new frontier in the understanding of reproductive problems or other biological changes, for example, a medical intervention may not be adequate; and even were it possible, dealing with the consequences individual by individual would overwhelm any health system.

If public health professionals are to effectively address the problems of chronic conditions, subtle neurological damage, obesity, and childhood developmental anomalies, they will be forced to confront huge industries that profit from, for example, the production of fast foods, high-calorie drinks, and tobacco. These health difficulties are not simply an issue for public health professionals; they are of course an issue for society as a whole. Public health individuals and institutions can press, but ultimately their success depends on political and economic forces larger than themselves. From the guarantee of an adequate water supply and sewer system to the passage of Medicare and Medicaid, successful public health reforms of the past have depended on social movements and legislative and/or executive action, and the same is likely to be true for effective action on a broad array of toxins, lead included.

THE SCIENCE AND POLITICS OF LOW DOSES

As the character of the lead-poisoning epidemic has changed over the past half century, especially with the elimination of lead from the manufacture of paint and from gasoline, and as the harm to children of nonfatal doses of lead has become more apparent, the focus of research has shifted to the effects of these smaller doses. Results indicate that, though the level of lead exposure may be low compared to what brings on acute episodes of lead poisoning, the effects are far from minor.

Children with even relatively low levels of lead in their blood (even below 5 micrograms per deciliter) have been shown to suffer disproportionately from behavioral problems in school, school failure, hyperactivity, trouble concentrating, difficulty with impulse control, lowered intelligence scores on standardized tests, higher rates of juvenile delinquency and arrests, and ultimately unemployment and failures in life. Further, children with lead exposure are more likely as adults to have physical problems like kidney and heart disorders. The scientific community and many political leaders now recognize that lead poisoning has been among the most important epidemics affecting children in the United States in the last century.

A particular tragedy of low-level lead poisoning is that its "symptoms" are easily confused with myriad other insults suffered by children who grow up in poor communities, whose housing is substandard and whose lives are shaped by poor education, social marginalization, and, in some instances, racism. In a 1990 article Herbert Needleman noted a stunning statistic that brings this issue home: more than half of all "poor black children have elevated blood lead levels," estimated at the time as exceeding 25 µg/dl.[25]

Consider, for example, Sam T., the youngest of his family's nine children, born in June 1990, just as the Kennedy Krieger Institute study was beginning in Baltimore.[26] The family lived in an apartment located in one of Milwaukee's poorest and most lead-polluted neighborhoods, but according to his medical record, Sam "thrived as a baby" and was developmentally normal at the ages at which he started to crawl, walk, and babble.[27] Like many lead-poisoned children, his problems began as a toddler, when he began to move more freely around the apartment, mouthing or sucking his fingers after touching the walls, windowsills, or other objects covered with lead paint or dust.[28] When Sam was fourteen months old, a routine check found his blood lead level to be 18 µg/dl, at that time almost twice the Centers for Disease Control's acceptable exposure limit, which had been reduced from 25 to 10 µg/dl in 1991. A few months later, his blood lead level had almost doubled, to 40 µg/dl, and it did not fall below 25 µg/dl at any time tested over the next two and a half years.[29] The family moved to a house nearby in an attempt to escape such a heavily leaded environment, but conditions there were no better. In the summer of 1993, when Sam turned three, his lead levels jumped significantly and he was hospitalized for five days while he received chelation treatments, the in-hospital chemotherapeutic blood treatment aimed at leaching lead from the body.[30] But by then it was too late to forestall damage.

When Sam entered kindergarten, teachers immediately noticed that he had problems. Within weeks, he was referred for speech and language therapy and was soon, according to the court record, "transferred to a different school because he needed a small, structured classroom."[31] In first and second grades, he had difficulties with reading, writing, and arithmetic and he suffered various language delays.[32] In his teenage years, a battery of neuropsychological exams indicated that Sam "had a number of deficiencies in various areas of brain function . . . : problem solving, planning, executive function, fine motor function, expressive language, aspects of visual-spatial construction, visual working memory, visual-spatial memory and verbal concept formation"[33]—an array of deficits consistent with what is known about damage from lead ingestion. "[Sam]'s injuries are permanent and irreversible," the examining physician concluded.[34] By his midteens Sam, who had been described as a normal, happy infant, had become a failure in school, a troubled young man who lacked the skills to escape the dangerous neighborhood in which he was raised.[35]

The lessons of America's continuing lead-poisoning epidemic are not confined to the tragedies of a few specific children like Sam T. Nor are its lessons limited to lead alone. Discovery by lead researchers of the impacts of early low-level lead exposure has been instrumental in revolutionizing our understanding of environmental danger and how we define what is a risk. As a result, our concerns regarding environmental dangers can no longer be confined to worries over cancer, heart disease, and the like. Researchers have identified that low-level exposures can result in biological changes with measurable and important consequences for individuals. Behavioral changes such as hyperactivity, attention deficit disorders, and even antisocial behaviors have been linked to low-level exposures to lead, mercury, and other heavy metals in infancy and even in utero. Morphological changes such as premature puberty and an increased proportion of female births have been linked to the rise in the use of plastics and bisphenol A and other "endocrine disruptors."[36]

Researchers into low-level exposures to a variety of substances have also challenged, even transformed, our understanding of what is toxic and what is toxicology. We can no longer take solace in believing that any substance can be used if a "safe" level of exposure is officially identified. Researchers have shown that for many synthetic materials introduced yearly into our environment, the developmental moment at which a fetus or child is exposed to a toxin is every bit as important as the amount to which he or she is exposed.[37] Many of these issues that challenge us today were first identified while studying lead and lead exposures. The modern history of this unfolding understanding and corresponding attempts to regulate lead may thus give us insight applicable to current debates over other toxic substances.

Sam T.'s story is similar to that of countless others, often who have ingested far less lead. In fact, from the 1970s to the 1990s a growing body of research indicated that as each lower "safe level" was agreed upon by the federal government, deleterious effects were found at a still lower level. Investigators such as Philip Landrigan at Mount Sinai Medical Center in New York, Herbert Needleman at the University of Pittsburgh, and Kim Dietrich and Bruce Lanphear, both then at the University of Cincinnati, showed that even quite small amounts of lead, between 1 and 10 micrograms per deciliter of blood, were associated with deficits similar to Sam's: lowered IQ, behavioral disorders, perceptual problems, and other effects that seriously undermined the ability of children to succeed in school or work environments. This shift in focus—from the impact of relatively high blood lead levels as the cause of severe, sometimes fatal neurological damage to the subtler behavioral and intellectual deficits associated with low-dose lead exposure—raised new concerns about lead's wide-ranging toxic effects and forced rethinking of what clinicians should attend to beyond textbook symptoms of severe lead poisoning. The growing scientific literature on lead's effects, as we will see, has been bitterly contested by the lead industry at every step and has resulted in some classic instances of attempted intimidation of university researchers and attacks on their scientific integrity.[38]

The extensive documentation of low-level effects over recent decades has led the Centers for Disease Control to progressively lower the blood lead levels considered to put children at risk. Until the late 1960s, most public health officials and physicians believed that 60 micrograms per deciliter of blood was not dangerous for children. But by 1978 the CDC had halved this figure, reducing it still further in 1985, to 25 µg/dl, and then in 1991 to 10 µg/dl.[39] Jane Lin-Fu, a leading lead researcher, has observed that today "we know that normal [blood-lead level] should be near 0, that unlike essential elements such as calcium . . . lead has no essential role in human physiology and is toxic at a very low level."[40] Most prominent researchers agree with Lin-Fu's assessment.[41] Indeed, the CDC's lead advisory committee, the scientific body that consults on the federal definition of lead poisoning, recommended in January 2012 that the level of concern for lead be cut in half, to 5 µg/dl. This was adopted by the CDC later that year.[42] The political implications of this recommendation are profound and contentious, however. As a result, the number of children considered at risk of lead poisoning rose dramatically, from an estimated 250,000 children with levels above 10 µg/dl to as many as 450,000 with levels exceeding 5 µg/dl, placing renewed pressure on government, industry, and public health officials to take action.

Lowering the overall exposure of children to lead entails eliminating the wide variety of ways that children come in contact with lead in their everyday lives. Newspapers are filled with stories of children who have been poisoned by the lead paint on imported toys, lead solder on children's jewelry, lead from pipes that deliver water to homes, lead in soil tainted by leaded gasoline that once powered cars, lead spewed from smelters in the United States and throughout the world, and, still most importantly, lead from paint that remains on the walls of nearly all houses built before 1960 or that was applied in many other homes until lead paint was banned in 1978.

Just as there have been disagreements over what constitutes a "safe" blood lead level, so too have there been debates about how best to protect children from lead in their homes. In 1991 the CDC, under the auspices of the U.S. Department of Health and Human Services, published its *Strategic Plan for the Elimination of Childhood Lead Poisoning,*[43] which some prominent researchers called "a truly revolutionary policy statement."[44] This document, building on an extensive period of reevaluation among researchers of childhood lead poisoning, proposed "a society-wide effort [to] virtually eliminate this disease as a public health problem in 20 years."[45] The document's publication led to a host of studies seeking ways to eliminate or at least broadly curtail lead poisoning in America. While some researchers developed protocols aimed at eliminating lead as a widespread urban pollutant through its complete removal, others sought more pragmatic solutions—pragmatic, that is, from the viewpoint of the politics of the times, not from that of families whose children were at risk of permanent brain damage—seeking to remove some if not all lead from the windowsills, walls, ceilings, and woodwork of older homes.

The debate in the early 1990s over what should be done developed in a dramatically altered political environment, as memories of the Great Society were replaced by a more conservative political culture. The rise of Reaganism after 1980, the growing power of corporations, the decline of the civil rights and labor movements, the end of the construction of low-income public housing, and the antigovernment rhetoric and attacks on what were considered liberal social reforms all undermined support for more far-reaching solutions to the lead-poisoning problem. As Herbert Needleman, a pioneer in the early studies of low-level lead neurotoxicity, put it: "Instead of asking, 'how can we develop a plan to spend U.S. $32 billion over the next 15 years and eliminate all of the lead in dangerous houses?' the question became, 'how little can we spend and still reduce the blood-lead levels in the short term?'" Opposition from industry, landlords, and others was so strong, and the countervailing voices so few, said Needleman, that "it was not long before the vision of the early 1990s, true primary prevention, eradication of the disease in 15 years, was replaced by an enfeebled pseudopragmatism," which came down to only partial abatement of polluted homes.[46]

One researcher's pseudopragmatism, however, is another advocate's realistic attempt to help children at risk. And one person's policy failure is another's public health success story. Those who have watched a century of children sacrificed on the altar of lead poisoning are aghast that we, as a wealthy industrial society, would continue to knowingly allow future generations of children to be exposed to lead. In contrast, those who have set their sights lower and labored to reduce rather than eliminate lead in children's environment, believing this to be the only "practical" course, celebrate dramatic declines in both blood lead levels and symptomatic children as among the great successes in public health history.

THE KENNEDY KRIEGER CASE AND
THE ETHICS OF LEAD RESEARCH

The lead researchers at Johns Hopkins's Kennedy Krieger Institute faced a troubling dilemma in the midst of this history: children living in Baltimore, the epicenter of the lead-poisoning epidemic for almost a century, were being poisoned because their homes had been covered with lead paint, which, when it deteriorated, the children inhaled or ingested. Despite the CDC's grand vision of eliminating lead from the home, it was highly unlikely that the money necessary for a dramatic federal detoxification program would be appropriated: during the Reagan and first Bush administrations, government social projects were defined as part of the problem, not a part of the solution. It was in this general context that the Environmental Protection Agency funded the Kennedy Krieger Institute: the federal government, and various lead researchers, were looking for relatively inexpensive, nonconfrontational, noncoercive methods of partial abatement so that landlords would reduce the lead hazard to children rather than either evade an abatement law or abandon their properties.[47]

"The purpose of the study," wrote Mark Farfel, the co-principal investigator with Julian Chisolm, "is to characterize and compare the short and long-term efficacy of comprehensive lead-paint abatement and less costly and potentially more cost-effective Repair and Maintenance (R&M) interventions for reducing levels of lead in residential house dust which in turn should reduce lead in children's blood."[48] "R&M," as Farfel later put it in a grant renewal request, "may provide a practical means of reducing lead exposure for future generations of children who will continue to occupy older lead-painted housing which cannot be fully abated or rehabilitated without substantial subsidy."[49] In the struggle to prevent lead poisoning, there was no question in the researchers' minds as to what was ultimately needed: the complete removal of lead paint. But "repair and maintenance" was a compromise they made in the hopes of doing at least some good in a difficult time.

The Farfel and Chisolm study was designed to test the efficacy of three different methods of lead reduction in older homes. The investigators then planned to contrast results with those of two control groups: one of children living in homes that had previously undergone what was thought to have been full lead abatement and the second of children living in homes built after 1978 and presumed to be lead free. For the study, more than a hundred parents with young children were recruited to live in the various partially lead-abated houses. The premise of the research was that children would now be in a safer environment, a home that was an improvement over the lead-covered homes that were generally available to poor residents of Baltimore. However, the blood lead levels of children in at least two of the homes rose over the course of the study.[50] It was the two sets of parents of these children who filed the lawsuits alleging that they had not been properly informed of the risks their children faced while participating in the study.[51]

To some, the Johns Hopkins study was an attempt by dedicated researchers to address the discoveries about the effects of low-level lead exposure and determine the cost of reducing harm to children living in leaded environments. This was the view the Baltimore City Circuit Court took in granting KKI's motion for summary judgment and dismissing the suit initially. But others, including the plaintiffs on appeal, clearly saw things in a different light. In reversing the lower court's decision and ordering the lawsuits to proceed to trial, the Maryland Court of Appeals in 2001, quite aware that the subjects of the KKI study were African American children, saw the case through the lens of a long history of ethical and social debate over the use of vulnerable populations in human subjects research, as well as through the lens of the ongoing environmental justice movement that joined the civil rights and environmental movements of the previous three decades. Since the 1970s, and particularly following revelations about the Tuskegee experiments, in which an initial sample of 399 African American men with syphilis were "observed" over a forty-year period from the early 1930s through the early 1970s and to whom state-of-the-art treatments were denied, historians, ethicists, and others had explored instances where scientific research has crossed generally accepted ethical and social boundaries. They had detailed the evolution of standards for human subjects research, the importance of informed consent, and other ethical issues involved in nontherapeutic and sometimes harmful experimentation.

The Baltimore study was organized in the wake of a dramatic rethinking of the use of human subjects in scientific experiments. During the preceding two decades researchers had become acutely aware of the ethical dilemmas presented by human subjects research, especially when it involved "vulnerable populations." The legacy of Nuremberg, the revelations about the Tuskegee experiments, and publication in the late 1970s of the "Belmont Report," the landmark federal report that expanded and codified the principles of ethical research with human subjects, all combined to cast doubt on the morality and ethical basis of the KKI research.[52] But this framework may be too simple, incapable of acknowledging the complexity of the issues at hand.

Two contending interpretations of the events in Baltimore indicate fissures in the public health community over the ethics and politics of the KKI study, echoing the debates over research on vulnerable populations that emerged in the 1970s, 1980s, and 1990s and the debates over what was feasible to accomplish in a conservative political environment. In one common interpretation, the KKI study was intrinsically unethical because the means of protecting children by complete abatement from lead poisoning were well known, and to knowingly subject children to lead by placing them in homes where only partial abatement had been performed put them needlessly at risk. In the main contending interpretation, research such as Farfel and Chisolm's on incremental improvements that could lessen exposures was necessary and important because, in the context of the social realities of housing and income inequalities in America, complete abatement on a large scale was a utopian idea. As two subscribers to this general interpretation explained, "Powerfully appealing egalitarian principles cannot be regarded as a sufficiently compelling reason to totally shut down research that offers a realistic prospect of improving conditions [in this instance, complete abatement] or to what many might consider a minimally just standard of living. . . . We contend that it is the failure to conduct such research that causes the greater harm, because it limits health interventions to the status quo of those who can afford currently available options [complete abatement] and deprives disadvantaged populations of the benefits of imminent incremental improvements in their health conditions."[53]

In this light, the history of the KKI research could be seen as a tragedy rather than a melodrama: a fight between two defensible conceptions of the public good rather than a fight between the forces of good and evil. Of course, this raises different questions: Are two defensible conceptions of the public good both ethically justifiable with respect to putting others knowingly in harm's way? Could not valuable research be—and have been—done on levels of abatement without putting children in harm's way, with a differently designed study? Lurking here, too, is another question that, as we will see, adds a further twist: was it justified to assume that partial and complete abatement could be conducted safely and effectively in the early 1990s?

The decision of the Maryland Court of Appeals to let the case go forward unleashed a storm of controversy and argument, not just about the KKI study but more generally about the ethics of what was called "nontherapeutic research" on children. Until the Maryland court decision, discussion about the use of children as research subjects, according to bioethicist Lainie Friedman Ross, had been largely "pragmatic." She notes that "unless research is done with children the advances of modern medicine cannot accrue to them or to future generations of children."[54] Following the KKI decision, the questions became more complex as ethicists began weighing in.

The first article laying out the issues raised by the court's ruling was written by Robert Nelson, a professor of anesthesia and pediatrics at Philadelphia's Children's Hospital, and published in late 2001. Nelson addressed three basic considerations relating to the use of children as vulnerable populations in research: (1) whether or not "the interventions or procedures of the research offered the prospect of direct benefit to enrolled children"; (2) whether or not the "interventions or procedures involved in the research provided greater-than-minimal risk"; and (3) whether or not the parents of the children were properly informed of the potential risks of the study. On each of these issues Nelson argued that the court had acted properly in remanding the case to trial. With regard to the first question, for half of the children (those already living in housing that was to be abated as part of the study) the study "offered the prospect of direct benefit," he said. But this was not true for those children who were moved into potentially more dangerous situations. Ethically, the partially abated home was a potential danger and therefore moving a child into it could not be considered a direct benefit. This was related to the second issue, whether the study presented these children with greater than minimal risk. Addressing this question was critical because the Belmont Report in 1977 argued, according to Nelson, "that a parent lacks the moral authority to expose a healthy child to more than minimal risk research." Because the KKI researchers did not know for certain how partial lead abatement would affect the blood lead levels of the children, "the risk of continued lead exposure compared to the standard or full lead abatement procedure is more than minimal." In addition, Nelson maintained, intentionally exposing children to lead by moving them into partially abated homes "cannot be considered as minimal risk" because "a 'reasonable parent' would not intentionally expose a child to environmental lead without making every effort to reduce or eliminate the lead exposure."[55]

Were the parents properly informed about the critical matters that might concern a parent of a young child exposed to lead? The KKI study consent forms offered to the parents, Nelson said, "did not contain information that the 'reasonable parent' would want to know," specifically, that the aim of the study was to evaluate "the effectiveness of three different methods of lead abatement," what the impact on young children would be of the resulting lead exposure, and what the risks were "of inadequate lead abatement."[56] Further, what action was reasonable to expect from public health and housing officials in this conservative political era?

In the end, Nelson concluded, the court of appeals's decision was consistent with the recommendations of the Belmont Report that "parents do not have the moral or legal authority to enroll healthy children in research that does not offer the prospect of direct benefit unless the risks of that research are no greater than the ordinary risks of daily life—a standard referred to as 'minimal risks.'"[57] In short, healthy children should not be encouraged to move into potentially dangerous situations.

Following the court's decision, the critical issue that emerged for researchers, policy makers, and the public alike was the meaning of "minimal risk" and, more specifically, the relationship between socioeconomic inequality and the everyday risks of being poor in American society. The KKI study and the court's response to it begged the question of whose life should be the standard of "the ordinary risks of daily life." Did the dangers inherent in being poor mean, for example, that the children in the KKI study, because their everyday experience carried with it greater potential for harm, could be exposed to greater danger than average middle-class children who lived in a safer environment?

"Two entirely different standards emerge [in interpreting the meaning of 'minimal risk'] depending upon whether researchers consider the daily or routine risks of harm encountered by *some* or *all* children," wrote Loretta Kopelman, a professor at the Brody School of Medicine of East Carolina University and a member of the Institute of Medicine's Committee on Research on Children. "With the first interpretation, or relative standard, the upper limit of harm would vary according to the particular group of subjects; with the second, or absolute standard, the upper limit would be the risks of harm encountered by all children, even wealthy and healthy children." Kopelman reminded readers of the terrible consequences and ethical quandaries of such interpretative variation. In the 1960s and 1970s, for example, mentally retarded children had been used as subjects in the infamous Willowbrook hepatitis studies in which children were given hepatitis using the rationale that the "disease was endemic to the institution [and thus] the children would eventually have gotten hepatitis."[58]

As the court of appeals's ruling sank in, its implications appeared more profound and troubling. In an article titled "Canaries in the Mines," Merle Spriggs, a medical ethicist at the University of Melbourne's Murdoch Children's Research Institute, gave perhaps the most cutting critique of the Johns Hopkins research: "The argument that the [KKI] families benefitted because they were not worse off can be compared with the arguments used in the infamous, widely discussed mother-child HIV transmission prevention trials in developing countries," Spriggs said, referring to medical trials sponsored in the previous decade by the U.S. government in which researchers, seeking an inexpensive, effective way of reducing HIV transmission between mothers and children in African countries, provided AZT treatments to some mothers while comparing them with untreated "controls" who received only a placebo. Some argued that the research was justified in part because the African women who received the placebo would not normally have received any treatment at all, though ethical concerns would have precluded the research from being conducted in the United States. Both the HIV transmission prevention trials and the KKI research, Spriggs pointed out, "involved the problematic idea of a local standard of care," an underlying assumption that "risky research is less ethically problematic among people who are already disadvantaged." If this "relativistic interpretation of minimal risk" was considered acceptable, it opened a Pandora's box of deeply disturbing issues and could virtually unleash the research community on poor people. She warned that such a stance "could allow children living in hazardous environments or who faced danger on a daily basis to be the subject of high risk studies."[59]

Above all, what the KKI research effort exposed was a fault line that divides poor people from the rest of Americans and extends far beyond the ethics of occasional research. No one would suggest that a middle-class family allow their children to be knowingly exposed to a toxin that could be removed from their immediate environment. But for decades, as a society we have accepted that poor children can be treated differently. We have watched for over a century as children have, in effect, been treated as research subjects in a grand experiment without purpose. How much lead is too much lead? What are the limits of our responsibility as a society to protect those without the resources to protect themselves? As we confront new information about environmental toxins like mercury, bisphenol A, phthalates, and a host of new chemicals that are introduced every year into the air, water, and soil, whose reach extends beyond the poor, the issues raised by the KKI story—and by the modern history of the lead wars more generally—are issues that, by our responses, will define us all.

The history of lead poisoning and lead research is paradigmatic of the developing controversies over a range of toxins and other health-related issues now being debated in the popular press, the courts, and among environmental activists and consumer organizations, as well as within the public health profession itself. Public health officials struggle mightily with declining budgets, a conservative political climate, and a host of challenging and new health-related problems. Today, the public health community continues to have the responsibility to prevent disease. But it has neither the resources, the political mandate, nor the authority to accomplish this task, certainly not by itself. It is an open question whether it has the vision to help lead the effort, or to inspire the efforts needed.

Whatever the limitations of the bacteriological and laboratory-based model that public health developed in the early part of the twentieth century in response to the crises of infectious disease, there is no arguing that this model provided a coherent and unifying rationale for the profession. But, as we witness the emergence of chronic illnesses linked to low levels of toxic exposures, no powerful unifying paradigm has replaced bacteriology. Some suggest that the "precautionary principle" can serve as an overall guide, arguing that it is the responsibility of companies to show that their products are safe before introducing them into the marketplace or the environment, that we as a society should err on the side of safety rather than await possible harm. By adopting this approach, public health would reestablish prevention as its primary creed. Others insist that a renewed focus on corporate power, economic inequality, low-income housing options, racism, and other social forces that shape health outcomes is most needed to counter the antiregulatory regime of early twenty-first-century America. These ideas, or a more unified alternative, however, have yet to galvanize the field or the broader public, at least in the United States.

In this book we look at the shifting politics of lead over the past half century and the implications for the future of public health and emerging controversies over the effects of other toxins. The developing science of lead's effects, the attempts of industry to belittle that science, the struggles over lead regulation, and the court battles of lead's victims have taken place against the backdrop of a changing disease environment and, in more recent decades, an emerging conservative political culture, both in the broader society and in the public health profession.

Researchers have shown over the last five decades that the effects of lead, at ever-lower exposures tested, represent a continuing threat to children, a tragedy of huge dimensions. In the coming decades, without substantial political and social change, we will be placing millions more children at risk of life-altering damage. This research, combined with declining public will and resources to remove lead from children's environment, has left the public health community and society at large with a difficult dilemma, not unlike that which Julian Chisolm and his young colleague Mark Farfel faced: Should we insist on the complete removal of lead from the nation's walls, through some combination of full abatement and new housing, and therefore a permanent solution to this century-old scourge? Or should we search for a "practical" way to reduce the exposure of children to "an acceptable" level?

If we choose the former, the danger is that, without strong popular and political advocacy and a public health profession rededicated to the effort, nothing will be done—complete abatement may well be judged too costly, and we may encounter an ugly unwillingness to address a problem that primarily affects poor children, many of them from ethnic and racial minority groups. If we choose the latter, and if the dominant political forces give at best only grudging support to this ameliorative effort, the danger is that the children of entire communities will continue to be exposed, albeit at gradually declining levels, to the subtle and life-altering effects of lead. Public health as an institution, in trying to define what an "acceptable" level is, could lose in the process its moral authority and its century-long commitment to prevention, yet with no viable coherent intellectual alternative. This is a conundrum that affects us all, for we console ourselves with partial victories, often framed as progress in the form of harm reduction rather than prevention. We have become willing to settle for half measures, especially when what is at issue is the health of others, not of oneself. Isn't this, so to speak, the plague on *all* our houses? In this sense, we are all complicit in the "experiment" that allows certain classes of people to be subjected to possible harm in the expectation of avoiding it ourselves.

2   From Personal Tragedy to Public Health Crisis

> All scientific work is liable to be upset or modified by advancing knowledge. That does not confer upon us a freedom to ignore the knowledge we already have, or to postpone the action that it appears to demand at a given time.
>
> BRADFORD HILL, 1965

By the mid-1950s the cat was out of the bag. Any doubt that lead exposure could permanently damage children was put to rest as researchers at Harvard documented continuing mental and neurological disorders among those ostensibly "cured" of acute lead poisoning, which was most often diagnosed after children showed a variety of symptoms, such as convulsions, muscle paralysis, "mental lethargy," vomiting on eating solid food, and dizziness. For generations it was well recognized that workers in lead-based industries suffered severe neurological damage from lead poisoning, and by early in the twentieth century women and children were often barred from working in the areas of pigment and paint factories where lead was used. Beginning in the early twentieth century recognition grew that children outside the factory were also at risk because of contact with lead paint in their homes. As the nation's cities grew exponentially following the Civil War, so too did the danger from lead paint that was used in and on the new houses.

By the 1920s physicians were remarking on the fact that children "lived in a lead world," and by the 1940s a huge literature had emerged that detailed the horrifying effects of this metal on children. But for both children and adults prior to the 1940s, the assumption had been that if the overt symptoms of lead poisoning passed, there would be no residual effects. During World War II, the two Harvard researchers—Randolph Byers and Elizabeth Lord, a pediatrician and psychologist, respectively, at Boston's Children's Hospital—documented the long-term effects of acute lead poisoning even after a child had ostensibly "recovered." From a group of 128 patients ranging in age from about ten months to four years who had been admitted with acute symptoms of lead poisoning over the span of a decade, the researchers followed twenty children who still lived in the

Boston area. All but one of the children who had returned home with no clinical symptoms of cerebral damage still suffered in "both the intellectual and emotional spheres" in school over the course of the study. These children's motor coordination was abnormal and their general intelligence appeared to have been permanently affected. A few of the children suffered "recurrent convulsions." One child at the end of first grade had "not learned to write or print his name or recognize any figure." Another six-year-old was described as "cruel, unreliable [with] impulsive behavior; runaway; unable to get on with other children or adults; excluded from school because of behavior."[1] In the decades since, researchers and clinicians have documented the huge numbers of children at risk, now with the understanding that lead causes permanent damage.

As the seriousness of this epidemic became increasingly apparent in the 1950s, public health officials in Baltimore, New York, Chicago, Cincinnati, Boston, and other large cities began to follow the scientific and medical literature on the effects of lead paint poisoning. Many cities passed ordinances that required warnings on containers and restrictions on the sale of lead paints for use on walls, woodwork, and other surfaces accessible to children. But their actions were piecemeal and uncoordinated.

Historically, health departments in the United States were local operations whose administrators rarely harmonized responses with each other, even in the face of the most dire public health threats. In the case of childhood lead poisoning, very few city administrators as late as the 1950s were even aware of the national scope of the problem, much less how colleagues in other communities were coping with it. While some of the larger cities began to establish registers to document the extent of the problem within their jurisdiction, there was no central source for information outside of the Lead Industries Association (LIA), the trade association of the lead industry. Nor did public health officials generally remember the controversy that arose about the potential hazards from lead when it was introduced into gasoline in the 1920s.

Since its creation in 1928, the LIA had downplayed health concerns for fear that they might undermine business, but that had not stopped the organization from tracking reported cases in the medical literature of death and disease among children exposed to lead paint. In the 1950s the LIA bragged that it possessed the most extensive archive of newspaper articles, reports, and general information on this toxic metal.[2] Though the U.S. Public Health Service (PHS) was nominally responsible for addressing the health effects of toxic metals, at the time this agency was largely focused on the problems of infectious epidemic diseases and their threat to the nation as a whole. The modern federal institutions that potentially might coordinate a national effort to inform local agencies of toxic threats and to coordinate remedial action were just being born. The U.S. Department of Health Education and Welfare, the predecessor to the current U.S. Department of Health and Human Services, which today oversees the PHS and the National Institutes of Health, was only established by Congress in 1954.

In the absence of federal and local knowledge and coordination on lead issues, from the 1930s through the 1950s the LIA assumed a central role in funding research on lead-related illness and framing national policy regarding childhood lead paint poisoning. The trade group resisted efforts by cities and states to regulate lead pigments in paint. Instead, in the 1950s it called for the establishment of limited, voluntary agreements among paint manufacturers to cap the amount of lead used in paints intended for indoor use. These recommendations the LIA misleadingly called "standards," and both the lead and paint industries hoped they would thereby inoculate pigment and paint manufacturers from state and local regulatory action. The lead industry, through the LIA, in effect set the agenda that public health officials and lead researchers would live by for the foreseeable future: and the LIA of course did not advocate the removal of lead paint from the walls of homes. Rather, from the 1950s onward it promoted the view that lead poisoning was a virtually insoluble problem, largely limited to black and Puerto Rican children living in slum dwellings, and that the elimination of childhood lead poisoning was a utopian dream.

Before the mid-1950s, the one exception to general ignorance about the extent of lead poisoning was in Baltimore, where in the 1930s the Department of Health had begun to track and even treat lead-poisoned children who appeared in its clinics. Baltimore was the first and only American municipality before the 1950s to develop, according to the pioneering research of historian Elizabeth Fee, "an extensive public health program on childhood lead paint poisoning."[3] The City organized health education campaigns, housing inspections, and lead-abatement programs, and it passed some of the nation's first paint-labeling laws. Baltimore's visionary commissioner of health, Huntington Williams, appointed in 1931, was instrumental in bringing the city's lead problem to the forefront of public health knowledge. Baltimore's early recognition of the issue's seriousness may also be traced to the identification of fifty-nine cases of lead poisoning among poor African Americans who had burned battery casings to keep warm in the early years of the Depression.[4] According to Fee, "Several patients developed acute encephalitis while others experienced headaches, vomiting, and dizziness."[5] The *Baltimore American*, too, described cases of lead poisoning and its dangers and communicated Health Department warnings about ingesting lead paint. "Parents should be on the lookout and remember that paints often contain large quantities of lead compounds and that the eating of considerable amount from paint materials may result in lead poisoning," read one such alert from the 1930s.[6]

By 1935, the Health Department had begun to offer free laboratory diagnostic tests to doctors who suspected that their patients were suffering from lead poisoning.[7] Department inspectors visited homes, took samples of loose paint, and tested them for lead. When lead was found, the agency ordered the paint removed.[8] During the first three years of the program, fifty-seven cases of acute lead paint poisoning in children were confirmed. Throughout the 1930s, the department documented paint as a prime source of childhood lead poisoning and used the new medium of radio to warn local residents of the often dire, even fatal effects of lead poisoning.[9]

The dedication of Williams and the Baltimore Department of Health to uncovering lead-poisoned children was quite remarkable, given the enormous effort such an undertaking required. It was nearly impossible to get children tested for suspected lead poisoning for several reasons: legal restrictions limited testing to occupational, not environmental, exposures; the tests themselves were difficult to carry out; and only a limited number of laboratories were capable of performing the extraordinarily time-consuming analysis needed.[10] As late as the 1950s, one technician could typically analyze only eight tests per day.[11]

By the early 1940s, it was abundantly clear to Baltimore's health officials that children were the prime victims of lead poisoning: according to Fee, in 1942 "86 per cent of the recorded deaths [from lead] were those of children, with an average age of death of two and one half years."[12] Recognizing that the problem was related to lead paint in the dilapidated slum housing of the city, Williams convinced the mayor to promote a city ordinance that would enable Baltimore to take action when harm seemed imminent. The Hygiene of Housing Ordinance was signed into law in 1941, authorizing the commissioner of health to order the removal or abatement of anything in a building or structure found to be "dangerous or detrimental to life or health."[13]

Baltimore's efforts were only successful in removing lead from a small number of buildings, but those efforts demonstrated that if you looked for lead poisoning among America's urban children, you generally found it.[14] Because of Huntington Williams's efforts, Baltimore provided the nation's most startling evidence on childhood lead poisoning. This in turn prompted Maryland to pass a Toxic Finishes Law in 1949, which, one LIA spokesman noted, "made it unlawful to sell toys and playthings, including children's furniture, finished with any material containing 'lead or other substance of a poisonous nature from contact with which children may be injuriously affected' unless such articles are so labeled as to show that the finish contains lead or other poisonous substance."[15] The LIA subsequently lobbied state officials to repeal the law and soon claimed success in 1950 when the governor signed the repeal: "The campaign to remove this 1949 enactment from the statute books of the state was brought to a successful conclusion," the association trumpeted to its members.[16] The law imposed a burden on its affiliates, the organization said,[17] while its health and safety director, Manfred Bowditch, complained privately that "these young Baltimore paint eaters were a real headache."[18] Not surprisingly, the lead industry favored placing the burden for preventing lead poisoning directly on the family. "The only seemingly feasible means of coping with the childhood plumbism problem is that of parental education," the LIA argued.[19] This ran counter to some of the oldest observations about childhood lead poisoning, dating at least to the first decade of the twentieth century when A.J. Turner, one of the first researchers to document childhood lead poisoning due to paint, argued that public health could not rely on parental education; legislation was needed to stem the epidemic.[20]

By the 1950s Baltimore institutions were dramatically affected by the ongoing lead crisis. Indicative is the experience at one hospital in Baltimore, as summarized by Mark Farfel: "Ninety per cent of the children between the age of seven months and five years seen at the hospital's outpatient clinics in a one year period in the early 1950s had blood lead levels greater than 30 µg/dl [micrograms per deciliter]."[21] In an attempt to curb the further spread of lead paint, Baltimore's health commissioner issued a regulation in 1951 that it would take other communities at least a decade to replicate: "No paint shall be used for interior painting of any dwelling or dwelling unit or any part thereof unless the paint is free from any lead pigment."[22]

Huntington Williams meanwhile had begun looking beyond the seizures and deaths of children to speculate that "unrecognized plumbism, lead poisoning, in children may explain many obscure nervous conditions and convulsions of undetermined etiology." His (correct) conclusion was that "lead poisoning is cumulative."[23] Even the LIA, in 1950, recognized that new problems were on the horizon: "As our hygiene activities have expanded, the magnitude of our industry's health problems become more and more evident."[24] In 1953, the LIA said it collected during the previous year "nearly 500 newspaper clippings featuring lead poisoning, often in sizable headlines," indicative of the greater role the press was playing in bringing the severity of lead poisoning to the attention of the general public. Internally, the LIA admitted that "childhood lead poisoning continued to be a major problem and source of much adverse publicity,"[25] yet it still opposed warning consumers of the danger its product posed to children.

The continual refrain from the lead industry—that childhood plumbism could only be addressed through the voluntary action of parents—quickly grew stale for anyone who routinely saw the effects of acute lead poisoning. J. Julian Chisolm, then a young physician associated with Johns Hopkins Hospital, had much firsthand experience with the group of children that by the mid-1950s were unfortunately labeled "lead heads" by the young residents at the hospital. Chisolm took issue with the industry's casual attitude toward what was obviously a serious medical problem affecting Baltimore's children. In a study of children at the Harriet Lane Home, he and his coauthor, Harold Harrison, had inspected sources of lead contamination in homes and found, like Henry Thomas and Kenneth Blackfan more than forty years before, that the prime "sources of lead were windowsills and frames, interior walls, including painted paper and painted plaster, door frames, furniture and cribs." Throughout the "dilapidated dwellings" where young children lived, Chisolm observed that "flaking leaded paint is readily accessible." He took umbrage that the industry blamed parents for the tragedy: "While the responsibility of parents to protect their children from environmental hazards is not denied, no mother can reasonably be expected to prevent the repetitive ingestion of a few paint chips when these are readily accessible."[26]

THE GROWING EPIDEMIC: FROM
BALTIMORE TO THE NATION

As early as 1951, the *American Journal of Public Health* acknowledged both the centrality of Baltimore and Johns Hopkins in the unfolding story of lead-poisoned children and the reality of lead poisoning as a nationwide problem. It chastised the public health profession for not recognizing the extent of lead poisoning, sarcastically asking "whether babies brought up in the shadow of 'the Hopkins' develop peculiar alimentary tastes not common elsewhere" and arguing that "if such is not the case, perhaps other health officers have been missing something."[27] This was indeed the case in Chicago, where Robert Mellins, a young Public Health Service officer, uncovered an epidemic of childhood lead poisoning in 1953. Mellins had been assigned to Chicago in response to the continuing polio epidemic that terrified the nation in the post–World War II era. His first day in Chicago, he learned from local health personnel about what they feared was an outbreak among the city's children of St. Louis encephalitis, a serious mosquito-borne neurological disease. Having been a medical student at Johns Hopkins in the late 1940s and early 1950s, Mellins was aware that lead poisoning was often mistaken for encephalitis, which led him to question the diagnosis and suggest the children be reevaluated. What he had come upon was, in fact, the first epidemic of lead poisoning in Chicago that would be recognized as such.[28]

In an internal summary of his LIA activities in 1952, Manfred Bowditch once again used the image of a "major headache" in what was emerging as a major national tragedy. Calling childhood lead poisoning "a source of much adverse publicity," he counted 197 reports of lead poisoning in nine cities, of which 40 were fatal, but acknowledged that this was an "incomplete" estimate, especially for New York City.[29] Others also began to notice the scale of the epidemic. Between 1951 and 1953, according to George M. Wheatley of the American Academy of Pediatrics, as reported in the *New York Times*, "there were 94 deaths and 165 cases of childhood lead poisoning . . . in New York, Chicago, Cincinnati, St. Louis, and Baltimore."[30] By the standards of the time, these were of course only the most acute cases, often life-threatening; lead poisoning that caused lesser damage was neither the focus nor in many instances even attributed to lead.

The LIA was caught in a bind. On the one hand, it had in its possession numerous reports from health departments demonstrating the widespread nature of the lead paint hazard. On the other hand, the association was fighting a rearguard action hoping to convince officials and the public that the number of lead-poisoning cases was exaggerated. To continue in this fight, Bowditch confided to an industry colleague, would be "prohibitively expensive and time-consuming."[31] Bowditch did not dispute that childhood lead poisoning could come from ingesting lead-based paint. But rather than concentrate on how to prevent lead poisoning—toward which a first step would be the elimination of lead from interior paint—Bowditch believed the LIA should focus on "securing more accurate diagnoses of lead poisoning or face the likelihood of widespread governmental prohibition of the use of lead paints on dwellings."[32] Robert Kehoe, the longtime head of the Kettering Institute at the University of Cincinnati, a research center established and funded by the Ethyl and General Motors Corporations in the 1920s, admitted in 1953 in a personal letter that the problem was not diagnostics but the paint itself. If the elimination of lead paint "for all inside decoration in the household and in the environment of young children . . .

is not done voluntarily by a wise industry concerned to handle its own business properly, it will be accomplished ineffectually and with irrelevant difficulties and disadvantages through legislation."[33]

By the mid-1950s, newspapers and public health departments in other cities had begun to report more systematically on cases of lead poisoning. The LIA responded by trying to divert attention from the lead industry's role in distributing a known poison, sometimes in the process even mocking the children who were poisoned. In a private letter to the editor of the *American Journal of Public Health*, Bowditch suggested that the high rates of lead poisoning in Baltimore indicated that there was "all too much 'gnaw-ledge' among Baltimore babies."[34] When he was being serious he was even more dismissive of the victims: the problem was not lead in the paint, it was the housing and the parents. In 1956 Bowditch wrote to a former head of the LIA, Felix Wormser, then assistant secretary of the interior—the federal agency responsible for regulating lead and other mining and metal industries—criticizing an article on childhood lead poisoning that had appeared in *Parade*, the nationally distributed Sunday newspaper supplement. "Aside from the kids that are poisoned," Bowditch complained, "it's a serious problem from the viewpoint of adverse publicity." The basic problem was "slums," he argued, and to deal with that issue it was necessary "to educate the parents." "But most of the cases are in Negro and Puerto Rican families, and how," Bowditch wondered, "does one tackle that job?"[35]

Bowditch was a bit more discreet in his statements to the LIA's general membership. At the association's 1957 annual meeting, he argued that "the major source of trouble is the flaking of lead paint in the ancient slum dwellings of our older cities"—though in saying this he obscured the fact that lead had been the main component of interior paint as recently as the early 1950s (and still constituted 1 percent of many wall paints for the next twenty years). "The problem of lead poisoning in children will be with us for as long as there are slums," he said. But then he absolved the LIA of responsibility, again arguing that the real problem lay with the ignorant children and parents. "Because of the high death rate, the frequency of permanent brain damage in the survivors and the intelligence level of the slum parents, it [the issue of lead-poisoned children] seems destined to remain as important and as difficult [a problem] as any with which we have to deal."[36]

But how could the problem be addressed? Bowditch was not optimistic: "until we can find means to (a) get rid of our slums and (b) educate the relatively ineducable parent, the problem will continue to plague us."[37] This argument, that it was inevitable that black and Puerto Rican children would be damaged by lead for the foreseeable future, set the stage for the next half century of lead-poisoning policy. With the lead industry unwilling to accept its responsibility for this epidemic or remove all lead from paint, and with only sporadic moves to restrict use of lead products and enforce the housing codes that did exist, doctors were forced to treat more and more children suffering from lead-induced acute symptoms of severe brain damage with powerful drugs, the "chelating agents" that when introduced into the blood stream could bind with lead, allowing it to be passed from the body through urination. The more sophisticated and progressive public health departments would sometimes visit children's homes and remove the lead from the walls. At best, this helped to prevent further injury, but such remedial actions did little to forestall the housing, pediatric, and public health crises that were emerging. The industry's proposition that lead poisoning was largely a problem of "flaking of lead paint in the ancient slum dwellings of our older cities" rendered it a disease of poverty and the socioeconomically deprived. As lead poisoning became increasingly defined as a problem of poor African American and Latino children in urban slums, in this pre–civil rights era there was no active political constituency capable of making it a pressing concern.[38]

From the very first, then, lead poisoning and housing were inextricably linked. For housing officials, removing lead paint was (and still is) an expensive procedure that landlords were often unwilling to undertake. And housing officials in the few cities that passed regulations to control lead often ignored these housing codes, fearing that the expense of abatement would prompt landlords to abandon their properties.[39] Further, effective enforcement required a huge army of inspectors, personnel that were unavailable to local departments of health with limited budgets. Finally, identifying dilapidated interiors was itself difficult because most poor tenants were unaware of their rights to a safe home even under the existing housing codes, or they were afraid they might be evicted if they filed a complaint. Even when buildings with peeling lead paint were identified, it might take months, even years for a landlord to be hauled into court, and even then the fines were generally minimal, leading landlords to forego expensive repairs and pay the eventual fine instead.[40]

Children suffered enormously as a result of this inaction. Until the 1950s, when BAL (British anti-Lewisite, or Dimercaprol) and CaEDTA (ethylenediaminetetraacetic acid) were introduced as chelating agents,[41] two-thirds of children who suffered convulsions and swelling of the brain due to lead ingestion died. With the use of chelating agents, the death rate was cut in half, but it was still almost one in three,[42] and those who did survive were often deeply damaged.

IT'S IN THE AIR: LEADED GASOLINE AND OTHER
SOURCES OF LEAD DANGER

Increased attention to paint as a source of lead in the environment was complemented in the early and mid-1960s by a growing body of evidence suggesting that significant amounts of lead were also entering the human environment through other means: contamination of the soil and air from insecticides; and fallout from lead-bearing compounds during smelting, mining, and fabricating processes and automobile exhausts. Pots and pans, water pipes made of lead or joined by lead solders, and cans sealed with lead solder—once hailed by the industry as symbols of lead's role in creating the modern environment—were now suspected as contaminants of the human food chain, as was beef, from the lead cattle absorbed in grazing. To explore these issues, the U.S. Public Health Service sponsored a conference in 1965 on environmental lead contamination, where it soon became clear that lead from gasoline was the most pressing concern because of its magnitude and dispersal throughout the country.

As early as the 1920s, public health leaders had worried that the introduction of lead into gasoline would, as the auto industry expanded, ultimately prove to be a serious source of environmental pollution.[43] A 1966 study of lead in the soot of New York City streets, for example, revealed the startling fact that its lead concentration was 2,650 parts per million (ppm).[44] Of particular worry at the time was the rapid expansion of the interstate highway system through the heart of most American cities: studies had found that much more lead was deposited from exhaust pipes when cars were moving at high speeds, thereby increasing the threat to urban populations.[45]

Yet since the 1920s the lead industry had sponsored research by Robert Kehoe that claimed that introducing more lead, even much more lead, into the environment presented no danger to people because, he argued, lead was a natural part of the human environment and people had developed mechanisms over the millennia to excrete lead as rapidly as they inhaled or ingested it. This rationale, that lead was a "natural" constituent of the human environment, became a mainstay of the industry argument from the 1920s forward. At the 1965 conference, Kehoe laid out the industry view of lead's dangers: the intake of lead "is balanced for all practical purposes by an equivalent output," so there was "an equilibrium with the environment." Did the lead that people absorbed in the course of their daily lives constitute a risk? "The answer," said Kehoe, "is in the negative."[46]

This fanciful model of lead's ecology was dismantled piece by piece as speaker after speaker at the conference, for the most part in a businesslike and respectful manner, questioned Kehoe's underlying assumptions. While the world of lead toxicology was still relatively small and dominated by a few recognized experts, new voices, influenced by the emerging environmental movement following publication of Rachel Carson's *Silent Spring* in 1962, were beginning to be heard. Criticisms of virtually every element of Kehoe's model were made throughout the conference, but only on the last day did they coalesce as a full-blown rejection of the industry's paradigm. Harry Heimann of Harvard's School of Public Health, who had had experience working in the PHS Division of Air Pollution, told the conference that he wanted to make some "comments based on my listening for the last two days, having some discussions with some people in and outside the room, and my experience as a physician who has spent most of my life in public health work." While he did not "mean to get into any acrimonious debate" and was "not intending to impugn anybody's work," Heimann confronted Kehoe directly. He announced that he felt compelled to "point out that there has been no evidence that has ever come to my attention . . . that a little lead is good for you." It was, he went on, "extremely unusual in medical research that there is only one small group and one place in a country in which research in a specific area of knowledge is exclusively done." Kehoe's experiments that were said to provide evidence that lead from gasoline and other airborne sources presented little danger to people would need "to be repeated in many other places, and be extended," before the scientific community lent them legitimacy. He also questioned Kehoe's assertion that no danger existed below a blood lead level of 80 micrograms per deciliter, a reading that often corresponded with convulsions in adults working in lead-paint and other factories.[47]

In addition to presenting a clear challenge to the paradigm that Kehoe and the lead industry had carefully propagated for more than thirty years, participants at the 1965 conference challenged the very basis of industrial toxicology as it then existed. In the words of one attendee, lead toxicology put "the whole field of environmental health . . . on trial."[48] Scientists had for too long accepted the industry argument that if workers who were exposed to various toxins, including lead, did not show symptoms of disease, the public had little to worry about, since consumers were exposed to much lower levels of these materials. A broad public debate was needed on what was, and was not, an acceptable risk; industry assurances of safety were not sufficient. The "public at large [needed to] be given a rational basis on which to decide . . . that lead should or shouldn't be taken out of gasoline, that pesticides should or shouldn't be used in various situations, that asbestos should be curbed."[49] Indeed, in the coming years, the field of lead toxicology would be transformed to address just such concerns.

In the mid-1960s, Kehoe was just one of several industry supporters repeating the mantra that the critical measure of lead's toxicity was the worker in the plant. Studies had shown that lead workers on average were absorbing less lead than earlier in the century, and industry touted this as proof that the public was protected as well. When Senator Edmund Muskie (D-ME) held hearings on air pollution in mid-1966, the LIA campaigned to undercut any criticism of the lead industry that might emerge. In addition to preparing articles and press releases to encourage "positive stories regarding lead and its uses," the LIA developed testimony for the hearings.[50] Felix Wormser, retired but still on retainer for St. Joseph Lead Company, testified on behalf of the LIA, asserting that "vast clinical evidence" showed that "the general public is not now, nor in the immediate future, facing a lead hazard." Leaded gas posed no harm at all and a vast literature and much research confirmed this view, he claimed.[51] Kehoe went on to testify that "the evidence at the present time is better than it has been at any time and that [lead] is not a present hazard."[52] His commitment to an 80 µg/dl blood-lead-level threshold blinded him to the possibility that, whatever this standard's adequacy for protecting adults, children, because of lead's effect on their developing neurological systems, might be at much greater risk at lower levels.

Though Kehoe's position aroused skepticism among some in scientific and political arenas, it still found considerable acceptance among the general public. Kehoe himself had told Muskie's committee that his laboratory was "the only source of new information" about lead in the factory and the environment and had "a wide influence in this country and abroad in shaping the point of view and activities . . . of those who are responsible for industrial and public hygiene."[53]

Storm clouds were appearing on the horizon, however. In 1967, the LIA commissioned the Opinion Research Corporation to conduct a survey of "public knowledge and attitudes on lead." The survey revealed that 42 percent of the public identified "lead among ten substances as being harmful to health." In fact, lead ranked second only to carbon monoxide in Americans' perceptions of risk. The only solace the LIA could garner from the survey was that the public relations damage seemed, for the moment, to be contained: in the public mind, lead's danger "seems to be associated primarily with paints." Only 1 percent of those surveyed identified leaded gasoline as being "harmful to health." Still, few people polled could identify any positive uses for lead, the LIA learned, a point that did not augur well for the future. That so many people believed that lead posed a health problem meant, in the words of Hill & Knowlton, the lead industry's public relations firm, "they could be expected to be receptive to—or are, in effect, preconditioned for—suggestions that lead emissions into the atmosphere may constitute a health hazard." Hill & Knowlton warned that with increasing attention to air pollution the public could soon view leaded gasoline as a threat to their health.[54]

As with early concerns about lead paint, the industry made it its business to promote the metal as good for society and to challenge assertions that lead in the atmosphere was dangerous. In a letter to its members in 1968, the LIA extolled the importance of its new publication, *Facts about Lead in the Atmosphere*, which it described as "one phase of the LIA's efforts to refute the many claims made in the technical journals and the lay press that lead in the ambient air is reaching dangerous levels." Such claims were "entirely without foundation," the association asserted.[55] Just as the National Lead Company, producers of the Dutch Boy brand of lead pigment and paint, had sponsored ads in the century's opening decades, bragging that "Lead Helps to Guard Your Health," among other supposed benefits, the LIA called lead "an essential metal that is too commonly taken for granted by the public."[56] The uses for lead were now of a decidedly more modern and technological nature, though. It was used as "the basic ingredient in the solder that binds together our electronic miracles and is the sheath that protects our intercontinental communications system. It is the barrier that confines dangerous x-rays and atomic radiation. It is soundproofing for buildings and ships and jet planes." And, it was, of course, the major component of batteries and an ingredient of the gasoline that ran the nation's automobiles.[57]

Perhaps more than any other figure of the middle decades of the twentieth century, Clair C. Patterson, a geochemist at the California Technical Institute who had trained at the University of Chicago and had worked on the Manhattan Project during World War II, challenged the dominant paradigm of industry-sponsored lead researchers and the control that the LIA exercised in how lead was perceived. Among the many articles Patterson wrote, one that he submitted to the *Archives of Environmental Health* in 1965 particularly outraged Robert Kehoe.[58] Patterson's research challenged their belief that lead was present in only trivial amounts and had always been present at about the same level in the environment. Although both Robert Kehoe and fellow researcher Joseph Aub were asked to review Patterson's paper before its publication, only Kehoe was willing to critique it directly.

In the article, Patterson documented the extensive pollution caused by the growing use of lead in the wake of the Industrial Revolution.[59] He had taken core samples of ice from the polar ice cap and measured them for metal content. The increase of lead over time in the core samples from Greenland paralleled the increase in lead smelting and, what was more telling, the consumption of leaded gasoline. The lead concentration of the ice had risen 400 percent in the two hundred years from the mid-eighteenth to the early twentieth centuries; but in just the ensuing twenty-five years, the period when leaded gasoline became the standard fuel for the exploding automobile industry in Europe and America, it rose another 300 percent.[60] Patterson estimated that the average level of lead in the blood of Americans was about 20 µg/dl, well below what in the early 1960s was considered the "danger point," 80 µg/dl, but still startling.[61] (Today, as we have seen, the Centers for Disease Control defines 5 µg/dl as "elevated.") In this, Patterson was directly contradicting Kehoe's long-standing argument that humans had been adapted to roughly current levels of lead for centuries.

Far from it being normal for Americans to have such elevated levels, Patterson claimed that most Americans bore an unnatural, and potentially unhealthy, amount of lead in their bodies.[62] Unlike earlier lead researchers, he was coming at the issue of lead poisoning from outside the small world of lead toxicologists who had largely depended on industry to support their research. It was as important, from industry's point of view, to tarnish the credibility of this "outsider" as it was to rebut the specifics of his argument. With an attack on Patterson's work, the industry began a campaign—which continues to this day—to undercut the findings of researchers who have dared suggest that low-level lead pollution has subtle impacts on the general population's health and specifically on children's mental development.

Kehoe worried that so many draft copies of Patterson's paper had already circulated that without a formal channel for rebuttal, Patterson's position might gain greater and greater credibility through word of mouth alone. In the end, Kehoe supported the *Archives of Environmental Health*'s decision to publish the piece, a move that historian Christian Warren ascribes to Kehoe's recognition that its publication was inevitable, and to his hope to thus obligate the journal to make room for a subsequent detailed critique.[63]

In addition to questioning Patterson's credentials, methodology, and interpretation of the data, his critics were most concerned about his conclusion that "the average resident of the United States is being subjected to severe chronic lead insult."[64] Through his argument, Patterson was undermining the industry view that relatively low levels of exposure were harmless and that the only Americans at risk were workers exposed to high

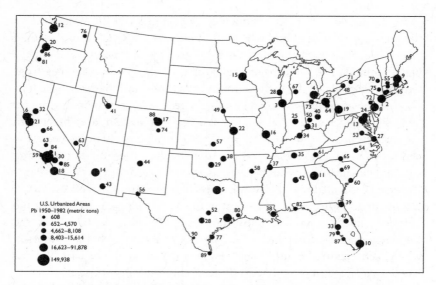

FIGURE 2.   Lead (Pb) deposited from leaded gasoline in U.S. cities, 1950–1982. Gasoline was a main source of lead that damaged many, particularly urban, children until the 1980s. The amount of lead in gasoline was gradually reduced from 4 grams per gallon to 0.1 gram per gallon in 1986. It was finally completely phased out of gasoline for automobiles in 1996. Source: Howard W. Mielke, Mark A.S. Laidlaw, and Chris R. Gonzales, "Estimation of Leaded (Pb) Gasoline's Continuing Material and Health Impacts on 90 US Urbanized Areas," *Environment International* 37 (January 2011): 248–57, available at www.sciencedirect.com/science/article/pii/S016041201000156X.

levels. He was questioning the industry view that one was either acutely lead poisoned or one was essentially unaffected by the substance.[65] Right after the publication of Patterson's 1965 article, Donald G. Fowler, the LIA's director of health and safety at the time, took issue with Patterson's "assertion that lead pollution in the air has reached 'alarming' proportions." Fowler dismissed the findings as "based on his [Patterson's] own geological studies . . . and his own interpretive extensions upon these studies into non-geological fields." Patterson's work, he claimed, ignored "the recognized body of clinical and biological evidence" and was "unsupported by any medical evidence." Fowler went on to declare that "lead is not a significant factor in air pollution" and "the public can rest assured that lead constitutes no public health problem."[66]

Patterson's critique of lead's ubiquity and its potential danger to the public came at a critical time for the industry. Historically, lead pigment had been the most economically significant market for lead producers, but it had begun declining in importance as latex and titanium pigments increasingly captured market share. As automobile sales mushroomed with the economic boom following World War II, the auto industry and the producers of batteries and leaded gasoline supplanted users of pigments as the major buyers of lead. Between 1940 and 1960, despite less frequent use of lead in interior paints, lead consumption increased from about 600 short tons to approximately 1,000 short tons per year. During this period, lead for use in gasoline increased eightfold, from about 25 short tons to just under 200; and lead used in batteries doubled, from 200 short tons to just under 400. Despite the increasing evidence of lead's destructive environmental effects, during the 1960s and the 1970s lead production increased substantially. In 1964, the United States consumed 1,202 short tons of lead. By 1974, this had grown by about 25 percent, to 1,550 short tons.[67]

Patterson was not alone in taking on Kehoe's paradigm. In 1966 Harriet Hardy, one of the nation's preeminent occupational health physicians, condemned the lead industry's threshold idea of harm based on adult lead workers; she argued it was inadequate as a means of protecting high-risk populations outside of the workplace. As coauthor, with Alice Hamilton, of the main textbook in occupational medicine, she argued that certain vulnerable populations—particularly children and pregnant women—might suffer the effects of lead at much lower levels of exposure than male workers did. Hardy also delineated the inadequacies in earlier definitions of lead poisoning, arguing that lead poisoning produced a host of subtle and difficult-to-define symptoms (such as fevers, lethargy, and joint pain), but no less damaging for that, which could easily escape the notice of physicians. "It is necessary to emphasize," she wrote, "that no harmful effect of lead is unique [to that poison] except perhaps the motor palsy of the most-used muscle group, as in the wrist drop."[68]

Hardy believed that the developing child was most at risk. Randolph Byers and Elizabeth Lord's research in Boston on long-term effects of acute lead poisoning, along with clinical observations by doctors such as L. Emmett Holt, John Ruddock, Charles McKhann, and Edward Vogt, supported Hardy's opinion that lead was more toxic to the young than to the adult population.[69] In contrast to Kehoe, who used adult males in his studies and in his model of classic lead poisoning, Hardy recognized that a much wider net had to be cast to understand the full range of lead's effects: "Prevention of diagnosable Pb poisoning in healthy male workers is important but not enough in our society." Lead was a known toxin, and there was "no available evidence that lead is useful to the body," particularly for women and children.[70]

In the coming years, the policy model that Patterson first proposed—that lead, a known toxin, should not be widely introduced into the human environment, and that Hardy expanded to specifically include women and children—would be embraced by those who pushed for the removal of lead from gasoline, and, hence, from the atmosphere.[71] This was an early statement of what, generalized, would become known as the "precautionary principle"—the basic idea behind public health, that, when considering the use of new or suspect chemicals, it is prudent to prove them safe rather than waiting to see if they are harmful to people or the environment. Hardy quoted Bradford Hill, the eminent English epidemiologist who, with Sir Richard Doll, demonstrated the relationship between cigarette smoking and lung cancer: "All scientific work is incomplete. . . . All scientific work is liable to be upset or modified by advancing knowledge. That does not confer upon us a freedom to ignore the knowledge we already have, or to postpone the action that it appears to demand at a given time."[72]

SOCIAL ACTION AND LEAD POISONING

Until the mid-1960s, lead poisoning—whether from lead paint, lead in gasoline, or lead in the factory—had remained, beyond the victims themselves, largely an issue for clinicians and researchers in a few major medical centers around the country, a small group of public health professionals, and an industry intent on protecting its market. But this changed as the civil rights movement galvanized the African American community and forced middle-class white Americans to acknowledge the extent of endemic poverty and racism. Michael Harrington's 1962 book, *The Other America*, and the civil rights–era sit-ins, Freedom Rides, voter-registration campaigns, and school-desegregation drives all made poverty and racial discrimination headlines in daily newspapers across the country.

As the War on Poverty took shape in the years following John F. Kennedy's assassination, the links between poverty, housing, and racism in the nation's cities became increasingly apparent to many Americans. Lead poisoning—particularly from peeling paint in slum housing—became a signature disease of poverty. In New York City, the number of children identified as lead poisoned, now defined as 60 or more micrograms of lead per deciliter of blood shot up from 20 in 1952 to 509 by 1965; in Philadelphia, from 2 in 1952 to 163 in 1965; in Chicago, from 33 in 1953 to 304 by 1966. This was not because more children were affected but because more public health authorities and doctors were now conscious of lead poisoning's existence and its array of symptoms.[73]

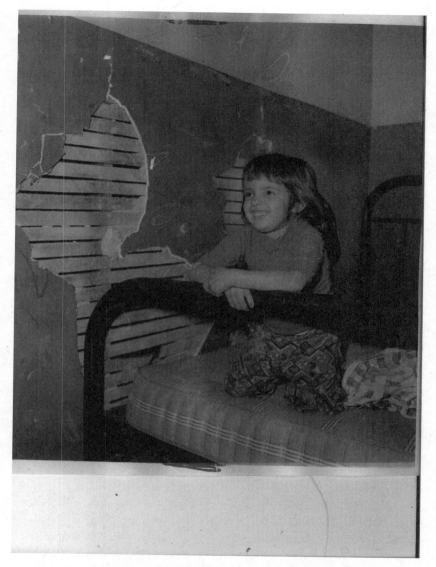

FIGURES 3A.   Children at risk, 1960s. During the War on Poverty, peeling and chipping paint became a symbol of urban blight and social inequality. Community activists and housing reformers were critical in pressing for improved conditions. Source: (a) *Chicago Tribune*, February 3, 1966, reprinted with permission;

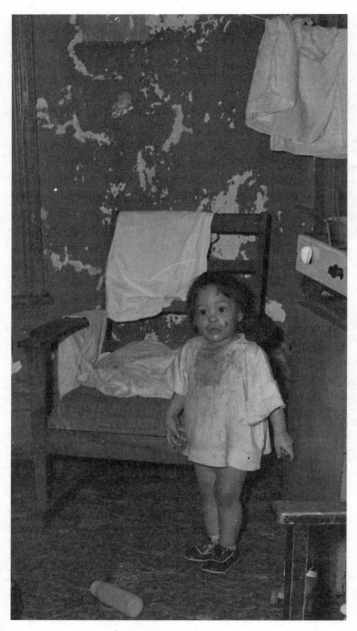

FIGURES 3B.   Continued_(b) New York City Housing Authority, Wagner
Archives, reprinted with permission.

Community groups such as the Young Lords in New York (a largely Latino organization), the Citizen's Committee to End Lead Poisoning in Chicago, the Black Panthers in Boston and Oakland, and the Harlem Park Neighborhood Council in West Baltimore, as well as others around the country, seized on this devastating disease, seeing it as a representation of the ills of a culture rather than as a product of nature. These groups began agitating for more testing of children, better enforcement of existing housing laws, poisoning surveillance and prevention programs by departments of health, and new laws to hold landlords accountable for lead hazards.[74] Sometimes, the lead tragedy actually led to civil disobedience, as it did in New York City in 1970 when the Young Lords seized unused mobile testing vans and began door-to-door screening for lead poisoning while others staged sit-ins at the Department of Health.[75] In 1969, Jack Newfield, an influential writer for the *Village Voice*, picked up the story and wrote a series of articles about lead poisoned children who had suffered irreversible brain damage, thereby putting enormous pressure on the city to strengthen housing codes against flaking and peeling paint.[76]

Community activism played an important role in bringing attention to lead poisoning and reducing its impact on poor communities, as Mark Farfel wrote in 1985, a few years before he would codirect the Kennedy Krieger Institute study: the "Great Society programs, including Medicaid, urban renewal projects, and food stamp and food supplement programs," led to the identification and amelioration of lead poisoning in subtle ways that were "difficult to quantify." Building on the public health model of an earlier time, in which social reform was viewed as essential to effective public health efforts, Farfel noted that "improved nutrition, access to medical care and new housing" were critically important in reducing risk to children. "Even the civil rights movement may have reduced risk for toxicity among blacks by opening some doors to better housing."[77]

Indeed, public health activists embraced numerous social causes in the mid-1960s and mid-1970s, building on the older tradition of allying with community organizations and consumer groups to effect changes in the delivery of services and health care. In New York City, the Health Policy Advisory Committee (Health PAC) gave young professionals both in and out of government a means of linking movements to combat poverty, poor housing, lead poisoning, racism, and other social ills to health and their professional identities. For at least a decade, Health PAC and other health professional organizations and other groups in the American Public Health Association—such as the Medical Committee for Human Rights, Physicians Forum, and Physicians for Social Responsibility—helped to build community health centers in poor neighborhoods in northern cities and southern rural communities, achieved a partial atomic test ban to reduce strontium 90 and other radioactive exposures, developed programs to improve housing condition in poor communities around the country, and pressured governments to organize services for the poor on Indian reservations and in urban neighborhoods.[78]

Throughout the country, large city health departments were pressed by community groups and concerned professionals to expand surveillance efforts and screening programs, which brought greater awareness of the extent of lead exposures and concern that Clair Patterson and Harriet Hardy were accurate in arguing that lead poisoning was a much more serious problem than previously assumed. According to one government expert, by the late 1960s several large cities, including Chicago and New York, "reported that 25 to 45 percent of one- to six-year-old children from high-risk areas had blood lead levels exceeding 40 μg per 100 ml."[79]

As doctors became more alert to the possibility of lead poisoning, the numbers of those acknowledged to be affected naturally increased. But the fatality rate didn't. In Chicago, in 1966, for example, a study of more than 60,000 children showed "a marked rise in cases reported [compared to the 1950s] and a sharp decrease in fatality rate."[80] In New York, like Chicago, the fatality rate among those diagnosed with lead poisoning declined from 27 percent in the 1950s to 1.4 percent in 1964.[81] Such drops in the fatality percentage were in part a function of increased surveillance and a lower threshold used to trigger a diagnosis of lead poisoning, which increased the pool with which the percentage was calculated but not the fatalities. But beyond that, it was widespread use of chelating agents that was responsible for this remarkable decline. An early champion of chelation therapy was J. Julian Chisolm, who would years later be the co-principal investigator of the KKI study so excoriated by the Maryland Court of Appeals.

As a young physician in the 1950s, trained at Johns Hopkins and at Princeton before that, Chisolm was in his generation almost unique in his ongoing professional focus on lead poisoning, particularly among African American children. In the early 1950s he received a fellowship to study the breadth of lead poisoning among Baltimore's children. He visited homes, collecting stool samples of young children to analyze their lead content, and found that the City had been grossly underestimating the extent of the problem. He recalled that his "first findings . . . were that children who ingested paint were getting more lead than even heavily exposed industrial workers."[82]

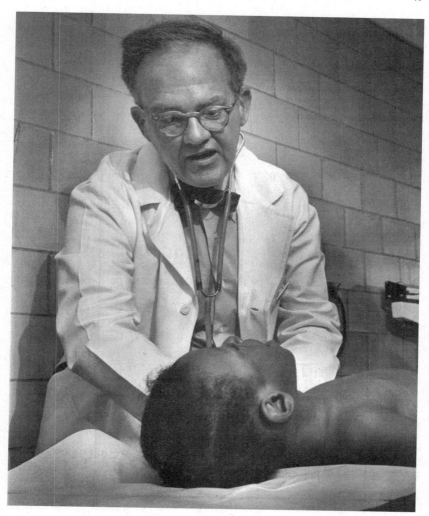

FIGURE 4.   J. Julian Chisolm examining a child, ca. 1972. Chisolm was one of the early pioneers who called attention to the lead-poisoning epidemic, and throughout his life he treated thousands of lead-poisoned children in Baltimore. Source: *Baltimore Sun*, March 14, 1972, reprinted with permission.

Chisolm's own background, perhaps, stimulated his commitment to and concern for African American children. Ironically, he came from a long line of southerners whose roots were in the South Carolina planter class. His great-great-great uncle, also named J. Julian Chisolm, was the leading surgeon for the Confederacy during the Civil War and author of the primary text for Confederate army surgeons.[83] That Chisolm moved to Baltimore after the Civil War, established the Presbyterian Eye, Ear and Throat Charity Hospital, and became professor of ophthalmology and dean at the University of Maryland School of Medicine in Baltimore.[84] J. Julian Chisolm Sr. (our J. Julian Chisolm's father), himself the son of a Presbyterian minister who presided over a Natchez, Mississippi, segregated congregation of African American and white parishioners, received his medical degree from Johns Hopkins early in the twentieth century and taught at the medical school there for many years.[85]

J. Julian Chisolm Jr., who died in 2001, was a tall, large man with "a round face and sort of wispy hair that wasn't very well combed," according to Ellen Silbergeld, his student and protégé. He was mild mannered "in a kind of old Maryland gentleman way," she remembers, and he "always wore a bow tie as the pediatricians in his day did," so that young children couldn't grab his tie. He could also be "very acerbic" to those who denied the importance of issues he cared deeply about. That the poisoning of African American children was one of these, Silbergeld said, "probably inhibited his promotion at Hopkins . . . to full professor until he was almost dead." His commitment to the children he treated from the neighborhood around Hopkins was unquestioned by his students and colleagues. He once told Silbergeld that he saw racism inherent in the society's lack of response to lead poisoning. "If this was a disease of white children," he told her, "we would have done something about this a long time ago." From these experiences came a life-long passion to address the effects of lead paint as the primary source of danger to children.[86]

Chisolm was working against the ingrained segregationist culture of Baltimore and Johns Hopkins at this time. Like other medical schools, Hopkins was an institution dominated by relatively wealthy, white, overwhelmingly male doctors and trustees. It was a "white enclave on a hill surrounded by" a largely poor African American community, recalls Connie Nathanson, now a professor of sociomedical sciences at Columbia, who worked in pediatrics at the Hopkins medical school from the late 1950s until 2002.[87] In the postwar period, plans were developed for 178 garden apartments for African American families who were being displaced by the urban renewal project close to the Hopkins medical school campus. Those same plans included housing for residents and staff at the university. As social scientist Stephanie Farquhar documents, the "planned 178 garden apartments for blacks were never built . . . though the garden apartments for Hopkins married staff and the residence hall for Hopkins' unmarried staff and students were."[88] Nathanson recalls that the "housing for residents and interns [was] surrounded by wire fencing that segregated it off" from the surrounding community.[89]

By 1969 the combined use of the two chelating agents, BAL and EDTA, according to Chisolm, "apparently reduce[d] the mortality from acute lead encephalopathy to 5%." It was a pyrrhic victory, though, for "the incidence of severe, permanent brain damage among survivors of encephalopathy continues to be 25% or more," he said. And "if survivors of an initial attack of acute lead encephalopathy are re-exposed to abnormal lead exposure the incidence of severe permanent brain damage is increased to virtually 100%."[90] Chisolm clearly understood the critical connection between treatment of children and the need to rehabilitate the housing where they lived. "The cornerstone of our current therapeutic program," he argued, "is prompt termination of environmental exposure to lead: no child with an increased body burden of lead is ever returned to a leaded home." Although it is not clear how often this was accomplished or who paid for this service, Chisolm wrote that after chelation therapy, children at Johns Hopkins clinics were either placed in suitable new housing or their homes were abated of lead. Chisolm understood that children having to be poisoned before remedial action was taken was both destructive for the child and expensive for society. "How much more intelligent it would be," he commented, "to spend our effort and substance on the *systematic* elimination of environmental lead exposure associated with old dwellings. Were this to be done, childhood lead poisoning could be largely eradicated in the United States."[91] Although the solution was obvious, the means of attaining it were not. In the late 1960s there were, for example, thirty million housing units nationwide still in use that had been built before 1950; of these, at least 90 percent were polluted by lead.[92]

3   Peeling the Onion
New Layers of the Lead Problem

The worth of the human brain is incalculable. The value we assign to
it will be defined by the intensity with which we pursue or avoid the
protection of its optimum development. Excess lead in the human
environment is man-made and is, therefore, preventable by man.

HERBERT NEEDLEMAN, 1977

Prior to 1970 and the establishment of the Environmental Protection
Agency, the federal government rarely regulated environmental toxins. But
by the late 1960s and early 1970s, environmentalists and public health officials were advocating such regulation to protect the food supply and
improve air and water quality. The Food and Drug Administration had
begun to expand its role in regulating foods and additives after a weed
killer, aminotriazole, feared as a carcinogen, was found in cranberries just
before the 1959 Thanksgiving holiday. Environmental activists and the
broader public also joined together to press for greater regulation following
publication of Rachel Carson's *Silent Spring* in 1962, with its vivid account
of the devastating effects of DDT and other pesticides on birds and other
wildlife, and then the revelation in 1966 that PCBs and other chlorinated
hydrocarbons were accumulating in animals—including *Homo sapiens*—at
the top of the food chain. Similarly, Congress began to pay more attention
to pollutants following passage of the first Clean Air Act in 1963.

By the late 1960s, environmentalists, politicians, community activists,
conservationists, scientists, and public health officials understood that lead
was one pollutant that challenged them all. It was in the air people breathed
and, as the previous decade had made clear, it was on the walls of the
nation's housing. With the new decade, physicians were more effectively
treating the symptoms of acute lead poisoning, public health personnel
were active in establishing more lead-screening programs to identify
children most at risk, and community groups and others were calling for
stronger housing codes and more effective enforcement for existing ones.
But as they seemed on their way to solving one problem, all through the
1970s they would discover new ones that were in some ways ever more
troubling, uncovering literally millions of children at risk of developing

life-changing neurological and behavioral problems from the slightest exposure to this devastating metal, while intense resistance from the lead industry continually tried to discredit the new research.

AN INADVERTENT ADVOCATE

Within the government, a federal official played an instrumental role in getting Washington to acknowledge the importance of childhood lead poisoning. Jane Lin-Fu came to her work by a circuitous route. Born in Singapore of Chinese parents, Lin-Fu spent her early years in Shanghai, where her father, a teacher educated in China and the United States, joined his brother Lin Yutang, then a rising journalist, to work as a journalist at *China Critic*, an English-language periodical. Her father, a Quaker, had a strong sense of social justice, and she still remembers how upset he was by the British treatment of Gandhi. Her mother was well-educated, pragmatic, a strict disciplinarian and a devout Christian. Jane was raised to believe she shouldn't worry what others thought as long as she was doing the right thing before God. "This upbringing molded me to be the free spirit who would take up social justice issues like lead poisoning, speak the truth about lead as I saw it, and not be intimidated by bureaucratic or academic authorities," she believes.[1]

In 1937, when the Japanese Army invaded China, her parents fled with her to the Philippines, where Jane later attended medical school before coming to the United States in 1955. She accepted an internship, followed by a pediatric residency, at Brooklyn Jewish Hospital, an institution that served many children from the impoverished neighborhoods nearby—in what was later referred to as the "lead belt." One summer, a two-year-old came to the clinic with a stomachache and vomiting. The physician thought the boy had summer flu but admitted him because he was quite dehydrated. On the ward, the child began convulsing and the attending doctor mentioned it might be lead poisoning. The event made a lasting impression on Lin-Fu.[2]

In the early 1960s her husband joined NASA and they moved to the Washington, D.C., suburb of Bethesda. She was a board-certified pediatrician, but she wanted a part-time job with the federal government so she could spend time with her children. In November 1963, just after John F. Kennedy's assassination, she was hired by Alice Chenoweth at the Maternal and Child Health Program in the Children's Bureau.

When Kennedy became president, the plight of his sister Rosemary led him to make a concerted effort to focus the nation's attention on the study and treatment of mental retardation. The Children's Bureau, a beneficiary of the subsequent funds appropriated by Congress for that purpose, helped develop statewide screening programs for phenylketonuria (PKU), a genetic disorder that causes mental retardation. Newborn PKU screening was a particularly exciting area then because, for the first time, severe mental retardation in children who suffered from this genetic disorder could be prevented through large-scale screening, early diagnosis, and dietary treatment.

When a colleague happened to ask Lin-Fu in 1965 what she knew about lead poisoning as a cause of mental retardation, the question triggered a flashback to that little boy who had convulsed from lead encephalopathy in Brooklyn Jewish Hospital a few years earlier. As she looked into the issue she was horrified to realize that her own training had not included lead poisoning, even though research indicated the prevalence of the problem in old, poor neighborhoods like the ones surrounding the hospital where she had done her residency. She was also deeply troubled that the Maternal and Child Health Program in the Children's Bureau, which was so active in preventing mental retardation caused by the PKU condition, was not doing anything about lead poisoning so common in young children living in dilapidated dwellings. "This is really unfair because poor children have no voice in society," she recalls thinking at the time. She could not understand how "we could ignore such a simple and readily preventable issue."[3] By December 1965, she had reviewed the existing literature on childhood lead poisoning and written a draft report on the subject that was intended as an internal memo. The Children's Bureau was so impressed, however, that it sent the draft to outside reviewers, including J. Julian Chisolm, and then published it. That became *Lead Poisoning in Children*, a widely circulated 1967 government booklet that was instrumental in drawing the attention of Congress and the public to the lead problem.[4]

It also attracted the attention of the lead industry. "When my booklet came out in 1967," Lin-Fu recalled, "the lead industry wanted to reprint it [with a gloss of their own accompanying it], and they hired Hill & Knowlton to contact me. . . . The industry found my early work useful because it emphasized that the [main] problem was lead paint, not all the other [lead-related] environmental issues [such as lead in gasoline, then the dominant interest of the lead industry]. . . . The lead industry kept sending public relations representatives to me to be my friend. They would call to chat and have lunch with me. They would be friendly and try to keep track of my work."[5] While the federal government distributed more than 28,000 copies of Lin-Fu's pamphlet, this effort, as historian Christian Warren puts it, "paled next to the efforts of the Lead Industries Association which distributed 61,000 copies [of Lin-Fu's work] . . . as part of its free booklet, 'Facts about Lead and Pediatrics.'"[6]

Lin-Fu's publication reflected the prevailing view of the time that lead poisoning was a problem mainly limited to "slums" and poor children, largely ignoring lead in gasoline, which exposed all children, rich and poor, urban, suburban and rural. People in public health and community organizations such as the Young Lords and the Black Panthers helped bring this scourge to public attention.[7] But even so, many practitioners simply did not recognize lead poisoning because the symptoms were nonspecific except in extreme cases. Others thought lead poisoning "went away" when titanium oxide replaced lead as the major pigment in interior paint in the 1940s.[8]

Arthur Lesser, a well-respected federal public health official who was director of the Maternal and Child Health Program in the Children's Bureau, said to Lin-Fu one day, apparently exasperated by her insistence about the lead issue, "You did not discover anything. We know lead poisoning was there, but this is a housing problem, not a public health problem. You screen children, diagnose them, treat them and send them home to eat lead paint again. Are you going to fix their houses and remove the lead paint? Obviously not. This is a housing problem—what do you want us to do?"[9]

THE EMERGENCE OF "UNDUE" LEAD ABSORPTION

While Lin-Fu remembers herself as naïve, someone who just tried to do the right thing, ignorant of the bureaucratic and political workings of the White House and Congress, she was in fact a very effective political infighter. Although she did not have a public health background, Lin-Fu saw lead poisoning from the position of a pediatrician and a mother of young children. In contrast to the kind of bureaucratic view Lesser expressed, she did not see why a housing problem causing such serious lead poisoning in children was not also a public health problem. As she put it, "It was a football bounced between housing and public health so it went into no-man's land."[10] This kind of tension over which agency should deal with childhood lead poisoning would continue to plague policy makers and advocates alike for decades.

Lin-Fu's pamphlet and her subsequent work on lead poisoning became the basis for the first statement on the subject by the surgeon general of the Public Health Service, Jesse L. Steinfeld. Lin-Fu remembers, "When we finally finished the draft of the guidelines [in the fall of 1970 for childhood lead-poisoning programs] and sent them downtown [to the Department of

Health, Education and Welfare secretary's office], the surgeon general was on duty that weekend, responsible for signing important papers for the DHEW secretary's office. He signed the paper and saw the significance of the draft, and it became the [basis for the] surgeon general's policy statement."[11] In November 1970, Steinfeld announced "guidelines for a nationwide campaign against lead poisoning" because "as many as 400,000 children" were estimated to have blood lead levels above 40 micrograms per deciliter—in 1970, a shocking number of children.[12] At the time, children were considered poisoned if their blood lead levels were over 60 µg/dl. This was the level at which many children, though not all, showed classic acute symptoms of lead poisoning—convulsions, coma, permanent neurological damage, and even death. According to the *New York Times*, Steinfeld recommended screening programs for "all children under six years of age living in old and poorly maintained houses."[13]

The surgeon general's policy statement was important, Lin-Fu recalls, "because a new concept of lead poisoning was contained in the document— that of 'undue lead absorption,' which was [seen as] an intermediate problem that preceded clinical symptoms. The document challenged the old concept and definition of lead poisoning—those with overt symptoms of profound neurological damage—and introduced the concept of finding children at the phase of undue lead absorption, defined at blood lead levels of 40 µg/dl and over."[14]

The federal government's acknowledgment that "undue" lead absorption was a danger to children was an important breakthrough. But it was not achieved without a struggle. The ad hoc committee that drew up the DHEW guidelines for lead poisoning, in case impending legislation became a reality, had included Jane Lin-Fu and other DHEW staff along with outside experts, including Julian Chisolm. "Chisolm opposed me [Lin-Fu] on this, as did the chairman of the committee. . . . He and Chisolm thought that I was being too aggressive and impractical to implement screening and follow-up, as New York City was finding 45 percent of its sampling above 40 micrograms." The chair challenged Lin-Fu: "How are you going to tell local public health officials that they have a lead problem in half of their kids?" And she answered: "That's their problem. Our job in the government is to tell them the scientific facts, the truth."[15] It was Chisolm who had originally written a paper stating that the upper limit of "normal" blood lead should be 40 µg/dl, she pointed out.[16] "When he refused to back up his own statement at the meeting, she recalls, "I knew that DHEW's committee would not let me say [in the draft guidelines] that the upper level of normal should be 40."[17]

As a compromise, Lin-Fu drafted a statement proposing that in cities with overwhelming lead-poisoning problems priority should be given to children whose blood lead levels were more than 60 µg/dl, followed by those with levels between 40 and 60, and then those with levels less than 40. Children of one to three years should be given priority over those of three to six years, and so forth. At the next meeting, Lin-Fu spread copies of the document around the table and said, "This is what I propose." Chisolm said, "If we include this statement on priority, then dropping to 40 µg/dl in the statement is OK." But the chair angrily said it was too radical: "I am leaving the government in three months and I don't really care what happens with this document. If you insist on the 40 µg criteria, after that statement is released, and when all the letters start coming in to the secretary's office, you will have to deal with this and answer those letters." "I will," Lin-Fu said without hesitation. "Deal," the chairman said, and the final draft included Lin-Fu's triage concept of dealing with lead poisoning and dropped the upper limit of what was considered the "normal" blood lead level from 60 to 40 µg/dl, with children having levels above 40 considered at risk from undue lead absorption.[18]

While Lin-Fu was fighting within the federal bureaucracy to convey a better understanding of and more action on low-level lead poisoning, a few senators and representatives were also trying to address the emerging lead-poisoning epidemic. Responding to pressure from community organizations in New York, Boston, and around the country and from local public health officials, Congressman William Ryan (D-NY) and Senator Ted Kennedy (D-MA) cosponsored bills in 1969 and 1970 to authorize $30 million in federal grants to combat lead poisoning. The Ryan-Kennedy Bill was passed on December 31, 1970, and signed into law as the Lead-Based Paint Poisoning Prevention Act by President Nixon in mid-January 1971. The act was composed of three parts: the first "empowered HEW [the Department of Health, Education and Welfare] to prohibit the use of 'lead-based paint' [paint with more than 1 percent lead pigment] in federally constructed or rehabilitated housing" but left unregulated the private housing stock; the second authorized the Department of Health, Education and Welfare "to make grants to cities establishing lead-abatement programs and . . . to establish screening and treatment programs"; and the third authorized the Department of Housing and Urban Development "to survey the scope of the lead-paint hazard and establish methods for abatement."[19] More broadly, the law set in motion surveillance of the lead problem nationally.[20] Thus, as early as 1970, lead paint abatement was considered essential to any attempt to deal with the lead problem. But it quickly became clear that the funds to address true removal would not be forthcoming anytime soon, fulfilling the prophesy of the Lead Industries Association that lead pollution would plague the country for the indeterminate future.

The administration and Congress initially refused to appropriate or even request the funds to implement lead-abatement or poisoning-prevention programs that were authorized by the Ryan-Kennedy Bill. As reporter Jack Newfield wrote in June 1971, six months after the law was passed, even though the appropriations bill for that fiscal year "included funds for every special interest: $3.5 million for dairy and beekeeper indemnity; . . . [and] $15 million for highway beautification . . . [there was] not one cent for lead poisoning.[21] The *New York Times* reported that as the cities "waited . . . the politics of embarrassment began. . . . The Administration asked for $2 million, which was raised to $5 million in the House and $15 million in the Senate, before the $7.5 million was agreed on in conference." Later that year, on August 14, 1971, Congress finally appropriated the agreed-upon amount.[22]

In its account of the politics of appropriations for lead poisoning, the *Times* identified a fundamental conflict embodied in the act and in lead-poisoning prevention programs in general: Should "prevention" measures apply only to children who were already poisoned? Or should abatement of lead-infested houses take place before children were damaged? This raised a fundamental question that would plague lead specialists and, the public health profession and society more broadly: Were children in effect their own "canaries in the mine"? As the *Times* put it, "what constitutes prevention . . . remains unsolved among public health practitioners. The few lead poisoning programs currently in operation around the country all look for children with high levels of lead in their blood and then clean up the environment that poisoned them." The newspaper noted that many in public health wanted a true prevention program, "a systematic clean-up of housing known to contain lead before children can ingest the paint." In the end, such a systematic program of detoxifying the housing stock might be slow, but it would be "more useful and less costly." The New York City Health Department had found that "93 percent of 2600 reported cases [of lead poisoning] last year could be traced to housing"; but in New York, as in Chicago, Baltimore, and other cities, "repair is only authorized in the dwelling unit in which the child has been poisoned even though other apartments in the same building may be equally hazardous."[23]

Meanwhile, the magnitude of the problem was becoming increasingly apparent as damage was found to be occurring to children at lesser levels of contamination than previously realized. In March 1972, Lin-Fu published an influential article in the *New England Journal of Medicine (NEJM)* that again called attention to the concept of "undue lead absorption" as a stage before overt lead poisoning and identified lead in dust and soil as a problem. She argued that the existing criteria, even for undue lead absorption, might still be too high. She pointed to numerous studies that led her to conclude that "the upper limit of normal [i.e., "safe"] should be no higher than 40 µg per 100 ml and may actually be lower."[24] After a review of the shocking statistics from New York City, Newark, New Haven, Philadelphia, Washington, D.C., Baltimore, and Chicago, among other cities, revealing the number of children who had blood lead levels above 40 µg/dl, she concluded that "in magnitude the problem of undue absorption of lead among children living in old neighborhoods is matched by few, if any, other pediatric public health problems."[25]

This was a truly stunning conclusion. At a time when measles, mumps, and rubella still posed a substantial threat to American children, a handful of public health professionals like Lin-Fu were identifying possibly a worse scourge. The *NEJM* article had a profound impact, she recalls, because she had "raised the question of subclinical neurological damage," such as behavioral problems, learning disabilities, reduced IQ, and perceptual difficulties[26]—"subclinical" at the time meaning merely that physicians of that era defined such symptoms as psychological or behavioral issues, not medical or biological ones.

THE TOOTH-FAIRY PROJECT

Jane Lin-Fu's analysis built on the findings of the blood lead surveillance programs that local public health departments across the country were implementing in the late 1960s and early 1970s. These programs were uncovering a huge number of children with blood lead levels above 40 µg/dl but who did not show overt clinical symptoms. Were the levels that were being found dangerous to the health of the child? What did these elevated blood lead levels mean for the neurological development of school-age children? Was there a way to estimate whether or not such children had experienced chronic, long-term exposure to lead? And if these children had experienced such chronic exposure, what impact had that had on their development?

These issues would take on special importance with the 1972 publication in *Nature* of a landmark article whose primary author, Herbert Needleman, a forty-one-year-old professor of pediatrics at the University of Pennsylvania, would become a lightning rod for the growing controversy over "subclinical" effects of lead on children. In the article, Needleman—along with his coauthors Irving Shapiro, a University of Pennsylvania assistant professor of dentistry, and Orhan Tuncay—began to develop a methodology and conceptual framework that would transform lead research by the end of the decade. In the early 1970s, blood lead levels were the diagnostic tool for defining lead poisoning. Without an elevated blood lead level, still commonly defined by most local health departments as more than 60 μg/dl, physicians generally assumed that a child was not poisoned. But Needleman's study raised the question of whether blood lead levels alone were an adequate measure of safety or harm. As Needleman and his associates explained, "Because elevations in blood lead are transitory, and decline once ingestion has stopped, blood lead levels are unsatisfactory indices of earlier exposure" and therefore inadequate for determining long-term exposure.[27] Or as Needleman later explained, testing for blood lead "represents a single static measurement of a number of dynamic processes."[28]

Needleman drew upon a method perfected by Barry Commoner, the environmental scientist and peace activist who, in the 1950s, had raised public awareness of the dangers of strontium 90, a by-product of atomic testing. At the height of the Cold War, as both the United States and the Soviet Union raced to develop ever more powerful atomic weapons, hydrogen bombs in particular, huge demonstration detonations had become commonplace. This testing released radioactive materials into the atmosphere that eventually settled to earth and were absorbed by children through ingestion of milk and other foods. Commoner and Anthony Mazzocchi, then a young organizer and official for the Oil, Chemical and Atomic Workers Union on Long Island, collected baby teeth to show that the radioactive material released in the distant testing grounds in Utah, the Pacific Islands, and Siberia soon became, in the words of the *New York Times*, "a lifelong component of the teeth and skeleton."[29] Needleman and his colleagues knew that calcified tissue, such as that found in baby teeth, likewise stored lead, and they hit upon the idea of using that as a means of measuring long-term exposure.

In a research effort whimsically called the Philadelphia Tooth Fairy Project, Needleman and his team allied with dentists in Philadelphia's "lead belt" to collect 69 baby teeth. In addition, they collected 40 teeth from suburban dentists. The results of their analysis were stark and startling: children living in poor urban communities had nearly five times the levels of lead compared to those living in the suburbs.[30]

Lead researchers had always known that lead in the blood was only a snapshot of a child's recent exposures to the toxic metal. They also knew that some of the lead that children ingested accumulated in their bones and remained there for years, even decades. There was little consensus about—and there had been no way of accurately measuring—the impact of lead that had accumulated over time, however. It was impossible to routinely do bone biopsies of living children with suspected, but asymptomatic, cases of lead exposure; and X-rays merely showed the presence, not the amount, of lead. Needleman's new methodology promised to provide some answers to the scientific conundrum of whether or not children's long-term exposure to lead was correlated with damage. The complexity and the terrifying dimensions of the lead pollution issue were, with Needleman's research, to soon become more apparent to the research community. No longer would scientists, physicians, and the public health community be able to take comfort in focusing only on the acute impacts of lead as measured by elevated blood lead levels.

Needleman's continuing work would eventually set off a firestorm of opposition from the lead industry. In October 1972, Needleman traveled to Amsterdam to present a paper at a symposium on environmental health aspects of lead that was sponsored by the recently established Environmental Protection Agency and the Commission of European Communities.[31] This meeting, Needleman later told journalist Lydia Denworth, was where he realized that powerful interests were going to oppose his scientific findings: "I woke up to the fact that it wasn't just that the truth will out."[32] The meeting brought together hundreds of representatives from twenty-one countries, including government officials, people from private industry, and independent research scientists. Forty-two came from the United States, of whom eighteen were industry representatives, some of whom took a very dim view of Needleman's work.

Needleman began his talk by discussing the difficult problem that relatively low-level lead exposure presented for researchers and clinicians alike. Lead poisoning challenged the older paradigm of what constituted health and disease. Lead poisoning was unlike acute infectious diseases that ultimately resolved themselves or resulted in observable, permanent damage. Unlike polio, for example, which left children (many of its victims), visibly disabled, children who were lead poisoned looked normal, exhibiting in all but extreme cases neurological, emotional, cognitive, and behavioral problems that initially might be easily overlooked. While IQ loss, dyslexia, hyperactivity, and behavioral problems could tragically change the direction and prospects of lead poisoning's victims, these symptoms were not commonly ascribed to the effects of lead. Except in acute cases of lead poisoning, it was also unlike other recent health crises. "When an agent produces dramatic symptoms, the establishment" of the cause, was "relatively easy." This was the case with thalidomide, a sedative prescribed in the late 1950s for women suffering from morning sickness that was found to cause birth defects. "Had Thalidomide produced mental retardation rather than phocomelia [the underdevelopment of various parts of the face, limbs, and body resulting in severe disfigurement], it would probably still be sold in Europe and the United States."[33]

Needleman was among the first to suggest that the effects of lead poisoning could be thought of as "a family of curves," starting with subtle biological change "at the lowest levels"; continuing with irritability, awkward gait, and fevers in the middle levels and comas and convulsions near the top; "and ending with death at the highest end of the scale." He reminded the audience that between 250,000 and 400,000 American children had blood lead levels in excess of 40 µg/dl and asked "how many of these children have behavior disorders, disturbances of cognitive function, or emotional disorders related to this body burden." The audience already knew that children living "in the urban American ghetto, and whose blood levels are consistently higher than their middle class counterparts, are known to have an increased prevalence of mental retardation, learning disabilities and behavior disorders."[34] Needleman challenged the scientific community to take the next step, to find out whether or not relatively low-level exposure to lead would produce damage. "If a means could be found to identify older children considered asymptomatic with elevated body burdens of lead, the measurement of their neuropsychologic performance, controlling for other factors known to produce developmental deficits, would allow the investigator to more accurately investigate the effects on their brains of sub-clinical exposure."[35]

Using statistical methods and the evolving tools of epidemiology—a field that once sought sources for the epidemics of infectious disease but was increasingly being used to uncover the epidemics of cancer, heart disease, and stroke among large populations—Needleman probed further into the effects of childhood lead poisoning. Like its role in establishing the relationship between cancer and tobacco use just a few years before, epidemiology was emerging as a critical tool in public health investigations. By comparing the relative risk of lung cancer among huge populations of smokers and nonsmokers in ways no clinician could determine by examining any single individual, Sir Richard Doll and Sir Austin Bradford Hill had opened the world's eyes to dangers of tobacco and had spurred the use of epidemiology and statistical methods to identify chronic conditions such as heart disease and environmental threats such as the bioaccumulation of chlorinated hydrocarbons like PCBs and DDT. Needleman was thus proposing to use the tools of epidemiology to uncover diseases among populations that no clinician could diagnose by examining any single individual. Certainly, epidemiology had been used before in the investigation of disease, and it had been particularly important in uncovering the statistical relationship between lung cancer and smoking, and between heart disease and diet, but Needleman was opening up a whole new realm of medicine and public health. His approach to looking at the impact on children of low-level lead exposures would challenge our thinking about, not only what constitutes an environmental disease, but also how society can protect its citizens from subtle, unseen, and even undefined danger from toxins.

Industry representatives who attended the Amsterdam talk were quick to pick up on the implications of this research, and quick to attack it, just as the tobacco industry had attacked Doll and other researchers who first identified smoking as a deadly habit.[36] Schrade Radtke, representing the International Lead Zinc Research Organization (ILZRO), the research arm of the lead industry, disdainfully dismissed Needleman's concerns, arguing that "the complexities of conception, birth and growth" were too numerous to "ascribe neuropsychiatric problems in children to one single element such as lead." In order for this data to have any meaning at all, he asserted, Needleman had to have "a full history of the condition of the mother and father at the time of conception," the "prenatal care and dietary history of the mother during the period of gestation," and be able to take into account possible birth and childhood injuries, dietary history, child abuse, and other factors. "Unless a complete and total medical history is provided, it is meaningless to ascribe causal factors to one single element."[37] All this additional information would have been nice to have, but the comment did not take away from the significance of the data that Needleman and his colleagues *had* gathered, despite the attempt of industry spokespeople to undermine the analysis. Further, the industry spokespeople ignored the point of epidemiological research: its particular strengths were in uncovering danger at the population level and not awaiting the fulminating symptoms of acute disease.

NEW RESEARCH AND NEW APPROACHES

Who was this man who would play such a controversial role in the study of the effects of lead? Born in Philadelphia in 1927, Herbert Needleman was the first person in his family to go to college. After attending Muhlenberg College in Allentown, Pennsylvania, he went to the University of Pennsylvania Medical School, interned at Philadelphia General Hospital, and then won a fellowship that enabled him to do rheumatic fever research at the Children's Hospital of Philadelphia. After a stint in the army, he returned to finish his training at Children's. "The experience that turned me toward lead is very clear in my mind," he recalled.

> I was working on the infant ward at the Children's, and a child was brought up from the ER with severe acute lead toxicity. I did what I'd been trained to do. I gave her EDTA [chelation therapy]. She was stuporous and very ill. Slowly she got better. It was a gratifying experience, and I felt very smug. I told the mother that she had to move out of that house: "You cannot go back to that house because if she has a second episode she's going to be retarded." This was what I'd been trained to do in medical school. She looked at me and said, "Where am I going to move to? All the houses I can afford are the same age." I suddenly realized that the issue was not just making diagnoses and treating them. The issue was in the life story of people.[38]

By the late 1950s, Needleman had become chief resident at Children's. As Lydia Denforth relates, "He enforced a new rule: In the summertime, any child with any possible symptom of lead poisoning—vomiting, anemia, staggering, and so on would be given a blood lead test. Assume lead poisoning until proven otherwise, he told his staff. Even so, the young doctors sometimes missed the signs."[39] The number of lead-poisoning cases diagnosed by blood test nearly doubled following Needleman's "new rule." And Children's Hospital became the center for the identification of Philadelphia's lead epidemic.[40]

After his years at Children's Hospital, Needleman established a pediatric practice in Philadelphia's suburbs. "I discovered that a lot of the parents who were coming in to see me, mothers, were coming because they were themselves anxious or depressed. These were suburban housewives, and in those days they didn't have jobs. A lot of my discussions were around psychological issues, so I took a psychiatric residency. In those days, the government was subsidizing general practitioners and pediatricians to go into psychiatry because they thought we needed more psychiatrists. I was going to be a child psychoanalyst." His child psychiatry residency at St. Christopher's Hospital, which served children from Philadelphia's poor communities, led him to make house calls. During his visits he was required to "size up the family, whereas in the clinic the mother would bring the child, the child would talk to a psychiatrist, the mother would talk to a social worker, and the father would somehow get evaluated. In a half hour in a home you learn much more than in that whole intake procedure." He grew unhappy with the training, though. "The theoretical basis of child psychoanalysis didn't satisfy me," he said. "I kept thinking, 'How many of

these kids who are coming in with learning problems have lead poisoning?'
The inner city we served at St. Christopher's had a lot of lead. People
thought that was a crazy idea."[41]

Shortly thereafter Needleman became the director of consultation education in the community psychiatry program in North Philly, also in the
inner city.

> I gave a talk at a black church one night to a group of adolescents—
> mostly boys. At the end of the talk, a kid came up to me and started
> telling me about his ambitions. He was a very nice kid, but he was
> obviously brain-damaged. He had trouble with words, with propositions
> and ideas. I thought, how many of these kids who are coming to the
> clinic are in fact a missed case of lead poisoning? My office looked out
> on a school playground. I watched the kids every morning line up and
> go to school. I said, "I'm going to go into that school and identify the
> children who have elevated lead and see what their IQs are." Then it
> occurred to me that the blood lead at 6 years of age might be normal if
> the exposure occurred at less than 2 years of age. So I began to think:
> "What can I use to read back in their exposure history?"[42]

He began to think about ways of estimating children's long-term lead
exposure, first considering hair lead levels and then fingernails. But both
had serious drawbacks. He knew that lead, when ingested or inhaled, accumulated in the bones, but how to discover its extent? "Then it occurred to
me there's a way to do a spontaneous bone biopsy. It's universal, spontaneous, and painless. You just have to catch a deciduous tooth."[43]

In the midst of the tumult created by Jane Lin-Fu, Needleman, and a
handful of others over the possible effects of children's blood lead levels
that were below 60 µg/dl, even below 40 µg/dl, researchers began investigating the association of levels of lead in children's blood with behavior
disorders, educational deficits, and other subtle biological and neurological
changes. In 1972, for example, Oliver David and his fellow researchers at
Downstate Medical Center, in the heart of the "lead belt" of Brooklyn,
where Lin-Fu had been trained, compared hyperactive children with a control group of nonhyperactive children and found that "hyperactive children
had significantly higher [blood lead levels and lead urine levels] than did
the controls. More than half of the hyperactive children had blood lead
levels in the range considered to be raised but not toxic [below 60 µg/dl]."
They concluded that there was "an association between hyperactivity and
raised lead levels; that a large body-lead burden may exert consequences
that have been hitherto unrealized; that the definition of what is a toxic
level for blood lead needs re-evaluation." Though this showed correlation

between lead burden and hyperactivity, not necessarily cause, to David and his colleagues the results were suggestive enough that "blood lead levels and . . . urine-lead levels should be routine investigations in cases of hyperactivity."[44]

Increased focus on blood lead levels that were elevated but below the standard of the time led to renewed questioning of an older discussion between industry and medical scientists over what constitutes a disease. To its workforce, industry had traditionally argued that only biological changes that interfered with the worker's ability to attend to his or her job constituted real disease, whereas labor advocates argued that other biological damage—such as shown by x-ray evidence that lungs were affected by dust or by blood tests that revealed exposure to toxins—should also be considered part of a disease continuum. Did a disease imply only biological change measurable through the use of the imprecise tools then available? Or could it encompass changes that were measurable at the biological level? In either case, did defining a biological change as a disease require some overt impact on the ability to work, function "normally," or live a normal life span? Were behavioral changes in and of themselves "pathological"? Hyperactivity, for example, might be a behavioral change, but did it imply a medical pathology? What, after all, was "normal" and what was "abnormal?" At this point, there was no consensus among researchers that lead caused hyperactivity or even that hyperactivity was truly a disease in the traditional sense. "Hyperactivity is a symptomatic state, not a disease," said David and his colleagues.[45]

This discussion in the early 1970s of what constituted a disease occurred at a critical moment in public health history: chronic illnesses had by the 1960s largely replaced infectious and acute conditions as the concern of medical and public health science. This was the moment, for example, when Nixon declared a war on cancer and when the environmental movement was drawing attention to chronic exposures to industrial poisons.[46] Much of the research on lead's effects for the rest of the 1970s—and until the more robust findings Needleman published in 1979—were devoted to exploring the question of lead's subtle but in many cases pervasive impact on children's lives.

These disputes came into focus during a conference called by the Environmental Protection Agency and the National Institute of Environmental Health Sciences (NIEHS) in October 1973 on low-level lead toxicity. Held in Raleigh, North Carolina, it brought together leading lead researchers, industry representatives, and government officials from both the United States and England.[47] The participants all concurred that high levels of lead exposure—that is, above 60 µg/dl—could result in severe damage to the child. But consensus broke down concerning the impact of lower levels of lead toxicity. John Rosen from New York's Montefiore Medical Center, Ellen Silbergeld, Needleman, and many others suspected that children were at risk for a variety of neurological and behavioral problems even in the absence of acute symptoms or high levels of exposure. But others disagreed. Henrietta Sachs, a pediatrician who headed a lead clinic in Chicago, for example, suggested that recent concern over low-level effects was misplaced. She argued that even children with elevated blood lead levels would find their levels return to normal over time "without lead poisoning having been detected. However, when he fails at school several years later, it is erroneously concluded that brain damage may result from low level lead toxicity."[48] Gary Ter Haar of the Ethyl Corporation—the producers of tetraethyl lead, the gasoline additive—argued that chips of lead paint were the critical danger to children. He and Regina Aronow of Detroit's Children's Hospital reported on the validity of recent reports concerning the importance of "dirt and dust contaminated with lead exhausted from cars" in childhood lead poisoning. Not surprisingly, they concluded that automobile exhaust was not the source of children's elevated blood lead levels.[49]

Until this time, those who believed and those who doubted the impact of comparatively low levels of lead exposure based their views on observational studies of lead-poisoned children. But Ellen Silbergeld, a young toxicologist and postdoctoral fellow at the Johns Hopkins School of Hygiene and Public Health, introduced a new kind of evidence to the debate. Initially interested in the physiology of lead, she designed experiments to trace the impact of lead on the nerves that control muscle function in mice. In the course of her experiments, she noticed that when "you opened the cage [of the mice injected with lead] they would bounce up . . . [and], if there was any noise, they would start running around in their cages," even during their normal sleep times.[50] At the time her sister worked at the Kennedy Krieger Institute as an art therapist with children and occasionally came over for lunch. "I showed her the hyperactive mice and she said, 'Well, you know with the hyperactive kids we give them Ritalin.' I thought, now this would be interesting; let's give them this. So I gave the hyperactive lead mice Ritalin and then I gave [it to] the normal mice. The normal mice began to act crazy and the lead mice became quiet," which was the classic reaction of normal and hyperactive kids to Ritalin. "That was really when we began to think we were onto something. These were at . . . way lower doses [of lead] from the classic animal model that involved [observable] physical brain damage."[51] Silbergeld followed up on these initial studies, detailing the relationship between lead and hyperactivity in mice, showing that mice pups exposed to lead from birth through their mother's milk were "more than three times as active as age-matched or size-matched controls." The resulting article, written with A.M. Goldberg, concluded that "lead produces an animal model of hyperactivity which may have clinical relevance and which may explain some cases of hyperactivity in children."[52]

Silbergeld was among the young generation of scientists and physicians who had emerged from the scientific, social, and political tumult of the 1960s and early 1970s. During this time, research had been freed of many of the constraints that had inhibited thinking for much of the twentieth century, as government funding, new federal agencies, and the social activism of students and scholars merged to create a new atmosphere of inquiry and opportunity. Throughout most of the history of lead toxicology specifically, and environmental and occupational health research in general, research concerns and ideas, not to mention funding, were limited by the simple fact that job opportunities, research labs, and even educational institutions were largely controlled by the very industries that produced the toxins and dangers of the workplace and consumer market. From the 1930s through the 1960s, groups like the Industrial Hygiene Foundation, which was founded in the mid-1930s by companies concerned with the growing number of lawsuits from workers suffering from silicosis, were the prime sponsors of much of the industrial hygiene research, for example. Trade associations such as the Manufacturing Chemists Association sometimes kept research secret if it indicated the dangers from, for example, vinyl chloride. Individual companies, such as Monsanto, shaped the research into their particular products, such as PCBs, often delaying recognition of these substances' dangers by years or decades.[53] But, with the rise of a new environmental and labor movement in the 1960s, along with the federal agencies born in the early 1970s—such as the Environmental Protection Agency, the Consumer Product Safety Commission, the Occupational Safety and Health Administration (OSHA), and the National Institute for Occupational Safety and Health (NIOSH)—traditional ties to industry began to erode.

Silbergeld's early career was formed in the cauldron of the social, scientific, and political changes overtaking students and graduate training itself. After receiving her undergraduate degree in history from Vassar College in 1967, she entered the Johns Hopkins doctoral program in environmental engineering sciences in 1972 as, she believes, its first female doctoral student.[54] During this time she interned at the Center for the Study of Responsive Law as one of the original "Nader's Raiders," whose work would emerge as a critical support for environmental and consumer advocates in the coming years. As the war in Vietnam galvanized the student movement and the broader American society, Silbergeld became all too aware of the societal issues involved in industrial and scientific work. In 1969, as the war escalated and as the nation absorbed the meaning of the assassinations of Martin Luther King and Robert Kennedy, the Days of Rage in Chicago during the Democratic National Convention, and the Tet Offensive in Vietnam, Silbergeld organized peace demonstrations of federal employees when she was a program officer at the National Academy of Sciences.[55]

Even with this background, she was unprepared for the reaction that her animal study of lead effects and hyperactive mice, along with her conclusion that the model might apply to humans, would set off: "It's amazing how naïve I was," she recalled in an interview with Lydia Denworth. "I gave my talk [at the Raleigh conference] and had no real notion of what to expect since I was just starting out in science. Somebody got up in the audience and launched right into me with a huge attack as if my science was suspect." Like Herbert Needleman in Amsterdam, she "realized [she] was in a different world." Compared to most scientific sessions, this one was unusually charged. "Scientists might ask questions, but they don't attack you as if you're doing something obviously evil. I thought, 'what in God's name is going on here?'" At the session break she met up with Needleman and Philip Landrigan, both of whom had experience with industry's wrath. Denworth writes that even thirty-five years later, Silbergeld remembered "the conversation vividly." Said Silbergeld, "They said, 'you might have wondered what was going on here. You probably don't know what's at stake.' Then Herb said, 'you're going to have to make up your mind. Do you want to be part of the debate or not?'"[56]

Silbergeld soon made her decision, after more encounters with lead industry representatives. They approached her when she was still a postdoc at Johns Hopkins and complimented her on her paper. When one visitor suggested that she needed to be more careful, since others might misuse her work to make claims she might not support, she grew suspicious. Soon afterward, "they went too far, even for me in my naïve state," Silbergeld recalled. Industry spokespeople suggested that she "might want to write to *Science* explaining what her paper was really about." When they told her they had already drafted a letter for her, she says, "the scales fell from my eyes. . . . I was converted. I could have called up Herb and Phil." and told them to "sign me up."[57]

As new research and researchers focused on lower levels of lead exposure, new technologies revolutionized the ability of people in public health

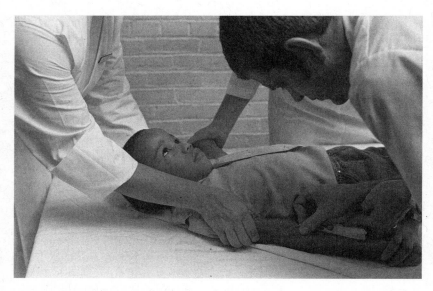

FIGURE 5. Three-year-old having blood drawn, ca. 1970. Until the finger-prick and other less intrusive tests for lead poisoning were developed, drawing the vials of blood needed for laboratory analysis was a potentially terrifying experience for young children. Source: Bettman/Corbis, reprinted with permission.

to grasp the true magnitude of the lead-poisoning problem. Mass screening programs had begun in the 1960s but they were extremely difficult to perform. Jane Lin-Fu recalled that "when mass screening began, blood lead determination had to be done on blood drawn by venous puncture," often leading to resistance from the child and enormous time and costs for the agency.[58] But, in 1973, the free erythrocyte porphyrins (EP) test became available, a measure that required only a finger prick.[59] "Unlike blood lead level which measures lead absorption," Lin-Fu noted, "EP is an index of lead toxicity"; in other words, instead of simply measuring the amount of lead in the blood, the EP test measured the lead's actual biological impact on blood. Since EP readings could be done within minutes, it was no longer necessary "to recall children with positive screening tests, thereby lowering costs and minimizing losses to follow-up," which could be substantial: one of every four children never returned for a more complete evaluation. In addition to its low cost and rapid results, the EP test aided public health officials in identifying children who had an iron deficiency, which, in turn, could increase a child's vulnerability to lead's ill effects.[60]

The two new technologies that were developed in the early 1970s—the EP test and the measure of lead in baby teeth— provided epidemiologists and statisticians with tools they could use to confirm the hypotheses and observations that Lin-Fu, Needleman, and others were generating about the extent of the public health crisis in lead. Further, the gathering epidemiological evidence and the growing data from Silbergeld's and other physiological studies allowed researchers to reconceptualize the problem of lead poisoning as a chronic disease with subclinical behavioral and neurological effects.

With these tools and fresh conceptions of the problem, researchers throughout the nation took up the challenge. In 1974, Hofstra University psychology professor Claire Ernhart and her graduate student Joseph Perino studied eighty African American preschool children whose blood lead levels were below the standard for lead poisoning at the time, which was still 60 µg/dl. They found, through the use of regression analysis, "that the relationship [between lead exposure and cognitive functioning] was significant and as lead levels increased general cognitive, verbal, and perceptual abilities decreased."[61] The children with blood lead levels above 40 µg/dl had trouble at the very least with reading, writing, and arithmetic. The next year, Brigitte de la Burdé and McLin S. Choate built on their own earlier work, which had shown a significant effect of lead exposure above 40 µg/dl on IQ, fine motor development, gross motor development, concept formation, and behavior.[62] In their new research, they evaluated the school performance of children with elevated lead levels through the third grade. These seven-year-old children had "more than twice . . . [the] deficits on neurological examination" as their controls.[63] Along with other studies, these papers pointed to permanent damage that was a result of a level of lead exposure—40 µg/dl—that only ten years before was considered by some to be "safe."[64]

But not all agreed with this emerging shift in outlook. In 1974, Richard Lansdown, a newly minted psychology PhD from England who went on to work as chief psychologist at the Hospital for Sick Children in London, stuck to the earlier view that lead was only a problem at high levels. Lansdown examined what he and his colleagues characterized as "the total population of children under the age of 17 living in a working class area exposed to undue amounts of lead." He found that the children's blood lead levels were directly correlated with the distance of their homes from a factory in their neighborhood, but he was unable to discern any "relationship between blood-lead level and any measure of mental functioning."[65]

The Lansdown article revealed a fault line among researchers and sparked a heated debate within the public health and research community.

It began mildly with a methodological critique of Lansdown's work by Oliver David. In a May 1974 letter to the editor of the *Lancet*, David pointed out that Lansdown's study did not include the most vulnerable population, children under the age of six, and thus the results were inconclusive.[66] The following month, more substantive critiques appeared in the journal. Two British researchers, D. Bryce-Smith of the University of Redding and H.A. Waldron of the medical school at the University of Birmingham, took Lansdown to task for what they believed were unsupported conclusions. Without data indicating the extent of past exposures, or a research design that would control for individual differences in susceptibility, it was impossible to eliminate lead as a causative agent. They cited, for example, the growing literature on the effects of blood lead levels from 17 to 40 µg/dl on the central nervous system, including the 1971 National Academy of Sciences report indicating that "subtle neurologic deficits and mental impairment are the more common outcomes" of lead exposure.[67]

Lansdown and his colleagues replied that they saw "no reason to reconsider our main conclusion at this stage," because it was "just not possible to incriminate lead as a cause" for the children's behavioral and neurological problems.[68] A month later, Bryce-Smith and Waldron again wrote to the *Lancet*, this time noting that a preliminary report of studies in El Paso's "Smeltertown" had led them to conclude that Lansdown was off base in exonerating lead as a subtle danger in children.[69] Edward B. McCabe, a researcher at the University of Wisconsin, rose to Lansdown's defense, arguing that children's blood lead levels of between 40 and 60 µg/dl were not a problem. He cited an industry-funded study as corroboration of Lansdown's work, asserting that "the question of the effect of moderate lead absorption" was "resolved."[70]

McCabe's university credentials lent credibility to his assertion, but a few months later some of the leading scientific and political figures in the country responded by raising broader scientific and ethical questions about his work. Herbert Needleman, then at Harvard Medical School and Boston's Children's Hospital; Samuel Epstein at Case Western Reserve University; Bertram Carnow of the University of Illinois School of Public Health; John Scanlon of Harvard Medical School; David Parkinson of Toronto's Hospital for Sick Children; Sheldon Samuels of the AFL-CIO's Industrial Union Department; Anthony Mazzocchi of the Oil, Chemical and Atomic Workers Union; and Oliver David of the State University of New York's Downstate Medical Center all threw down the gauntlet to the lead industry: why, they asked, was there such a sharp "divide between those who are alarmed that 'low-level lead' exposure is accompanied by adverse health effects, particularly in neuropsychological performance, and those who argue that no case has been made for low-level lead exposure as a hazard"? In examining the research done up to the mid-1970s, the authors "could find no statement, report, or study by an industry-sponsored scientist, whether in-house grantee, or academic consultant, which frankly acknowledges that low-level exposure is hazardous." It was only those who worked in universities or government agencies who were authors of "reports of toxicity due to low-level lead exposure." Edward McCabe himself seemed to be an exception, since the affiliation he gave for his letter to the *Lancet* was the Department of Pediatrics of the University Hospitals in Madison, Wisconsin. But the authors noted that he was not as independent as it might seem: three months before its appearance in the *Lancet*, "his text was first published almost verbatim as an International Lead Zinc Research Organization In-House Report, dated July 16, 1974," where he was identified as "Edward McCabe, Pediatric Consultant, ILZRO."[71] (What was not known at the time was that ILZRO described McCabe's role as "providing testimony for ILZRO and LIA as needed before various governmental groups" and that he provided these services until at least the early 1980s.)[72]

In fact, despite the effort by the lead industry to create doubt, study after study in the mid-1970s was adding to the evidence that levels of lead well below the Center for Disease Control's then-current recommendation of 60 µg/dl caused irreversible and serious damage to children.[73]

LEAD SMELTERS AND AIR POLLUTION

The El Paso study that Bryce-Smith and Waldron had referred to focused on how children's health was affected by air pollution from a lead smelter in that Texas city.[74] The study, conducted by Philip Landrigan, Stephen Gehlbach, Bernard Rosenblum, and others, would become one of the most important building blocks in the developing consensus that comparatively low levels of lead exposure, specifically from lead particles in the air, could have a harmful effect on children. And the principal author of the study, Philip Landrigan, would emerge in the following decades as one of the nation's most prominent environmental scientists.

Born in Boston in the early 1940s, Landrigan attended Boston College, a Jesuit university just outside of the city. He entered Harvard Medical School in 1963, planning to be a surgeon, but he "hated" the hierarchical, "top-down and abusive" culture he experienced in the surgical service. When he took his pediatrics rotation a few months later he found the human interactions and the medical care much more to his liking and decided to pursue a career in pediatrics. In 1967, in the midst of the Vietnam War, when Landrigan was an intern at Case Western, he was summoned to the Army Induction Board in Cleveland for a preinduction physical and realized "it was only a matter of weeks before I was going to be called up" for mandatory service as a doctor in a war he, like millions of others, opposed. With the help of the chief of service at Case Western, Landrigan was able to arrange an alternative to war participation by joining the nation's Public Health Service and working for the CDC in its immunization branch.[75]

The Smeltertown study then originated almost by chance. Landrigan had been "chasing outbreaks of measles and rubella during the winter of 1970," as he put it, when "we got a strange call from the health officer, Bernard Rosenblum, in El Paso, Texas." Rosenblum had partnered with the city attorney of El Paso, John Ross, and identified what they called "a lead problem." Rosenblum had been concerned that the ASARCO smelter on the edge of the city had been emitting sulfur dioxide, "which was causing respiratory distress to kids." When they looked at company documents detailing emissions from the plant, they noticed that over the previous three years ASARCO had also emitted large quantities of lead.[76] In fact, the smelter, which had been operating since 1887, had emitted "1012 metric tons of lead, as well as 508 metric tons of zinc, 11 tons of cadmium, and 1 metric ton of arsenic into the atmosphere through its stacks in the years 1969 through 1971."[77]

Landrigan's boss at the CDC, Lyle Conrad, told him to go to El Paso to investigate, even though the CDC at the time was almost solely concerned with infectious disease outbreaks and "was not doing environmental health."[78] The model Landrigan and his colleagues designed for the study was straightforward. They drew three concentric circles around the smelter in the summer of 1971 and measured the blood lead levels of children within each of the study areas. They found blood lead levels at or above 40 µg/dl "in 53 per cent of the children one to nine years old living within 1.6 kilometers of the smelter." That percentage went down the farther away from the smelter they tested, which led them to conclude that "the smelter was the principal source of this lead."[79]

A year after Landrigan and his colleagues began their study, ILZRO's Lead Environmental Health Committee, whose membership included Jerome Cole, who would emerge as the leading spokesperson for the lead industry for the next two decades, voted in September 1972 to appropriate $25,000 for its own epidemiological study of El Paso. ASARCO and the tetraethyl lead–producing companies in ILZRO each also contributed a like sum. A leader of one of the major mining and smelting companies, St. Joseph Minerals Corporation, located in Herculaneum, Missouri, in the middle of the largest lead mining and smelting area of the country, explained the importance of this proposed study to those at the committee meeting: "It is hoped that the study will disprove the 'lasting effect' premise of low grade lead absorption in children, [and] if so then we are ahead in the game."[80]

The result was ILZRO's support of a study by James McNeill, a pediatrician who worked for ASARCO in El Paso, and a colleague, J.A. Ptasnik. The study compared blood lead levels of children who had once lived around the smelter with others who had not. The study, which was rejected by the *New England Journal of Medicine* and never found a home in a peer-reviewed journal, was presented at a World Health Organization symposium on the effects of environmental pollution on health. It claimed there were no differences between the groups and concluded that "children who are healthy, well nourished, and not anemic may carry significant elevations of blood lead levels in the range of 40 [micrograms per deciliter blood] to 80 over a period of years without apparent deleterious effects." Jerome Cole was blunt in describing one of the industry's motives in supporting this research, believing that it would "cut [Landrigan] off," preempting his study.[81]

Landrigan, meanwhile, having established in 1971 that children living close to the smelter had elevated blood lead levels, returned to El Paso in 1973 to study possible longer-term effects in the children. Almost immediately he ran into trouble. The El Paso Board of Health "disinvited" the CDC team of ten medical officers and twenty support staff. Bernard Rosenblum "had overstepped his bounds" when he made contact with the CDC, the Board of Health claimed; the team should "go back to Atlanta." Landrigan then contacted Texas attorney general John Hill, who intervened, saying there was no legal reason the CDC should terminate the study. After that "there was no further interference" from the local authorities, Landrigan recalls.[82]

But soon thereafter, Landrigan received an invitation to lunch with Jack Duncan, ASARCO's attorney. Duncan invited him to the Cattleman's Club, an exclusive restaurant at the top of the El Paso Natural Gas Company building, the tallest building in the city. He remembers having steaks for lunch, an unusual treat for a young government employee. "We went over to the window overlooking the city after the meal," Landrigan recalls, "and Duncan said, 'Doctor, we're really proud of this city; we're really trying to keep the Mexicans happy.' He paused, and then said, 'Is there anything we can do to make your stay in El Paso more pleasant?'" Landrigan answered, "Everything is fine.... But Duncan kept repeating the question. 'Really, Doctor, is there anything we can do make your stay here more *pleasant?*'

It wasn't until I got back to my office and told the story to my friends . . . that I began to understand what I had been offered."[83]

Two years later, in 1975, Landrigan and his colleagues published the results of their study of low-level lead absorption among El Paso children in two prominent publications: the *Lancet* and the *New England Journal of Medicine*.[84] They showed that the IQs of children with blood lead levels between 40 and 68 µg/dl were significantly lower than those in a control group of children with lower blood lead levels and that the high lead group performed poorly on a simple finger-wrist tapping test, which indicated peripheral neurological damage.[85] With research later conducted by Joseph Graziano in Kosovo, Yugoslavia, this confirmed the suspicion that Jane Lin-Fu had first stated in 1972 and others were now reporting: that lead dust, whether from smelters or from burning leaded gasoline, was a significant source of lead poisoning.[86]

THE POLITICS OF AMBIENT AIR

The smelter issue was important, since thousands of children were poisoned who breathed in, played in, and even ended up eating lead dust from the dozen or so lead smelters around the country. But the lead particulates coming out of the country's millions of tailpipes dwarfed these localized tragedies.

In the 1960s, as Americans bought an unprecedented number of cars, tetraethyl lead, the gasoline additive introduced in the 1920s as an antiknock agent that increased the power and efficiency of the internal combustion engine, replaced lead pigments as a major source of industry profit. To protect this increasingly important outlet for lead, the Lead Industries Association decided as a "primary objective" of their Policy and Program on Childhood Lead Poisoning "to keep attention focused on old leaded paint as its [lead poisoning's] primary source and to make clear that other sources of lead are not significantly involved."[87] Despite the lead industry's efforts, however, the nation's first Environmental Protection Agency administrator, William Ruckelshaus, decided in 1971 that tetraethyl lead was "a threat to public health."[88]

By 1972, the EPA proposed regulations that would cut in half the amount of lead allowed in a gallon of gasoline and make it mandatory for gas stations to offer unleaded gasoline as an option. Under pressure from the lead industry, the EPA did not follow through on its first proposal, but the burgeoning environmental and consumer movements forced the issue. In 1973, David Schoenbrod, the staff attorney for the Natural Resources Defense Council, filed suit against the EPA, arguing that the agency had allowed "unreasonable delay" in fulfilling its responsibility to regulate lead as a dangerous air pollutant.[89] With increasing attention given to air pollution and lead in dust from engine exhaust, in December 1973 the EPA finally did act. Using the authority granted by the 1970 amendments to the Clean Air Act, the EPA called for a five-year reduction in lead from 2 grams per gallon to 0.5 gram per gallon by 1979.[90]

Ironically, it was the automobile industry's decision to introduce the catalytic converter in response to the federal Clean Air Act that had a greater impact than government regulation on reducing the amount of lead in gasoline. These converters—meant to reduce sulfur emissions, then seen as the major source of urban smog—were fouled by lead. According to Joseph C. Robert, the historian of the Ethyl Corporation, the president of General Motors, Edward N. Cole, in January 1970 "announced in Detroit at a meeting of the Society of Automotive Engineers . . . that to achieve the desired air quality in the engine exhaust as scheduled by federal regulation General Motors planned to install a catalytic converter." Cole told the group "that since leaded gasoline was incompatible with the platinum catalyst, leaded gasoline would have to phase down or out." This statement was "a bombshell . . . here was General Motors, which had fathered the additive [tetraethyl lead], calling for its demise!" The industry was shaken, for GM was essentially abandoning the Ethyl Corporation and accepting the "annihilation of the lead antiknock business."[91] The EPA's eventual action to phase out and eliminate lead in gasoline in the 1970s and 1980s simply hastened the process that had begun with little consideration for the lead issue itself.[92] This is not to say that the EPA's efforts to eliminate lead from gasoline were unnecessary or irrelevant; there was no guarantee at the time, as Paul Mushak (professor in the Division of Environmental Pathology, University of North Carolina School of Medicine) and others have pointed out, that industry scientists would not develop a catalytic converter unaffected by lead.[93]

The lead industry did not give up without a fight. In January 1975, at the American Association for the Advancement of Science meeting in New York, Gary Ter Haar, the senior research associate for the Ethyl Corporation, outlined the lead industry's position. Asserting that "lead is naturally present in the environment and most of it is found in soil," he claimed that "in general, most studies have shown that neither the lead emitted from automobiles nor from an industrial point source have an impact on the health of man."[94] Instead, he argued, "the overwhelming problem of lead in children is the eating of leaded paint." Citing the earlier testimony of Julian Chisolm before Senator Joseph Biden's (D-DE) Panel for Science and

Technology for the Senate's Public Works Committee, Ter Haar maintained that there was "no problem with lead in children in new public housing areas located between two expressways in the city of Baltimore, Maryland." According to Ter Haar, this and various studies exonerated lead in gasoline as a cause of childhood poisonings. Pointing his finger at lead paint, he argued that "the majority of lead problems in children will disappear if lead paint containing high lead is removed from a child's environment."[95]

The Ethyl Corporation, along with DuPont and other lead interests, fought back against the government's threat to their industry in the hope that a timely technological innovation would allow them to use lead with catalytic converters after all and, more generally, to weaken government attempts to regulate industry. In May 1975 they sued the EPA in an attempt to curtail the agency's right to regulate lead in gasoline based on a supposed threat it posed to humans or to the environment. They argued that the "will endanger" standard for EPA action demanded that the agency provide "a high quantum of factual proof" that lead pollution actually caused harm, rather than simply a "significant risk of harm."[96] The U.S. Court of Appeals of the District of Columbia rejected the industry's argument in a forceful and detailed decision in March 1976, laying out what became known as the precautionary principle, the idea Bradford Hill and Harriet Hardy had expressed in the early 1960s, that when there is a serious *potential* for harm, society has an obligation to act, even in the absence of definitive proof.

The court held that modern industrial society posed new threats to humans and to the environment that were difficult to evaluate and might take decades to manifest themselves. "Man's ability to alter his environment," the court ruled, "has developed far more rapidly than his ability to foresee with certainty the effects of his alterations." But it was "only recently that we have begun to appreciate the danger posed by unregulated modification of the world around us." The EPA, created only six years earlier, was a modern response to this new reality and was established as a "watchdog . . . whose task it is to warn us, and protect us, when technological 'advances' present dangers unappreciated or unrevealed by their supporters." The EPA and other regulatory agencies were "unequipped with crystal balls and unable to read the future" but were "nonetheless charged with evaluating the effects of unprecedented environmental modifications, often made on a massive scale." The agency was charged, by necessity, with the responsibility to act in spite of "conflicting evidence, and, sometimes, with little or no evidence at all."[97]

The court was struggling with the new challenges that pollution posed to our ideas about science and, more specifically, with what environmental science needed to address—and the responsibility of government in these new circumstances. Unlike the infectious diseases, in which specific bacteria or viruses were responsible for specific diseases, the chronic diseases and conditions that began to dominate health concerns in the middle decades of the twentieth century defied the methodologies and models that had led to the earlier "conquest" of infectious diseases.

Cancers, heart disease, stroke, and other chronic conditions, from asthma to emphysema, were products of complex environmental interactions and exposures that required new ways of thinking about danger and risk, and about the responsibilities of public health agencies. Prevention could not await one "single dispositive study" that definitively identified the cause of damage, the court pointed out. "Science does not work that way." Rather, science was a product of "suggestive results of numerous studies"; "the more supporting, albeit inconclusive, evidence available, the more likely the accuracy of the conclusion." The court rejected the lead industry's argument that you needed "one [definitive] single study or bit of evidence" to reach a conclusion, deciding instead that the EPA had a right, even an obligation, to act to prevent the possibility of future harm.[98]

Despite the court's decision affirming the EPA's authority, the lawsuit actually led the agency to adopt a more cautious, perhaps weak approach. In this, industry may have lost the battle but, at least temporarily, not the war: the lead industry's broader strategy included using the courts and the threat of lawsuits to put regulatory agencies on the defensive. And this could be effective.

In November 1976, for example, the EPA prepared its *Air Quality Criteria for Lead* draft for public comment, which was the document mandated by the Clean Air Act for the EPA to establish regulations "to protect the public from the adverse effects of air pollution."[99] The document would form the basis for future regulation of the tetraethyl lead industry and therefore, of the gasoline producers. But the EPA's draft raised the ire of both advocates and industry alike because it suggested that the status quo be maintained—specifically, the then-current ambient air lead standard of 5 micrograms per cubic meter ($\mu g/m^3$).[100] The agency's proposal was immediately denounced by environmental activists as "an apologia for lead."[101] The EPA's Science Advisory Board meeting in January 1977 was the scene of a major confrontation. "It was a couple of days of severe fighting," Herbert Needleman told Lydia Denworth. "The good guys in one corner, industry in the other," remembered Sergio Piomelli, the Columbia University physician who pioneered research into the relationship between lead and the synthesis of blood. "We fought on the document page by page, word by word."[102] David Schoenbrod, of the National Resources Defense Council, described the scene to Denworth this way: "The effect was electric. The chairman [of the science advisory meeting] went around the room. One by one, they agreed with doctors Needleman and Piomelli." The draft was set aside.[103]

While Paul Mushak, Needleman, and Piomelli were disturbed by the draft report's refusal to acknowledge the true harms caused by low-level lead exposures, the industry took exception to the draft because it accepted that lead could have chronic effects on children. In comments to the EPA on the original draft, the LIA and ILZRO argued that any blood lead levels below 80 µg/100 g—levels associated with seizures among children—were clinically insignificant. The groups fell back on a long-standing industry argument that "considerably more work needs to be done in this area" but held fast to the position that on the basis of what was then known, "it is inappropriate to conclude that lead causes any neurological effects at blood lead levels in the 80 µg/100 g range."[104] In its critique of the draft's section on lead in dust or dirt, the lead industry took aim at the scientific basis for regulating what was still a mainstay of the industry: lead in gasoline. Despite decades of accumulating research on air pollution and lead, the industry maintained that "there is no evidence that lead in dust from automotive emissions contributes significantly to the lead levels of children."[105]

Given this broad dissatisfaction with the draft, the EPA called on Paul Mushak, the neurobiologist Lester Grant, and the pathologist Marty Krigman to help rewrite it. They worked feverishly from April to December 1977 in a "series of hectic and around the clock meetings," as Mushak recalls them. "The control . . . and preparation of the criteria document was taken out of the hands of industry-friendly bureaucrats and put in the hands of scientific folk" including Herbert Needleman, Sergio Piomelli, Philip Landrigan, Ellen Silbergeld, and Sam Epstein. Not unexpectedly, Mushak recalls, "industry mounted a lot of resistance to the drafts as they were prepared. . . . They said they were not disputing that lead could be toxic but the arguments were about how far down you found these toxic effects." A small group of scientists also disputed the nature of the toxic effects, and posed a broader question: "what is an adverse effect?" Industry's position was that, in Mushak's words, "unless you were injured to a specific degree you were not injured."[106]

Needleman, along with Harriet Hardy and others, pointed out that physicians have consistently refined definitions of disease to include subtle biochemical changes as they became known. Laboratories, microscopes, and new technologies played a role in this process. In the late nineteenth century, for example, the diagnosis of leukemia was based on overt clinical symptoms; by the late twentieth century it was based on a blood test. "If practitioners were to await the appearance of a gross physical change as an indication of adverse health effects," said Needleman, "they would, in many cases be guilty of practicing inferior medicine, if not out-and-out malpractice."[107] Lead poisoning was the same. Waiting for symptoms to appear was irresponsible, and for society to allow children to be exposed to a known neurotoxin in the air was irresponsible. This argument carried the day.

In the first weeks of 1978 the EPA, based on the air quality criteria document, proposed to reduce the ambient air lead standard substantially, from 5 to 1.5 $\mu g/m^3$. Because gasoline lead was such a significant contributor to air lead levels, this standard would require a drastic reduction and eventual elimination of lead in gasoline and major reductions in emissions from lead smelters.[108]

Within days of the EPA's notice, the lead industry called a special meeting of the LIA Environmental Health Committee at New York's Lexington Hotel. Fourteen companies—including DuPont, St. Joseph Lead Company, ASARCO, National Lead, and PPG (the Pittsburgh Plate Glass Company), the largest producers and users of lead products in the nation—met on January 16, 1978, with the staff of the LIA, ILZRO, and the public relations firm Hill & Knowlton to plan a campaign to get the EPA to change the document to industry's liking. The meeting mapped out three lines of attack. First, industry representatives planned to interject doubt about the scientific basis for lowering the ambient air lead level. They believed that through legal action they could convince the courts that the EPA's science was flawed and that the ambient air lead standard should be between 4 and 5 $\mu g/m^3$ rather than the 1.5 suggested by the EPA.[109] Second was to challenge the document by arguing that the economic impact of the EPA rulings would be devastating, leading to "the shutdown of mines, mills and smelters, closing of small battery manufacturers," and other economic ills.[110]

The third line of attack would be an intensive Hill & Knowlton lobbying and public relations campaign aimed at members of congress; local, state, and federal officials; and the broader public that would emphasize the economic and political fallout from the EPA action. "Individuals, industry and companies should prepare press releases for use in local newspapers and use the LIA derived Health and Economic arguments to show the impact on . . . local industry." Such a press release should indicate the "combined cost being absorbed by the industry" for various OSHA and EPA air and water regulations. "This data should also be discussed with local legislators so they can be aware of the very real threat to employment, tax base and the like within their own geographic subdivision."[111] In addition, the industry would mobilize experts to testify in February at the EPA hearings on the proposed standards, testimony the LIA would use to bolster its case that children's blood lead levels were not dangerous below 40 micrograms per deciliter of blood.

The hearings brought together the two opposing camps: the lead industry and its experts, who argued for less regulation; and the CDC, environmental scientists, and lead researchers such as Philip Landrigan, Sergio Piomelli, and Herbert Needleman, who argued for much more stringent control over environmental lead.[112] Among those appearing on behalf of the industry was Julian Chisolm himself (whose time was paid for by the industry),[113] then emerging as the dean of the lead research community. Chisolm worried that the new research on low-level lead exposures and their subtle biological and behavioral effects would shift attention from what he considered the most important problem—acute neurological damage, convulsions, and in some cases death resulting from children ingesting lead paint chips. Using the testimonies of Chisolm, Edward McCabe, and Jerome Cole, the LIA argued that the lead standard should "be based on the earliest adverse health effect of lead in children: a decrease in hemoglobin which can be detected well before clinical anemia results," which, according to the LIA, occurred at no lower than 40 µg/dl.[114] But the scientific evidence of low-level effects won the day as researchers pointed to the potential damage that awaited children who were slowly accumulating lead in their bodies. On September 29, 1978, the EPA adopted a National Ambient Air Quality Standard for lead of 1.5 µg/m^3 as a ninety-day average.

A WIDENING VIEW OF DISEASE

By the late 1970s, the lead industry was growing isolated and its embrace of the traditional paradigm of lead poisoning as a discrete disease limited to its acute, sometimes fatal form was dissolving. In its assessment of the dangers of lead exposure, the federal government, through the CDC, began to consider studies of biological and behavioral changes previously deemed "subclinical." This in turn had a ripple effect on other parts of the medical community. The CDC issued a statement, published in late 1975 in *Pediatrics*, titled "Increased Lead Absorption and Lead Poisoning in Young Children," that was "developed with the assistance of" Julian Chisolm, Jane Lin-Fu, Sergio Piomelli, and others. The CDC continued to distinguish "lead poisoning" from "undue or increased lead absorption," but the statement broadened the CDC's definition of toxicity to include "subclinical manifestations

of biochemical derangements ... as well as overt clinical manifestations."
The CDC now suggested that "undue or increased lead absorption" occurred
at "blood lead levels [of] 30–79 µg/dl," a substantial lowering from the surgeon general's statement of only a few years earlier that had identified
40 µg/dl as the lower threshold of evidence of undue lead absorption.[115] The
CDC now recommended that "all children ages 1 through 5 years ... who
live in, or frequently visit, poorly maintained housing units constructed
prior to the 1960s, should be screened at least once a year."[116] In addition, in
September 1977 the Consumer Product Safety Commission, created
in 1972, acted to ban the sale of residential paints with more than a trace
amount (0.06 percent) of lead pigments and driers, further limiting the lead
industry.[117] In 1978 the CDC officially lowered the definition of "undue"
lead absorption from 40 to 30 µg/dl.[118] It incorporated a new conception of
disease and danger, declaring, "Lead toxicity is defined as biochemical ... or
functional derangements caused by lead. Undue lead absorption refers to
excess lead in the blood with evidence of biochemical derangements in the
absence of clinical symptoms."[119] In other words, even if it was invisible to
the clinician, parent, and victim, lead was destroying lives.[120]

Concern among public health experts and others in the 1970s about the
subtle but often significant impact low-level lead exposure could have on
behavior and biological processes amplified the growing attention to potential pollution and disease threats from substances other than lead. Studies
of the effects of lead, among the oldest recognized threats to human health,
were also transforming how epidemiologists, environmental scientists, and
consumers understood disease more generally. Growing awareness of the
threats from DDT, PCBs, saccharine, DES (a potentially cancer-causing
estrogen mimicker), and other products being introduced widely into the
human environment from the 1940s onward was leading to new models for
understanding what constituted disease, threats to human health, and
acceptable proof of harm. Increasingly the nation's scientists and environmental advocates argued that disease was more than physical impairment
and shortened lives. Rather, biological changes that affected behavior, psychological well-being, reproduction, and intelligence needed to be included
in our estimation of danger from a new industrial environment. The evolving science of low-level lead exposures, along with the political and social
movements around childhood lead poisoning, would provide support for a
growing social debate that would ultimately transform our ideas about disease, science, and, for the professional public health community, epidemiology. The lead issue was perhaps the most developed early challenge to the
still dominant paradigm of disease, that of acute and chronic diseases with

generally obvious clinical manifestations, which is today represented in the debates over endocrine disruptions and other impacts of low-level exposures.

New technologies developed post–World War II played a role in this growing public awareness of environmental toxins. For example, gas chromatography, a new means of measuring chemical presence in tiny amounts, revealed the terrifying extent of PCB and DDT pollution in the mid-1960s. After substantial resistance from the major producers of these chlorinated hydrocarbons, the use of DDT as a pesticide and the production of PCBs for use in carbonless carbon paper, paints, plastics, and other consumer products were stopped in 1971 and totally banned in 1979. Specifically for lead, a series of new technologies—most importantly, atomic absorption spectrophotometric methods for determining blood lead levels—provided lead researchers with the ability to quantify their hypotheses based on clinical and epidemiological evidence of the dangers of lower and lower blood lead levels.[121]

By the end of the 1970s, then, the federal government, through its regulation of lead in paint and gasoline, had taken significant steps to limit the introduction of more lead into the children's environment, and the lead research community had developed techniques for estimating low levels of lead in blood with tests requiring only a pin prick and a local laboratory. Further, researchers had begun to measure the subtler effects of elevated but comparatively low blood lead levels. Investigators now generally understood the limitations of these blood tests in estimating long-term exposures to lead and their biological effects, and Herbert Needleman with his colleagues had developed a method of measuring lead in baby teeth as a means of estimating long-term exposure during early childhood.

In a seminal article published in the *New England Journal of Medicine* in the last year of the decade, Needleman and his coauthors set forth a remaining question, in the spirit of the broadened notion of disease that had been gaining traction: "The neurotoxic properties of lead at high dose are well known and not a subject of general controversy. A source of considerable debate, however, is whether or not blood lead levels below those associated with obvious symptoms have adverse effects on the brain."[122]

In the article, Needleman and his colleagues reported on the correlations they had found between elevated lead in teeth and behavioral, intellectual, and subtle neurological damage to children. Needleman and his colleagues collected baby teeth from 158 first- and second-grade children in schools in the Boston-area communities of Somerville and Chelsea, and in a double-blind study researchers examined the children's performance based on several measures. Compared to children with relatively low dentine lead levels, those with higher dentine lead levels did not perform as well on intelligence, fine motor, auditory, and other neurological tests or in teacher evaluations of their behavior and performance in class. Using behavioral ratings by teachers themselves, Needleman and his colleagues looked for statistical correlations between lead accumulation and behavior. Children with more lead in their bodies were more easily distracted, less able to work independently, more disorganized, more hyperactive, more impulsive and excitable, and more easily frustrated by difficulties. These children also found it more difficult to follow simple directions and, in general, functioned less well in the classroom than other children of the same age.[123] In short, the lead that children accumulated over time produced "disordered classroom behavior."[124] Those with elevated dentine lead levels showed the effects of lead accumulated over time rather than a "snapshot" blood lead level—which might be high as a result of an acute exposure, or low because exposure was far in the past or because seasonal or other factors had limited the release of lead from the bones.

Many lead researchers recognized immediately the significance of Needleman and his colleagues' work, as previous studies of the neurotoxic effects of lead had been suggestive but not definitive.[125] And major newspapers around the country reported on the importance of the research. In a *New England Journal of Medicine* guest editorial, Jane Lin-Fu commented that the findings were "particularly ominous" because the effects of lead were so subtle and thus easily overlooked by clinicians and other researchers.[126]

The importance of the *NEJM* publication and the reception it received was not lost on the lead industry. Needleman's acceptance by much of the research community as the premier research scientist on the toxicity of lead would bring on a decade of attempts by the industry to both stifle his current work and discredit his past efforts. The lead industry's reaction to the Needleman study marked a major turning point in its attempts to shape lead toxicology, however. No longer was it sufficient to guide research direction through grants and contracts, the lead industry realized, and no longer was it possible to bury critical research through discrete funding of counterstudies and overwhelming public relations efforts. The LIA's Jerome Cole set the tone for the effort to demean and discredit Needleman's research. In a letter to the editor of the *New York Times* in mid-1980, he claimed that scientists had largely rejected Needleman's argument that low levels of lead could affect children: "This study provoked a storm of criticism from scientists around the world," Cole alleged, "a fact that has not been publicized."[127]

What the industry did not understand was that by the end of the 1970s Needleman's work was so well received because it built upon nearly a decade of suggestive research, new research technologies, and greater attention to and information on chronic conditions and low-level exposures. Along with new centers of power in federal agencies and in nongovernmental organizations that gave lead science a larger voice, a changing social environment and growing distrust of industry sponsorship combined to change the questions scientists were now asking and the issues that increasingly concerned them.

4 The Contentious Meaning of Low-Level Exposures

> A price must be paid for what we have done to our environment in the past. The crucial question is: Shall we pay it in controlling our environment or shall we pay it in terms of the health of thousands of children in our lifetime and millions in generations to come.
>
> JANE LIN-FU, 1982

The struggle over who would control the science and meaning of lead exposures continued into the 1980s as the lead industry recruited allies and sought to undermine the emerging scientific model that made its product the focus of regulation and increasing scrutiny. The election of Ronald Reagan in 1980 presented a wide range of polluting industries, lead included, with a fresh opportunity and a new lever to influence science and government policy, however. After a decade during which business leaders were caught off guard by the rising environmental movement, industry in the early 1980s sought to undermine the emerging scientific consensus about the import and impact of toxins in general and lead exposures in particular. In addition to trying to influence the Centers for Disease Control and the Environmental Protection Agency directly through pressure on individual administrators, gain more of a say in research funding decisions, and find greater representation on scientific bodies, industry turned to the highest levels of the Reagan administration itself for regulatory relief. Reagan had made clear, both in his election campaign and in his early appointments and actions, that defunding selected government programs and lifting the "regulatory burden" from private industry were high priorities. This shift in governing ideology from the Carter years, and to some extent even the Ford and Nixon years, was not lost on the lead industry. Here was a new opportunity to shape the political environment within which science was operating and, the industry hoped, reframe the conversation among policy makers, the public, and scientists themselves about what constituted risk and harm, and, ultimately, as we will see in later chapters, about who should bear the responsibility to remedy the legacy of decades of environmental pollution.

The Reagan revolution came none too soon for the lead industry. In the words of Jerome Cole, vice president of the International Lead Zinc Research

Organization, "For the past decade or so the lead industry has seen itself as an industry under siege." In January 1981 Cole traveled into the heart of the scientists' own trade group of sorts, the American Association for the Advancement of Science's annual meeting, to confront what the lead industry considered the cause of its nightmare: the industry, he argued, believed it had come close to losing the battle of ideas, and he denounced the scientific community whose "literature is littered with reports of study after study which associate, often on the basis of very meager data of questionable validity, a variety of societal ills to lead."[1]

What it could not win in the realm of science and ideas, the lead industry and its supporters sought to win in the new regulatory arena. Shortly after Reagan was inaugurated as president in January 1981, he nominated Anne Gorsuch for the post of EPA administrator. A member of the Colorado state legislature and a former corporate attorney, she came to Washington, she later said, "as part of a new Administration that brought a different approach to solving the problems of government. One of the tenets of that approach was what we now call the New Federalism, or the idea that there were any number of services being provided by Uncle Sam that could be better provided by the states themselves. Under that theory, while at EPA, we were the only agency in Washington that was truly practicing New Federalism."[2]

What Gorsuch characterized as an attempt to return power to the states was seen by environmentalists and many in Congress as a wholesale abandonment of the EPA's mission to protect the environment and reduce the influence of corporate America on critical environmental decisions. In her short tenure at the EPA—twenty-two months—Gorsuch drastically reduced not only the agency's budget and staff but also the number of lawsuits brought against industry polluters and the enforcement of critical legislation such as the Clean Air Act. Many reacted to her initial actions with disbelief and outrage, and Congress, after investigating misuse of federal Superfund appropriations, moved against her. In 1982, it cited Gorsuch for contempt for her refusal to provide documents in their investigation of possible misuse of $1.6 billion in Superfund money.[3] Despite Reagan's support for her policies and her probusiness orientation, Gorsuch had become a tremendous distraction to the administration, and in March 1983 she resigned. In an attempt to quash the continuing suspicions of his new administration and of the EPA itself, the president appointed in her place William Ruckelshaus, who had served in the Nixon administration initially first as EPA administrator and later as deputy attorney general. Ruckelshaus was held in esteem by many in Congress for his refusal to follow Nixon's command to fire Special Prosecutor Archibald Cox during the Watergate crisis.

During Gorsuch's brief reign, the lead industry believed it had a powerful ally in the EPA, while others correspondingly feared that the agency would seek to reverse its decisions that had reduced the level of lead allowed in gasoline and had introduced "unleaded" gasoline at all gas stations.[4] As Ruckelshaus put it soon after he took over the agency, "These concerns were apparently based on reports of private meetings between EPA and industry prior to decisions regarding the lead phase-down regulations and related matters."[5] Following Gorsuch's resignation, Ruckelshaus tried to cleanse the EPA's image by distancing it from the lead industry.

Under Ruckelshaus, the EPA formed a Special Expert Review Panel to evaluate the relationship between lead in gasoline and blood lead levels in children. The EPA had solicited expert opinions, including those of industry, in its early examination of the subject, but Ruckelshaus created the review panel to take a fresh look at the issue and come up with recommendations. The members of the panel were picked for their independent scientific judgment and were asked to sign a statement affirming that they were "neither affiliated with nor receiving nor expect to receive any form of financial or other support from any lead industry firm (or research organization) or any other industry-related commercial or research entity likely to be affected by standard setting or other regulatory activities potentially influenced by the present findings and recommendations of this Review Group."[6]

The specificity of the statement and the obvious attempt to distance the agency from special interests angered the lead industry to the point that Jerome Cole, who was now ILZRO's chief operating officer, contacted Vice President George H.W. Bush, in his role as chair of the Presidential Task Force on Regulatory Relief, to "protest" the statement. "The requirement by the EPA that scientists sign such a statement undermines by inference the perceived integrity of many fine, well-qualified scientists," Cole said. Revealing the breadth of the industry's reach into the scientific community, he pointed out that the industry had been supporting research by scientists for years and had, he claimed, provided "critical" information needed for developing national policy.[7]

The stringent disclaimer required of the review panel "was a special case, rather than a general Agency procedure," Ruckelshaus told Bush when he saw Cole's letter. He "assured" the vice president and Cole "that industry-associated scientists will continue to be able to participate fully, along with other interested parties, in the remaining stages of the review, and, if appropriate, revision of the ambient standards for lead."[8] Cole reported what he perceived as a victory to his board of directors and ILZRO's Environmental Health Committee (also called the Lead Environmental Health Committee): "Given the political problems faced by the EPA and Mr. Ruckelshaus, I believe the response was adequate and I was pleased to see that ILZRO-supported scientists will be given appropriate consideration based on their scientific credentials in future activities associated with EPA's standard setting activities."[9]

This was but one skirmish in a much broader war that the lead industry had been waging against any efforts of the EPA and other federal agencies to strengthen regulations governing lead. When, on September 29, 1978, the EPA adopted a National Ambient Air Quality Standard for lead of 1.5 micrograms per cubic meter as a ninety-day average, the industry filed suit in the U.S. Court of Appeals for the District of Columbia.[10] Cole, representing ILZRO and the LIA, argued that the EPA had established a standard based on faulty science that would not protect children's health but would be "ruinous for the industry."[11] In the subsequent decision in 1982 the D.C. circuit court upheld a further appeal of the EPA's ruling saying, as Paul Mushak, lead toxicologist at the University of North Carolina, put it, that it "would defer to the expertise of the EPA unless it could be shown that the agency had acted arbitrarily."[12] The *Wall Street Journal* chimed in to criticize the EPA for adopting the stronger limit and caving in to environmentalists' "scare" tactics. The editorial claimed there was considerable doubt in the scientific community about the validity of studies that saw danger in children being exposed to "minute doses" of lead. More—not less—lead was necessary in gasoline, the *Journal* went on. "Ghetto children," said the editorial, would be better served by increasing the amount of lead in gasoline, thereby promoting a "more efficient economy, capable of producing more wealth and more jobs."[13]

But lead researchers and public health advocates believed there was another way to aid poor children. In the 1950s and 1960s, the regulatory struggle was to reduce the lead content of paint and then to remove from children's environment the most obvious source of lead—peeling, flaking chunks of paint in the home. By the mid-1970s, as we have seen, there were fewer children convulsing, lapsing into comas, and dying, but screening programs had revealed an array of behavioral, intellectual, perceptual, and subtle neurological problems associated with elevated blood levels, such as slow learning and reduced IQ, reading difficulties and hyperactivity. These symptoms had largely been masked by an earlier focus on acute and obvious brain damage. Equally disturbing, epidemiologists in the 1970s had been finding evidence of deficits or biological abnormalities associated with lower and lower levels of environmental toxins, which meant that more and more children were at risk than previously realized. As a result, by 1980 the CDC had reduced the level of concern—the amount of lead in a child's blood that signaled potential harm—from 60 to 30 micrograms per deciliter.

The implications of lead's diffuse but often considerable effects on the neurological development, intelligence, behavior, and long-term well-being of America's children was a terrifying challenge to a public health community whose goal historically had been prevention of disease. Surveys revealed that many children who did not live in obviously dangerous houses still had blood-lead levels above 30 µg/dl.

THE WIDENING BREADTH OF THE LEAD EPIDEMIC

From the early 1970s through the early 1980s, researchers and public health advocates at the city, state, and federal levels emphasized screening children for lead poisoning and eliminating lead from paint and gasoline as the twin pillars of lead-related public health policy. If these traditional sources of lead pollution could be eliminated, and if poisoned children could be identified and treated, and their homes detoxified, lead poisoning as a threat to America's children could finally be all but eliminated. But the task appeared daunting indeed. One reason was the paucity of information on the problem's extent.[14] The U.S. General Accounting Office (GAO, now the Government Accountability Office) reported that as of 1980 "the following issues remain[ed] unsolved": "No reliable data exists on the total number of children with unsafe levels of lead in their bodies. The extent of lead-based paint in homes and, in particular, HUD-associated housing is still an unknown." In addition, the GAO asserted, "the relative contributions of ingested paint chips versus other sources of lead are not known."[15]

It had also become increasingly clear in the 1970s that lead poisoning was not confined to poor children. "Affluent Kids Also Harmed by Toxic Lead," the *Wall Street Journal* headlined in 1981. "Lead poisoning has started turning up in the homes of the affluent," the article noted. "A professional couple in a partly renovated neighborhood noticed that one of their eight-month-old twins was growing more slowly and eating less than the other" because the first child "had swallowed enough toxin . . . to cause slight learning disabilities." Vernon Houk of the CDC told the reporter that "lead toxicity is not, as once thought, confined to lower income urban areas." The threat was not just from lead paint but from the lead in gasoline as well. And Devra Davis, director of toxic substances for the Environmental

Law Institute, warned parents that "lead diseased middle class children can go unchecked by both parents and pediatricians."[16]

These concerns were given further support by the results of the second National Health and Nutrition Examination Survey (NHANES II), conducted between 1976 and 1980 and released in 1982. The survey, first conducted in the early 1960s, was an effort to document the health status of the American people. Since much public health data were collected by individual states and independent bodies such as insurance companies, hospitals, and physicians using varied criteria, NHANES was an attempt to provide consistency in developing an overall picture of the nation's health status and health problems. Thanks to Kathryn Mahaffey, then project manager for lead contamination of food at the Food and Drug Administration, the CDC and the National Center on Health Statistics in 1976 included blood lead levels in the survey for the first time.[17] The resulting survey data showed that one of every twenty-five children between six months and five years of age had "blood lead levels that exceeded the accepted limit of 30 µg per deciliter," in the words of Jane Lin-Fu. This meant that "780,000 children under six years old were poisoned." While "elevated blood lead levels were found in 2 percent of white children," she reported, lead affected "12.2 percent of black children." Only 2.1 percent of rural children were lead poisoned in contrast to 11.6 percent of "inner-city children." The survey also revealed the pernicious effects of class on this problem: "1.2 percent of children from families with an annual income of $15,000 [$34,000 in 2012 dollars] or more" were affected, "but 10.9 percent of those from families with an income under $6,000 [$13,500 in 2012 dollars]."[18]

Shocking as these data were, new analyses provided an extraordinary moment of hope and spur to action. In 1983, the *New England Journal of Medicine* looked at the reports of lead poisoning by year and noted that between the start of NHANES II in 1976 and its completion in 1980, there had been a dramatic nationwide reduction in children's "average blood lead levels from approximately 14.6 micrograms to 9.2 micrograms per deciliter, a decline of 37 percent."[19] This decline was attributed to the reduced lead in gasoline, a result of the EPA's 1973 decision to lower the lead content of gasoline over time and the auto industry's turn to using catalytic converters that required unleaded gas.[20] This suggested that if there was political will to further reduce the sources of lead in the environment, such action would have demonstrable and dramatic effects on children's blood lead levels—and on their ultimate well-being. But that moment would pass.

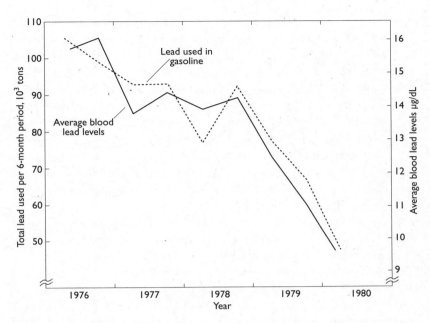

FIGURE 6.   Blood lead levels decline dramatically with reduction of lead in gas, 1976–1980. Declining blood lead levels continued to today following the complete removal of lead from gasoline and improved abatement techniques. Source: U.S. EPA, *Air Quality Criteria for Lead*, vol. 3, EPA-600/8-83/028cF (Washington, D.C.: U.S. EPA, June 1986), 11–43. See also David Jacobs, "Environmental Health Disparities in Housing," *AJPH*, 1012 (Supplement 1, 2011), p. S117.

NEW RESEARCH, NEW CONCERNS

If the news that reducing the lead in gasoline had succeeded in lowering average blood lead levels was a source of great satisfaction, the news that hundreds of thousands of children were still at severe risk from lead in their blood was extremely troubling. This became more disturbing when, in the early 1980s, more biological evidence came to light showing that "normal" blood lead levels in urban children were, in fact, potentially more dangerous than previously thought.

Sergio Piomelli, Carol Seaman, and others at the NYU Medical Center and the New York City Department of Health's Bureau of Lead Poisoning Control and Laboratories published a report in 1982 with broad implications for urban children because it challenged the long-held industry position, first promoted by Robert Kehoe, that lead was not only a normal but an innocuous component of the human environment. The study population consisted of more than 2,000 children between two and twelve years of age in New York City whose blood lead levels had been obtained by the city's Health Department. Piomelli and his colleagues found that even the level of lead considered "safe" at the time—30 µg/dl—interfered with heme synthesis (blood production), leading to suspicion of lead's broader pathological impact because blood production was "so essential to all of the body's tissues."[21] The findings were more evidence in support of what by the early 1980s was an emerging consensus in the scientific community that lead, even at levels of 30 µg/dl, caused serious physiological problems: anemia and damage to the ability of blood to carry oxygen, interference with the nervous system and brain chemistry, kidney and endocrine disruption, and changes in the ability of the liver to detoxify foreign substances, among others.[22]

What were public health professionals to make of this recent research? What was the significance of these biological changes? Specifically, did the blood lead levels that were considered "normal" at the time—30 µg/dl or below—constitute disease if they resulted in the kind of changes described? This was a continuation of the debate about what constitutes disease that had begun in the 1970s. In the words of Paul Mushak, "When does a biochemical perturbation become an adverse health effect?"[23] Evan Charney, then a researcher at Sinai Hospital in Baltimore, pointed out the "vexing issue": "Are the tens of thousands of overtly asymptomatic children we now identify with mildly elevated blood lead levels [30 µg] already suffering from a disease, or do they just represent a high risk group on whom preventive efforts can be focused to avert serious encephalopathy?" If it was the latter, "these children merit only careful monitoring, [and] the situation is in fact under good control; we have reduced the 'disease' to a rarity." However, if these "mildly elevated" blood lead levels were affecting children's development and functioning, "these children are already damaged, [and] there is a serious epidemic in this country." Were the programs that had been successful in uncovering and testing symptomatic lead poisoning in the 1950s, 1960s, and 1970s now, as Charney put it, "woefully inadequate to prevent or treat sub-encephalopathic lead poisoning" because the threshold had been set too high?[24]

The growing body of literature on the impact of what were thought to be low levels of lead exposure threw into high relief problems that researchers in a host of fields were encountering vis-à-vis the conception of toxicology. Historically, toxicology had as one of its major conceptual tools a belief that any material could be made safe by lowering its level below an established threshold, whether it be arsenic in the water, particles of sulfur in the air, or chemicals in the food supply. In this light, an important job of toxicology was to establish a "safe" level. In the 1950s, the Delaney Amendment to the Food and Drug Act had challenged this fundamental belief in thresholds. Passed in 1958, the amendment said that, when it came to carcinogenic substances in the food supply, there was no "safe" level. And during the 1960s and 1970s, improved technologies that enabled measurement of smaller and smaller levels of toxins had laid the groundwork for the debate that emerged in the 1970s and early 1980s as to whether existing thresholds set for lead and other toxins were adequate to protect the public's health. As surveillance of toxic materials became cheaper and more widespread, and as biological effects were found for lower and lower exposures, the triggers for concern, the thresholds, were lowered as well. Vinyl chloride, acrilonitrile, and other chemicals could now be measured in the water we drank, the air we breathed, and the food we ate; asbestos fibers could be found in the air of the schools our children attended; PCBs and DDT could be found in fish, shrimp, birds, and humans as well. But the underlying question remained: did these lowered thresholds really represented safety?

FROM SCIENTIFIC DISCOVERY TO REGULATORY CONFLICT

The polite technical debate that occurred in hundreds of articles and studies in scientific and medical journals of the 1970s and early 1980s aimed at reaching a consensus that could inform changes in public policy. For the most part, despite disagreements over the speed and adequacy of reform, the federal government had responded to the emerging data in appropriate ways: it had eliminated lead from paints, it had lowered the ambient air quality standard for lead, and it was in the process of lowering the amount of lead in gasoline. Most significantly, it had cut in half, from 60 to 30 µg/dl, the blood lead levels considered acceptable in children, which led to greatly increased awareness of the problem of lead poisoning among all groups in society.

But by the mid-1980s, any semblance of comity had vanished. What occurred instead amounted to a war in which the discourse was neither refined nor respectful and where scientists were forced to choose sides. In the end, this would be a Waterloo for industry science (though not for industry itself, of course). The lead industry in this period would abandon its effort to win the scientific argument over lead's effects on its merits and revert to attempting character assassination and manufacturing uncertainty about the emerging scientific consensus.

Should the federal government act to further reduce children's exposure to lead or should it leave well enough alone? That was the question of the moment. On the one side were the vast majority of research scientists who were finding actual and potential biological damage associated with blood lead levels previously considered "normal." On the other side were the lead industry and its antiregulatory supporters who argued that in the absence of absolute proof of harm, the government should take no action. The fierce battle that ensued in large part played out in what was then an obscure committee of the EPA, the Clean Air Scientific Advisory Committee (CASAC), a special congressionally mandated subcommittee of the EPA Science Advisory Board (SAB) tasked with reviewing criteria for pollutants such as lead, a committee that had no regulatory authority but did have tremendous influence. The Clean Air Act of 1970 authorized the establishment of National Ambient Air Quality Standards (NAAQS), which were to be revised every five years in light of new scientific evidence; and it was CASAC that was charged with evaluating the relevant research that had appeared since the previous standard and revising the criteria that would inform the new NAAQS for lead.

In April 1984, the EPA Science Advisory Board's CASAC met at Research Triangle Park in North Carolina ostensibly to discuss the narrow issue of the validity of the new lead research—especially Herbert Needleman's recent findings on the low-level effects of lead. But everyone was aware of the implications of these discussions: CASAC's recommendations would significantly influence the EPA decision in the 1980s about whether to phase out lead from gasoline once and for all. [25] CASAC's mandate was to consider the levels of lead that should be allowed under the Clean Air Act based solely on health effects, not on economic feasibility.[26] However, there was still plenty of room for disagreement and contention because, by statute, "other parts of the Act . . . allow the [EPA] Administrator to look at particular options with costs and benefits in mind."[27]

ATTACKING THE MESSENGER: THE LEAD INDUSTRY AND HERBERT NEEDLEMAN

The central part of the CASAC's charge was to evaluate whether there was damage seen with some regularity at blood lead levels below 30 µg/dl. If the literature documenting this danger was confirmed by the committee, it would indicate that the allowable amount of lead in gasoline should be further lowered, a prospect that threatened the already hobbled lead industry. In its efforts to derail further regulation of leaded gasoline, the industry itself sponsored studies that it hoped could refute or at least undermine research that implicated even low levels of lead as dangerous.

By supporting scientists who came to different conclusions about the effect of lead on children, the industry still hoped to create doubt and in that way forestall further regulation of industry practices. At the center of the scientific and medical argument for the reduction of lead were Herbert Needleman's studies, especially his 1979 analysis of the correlation between dentine lead levels and children's behavior and intellectual development.[28]

Long before CASAC met in April 1984, the conflict over Needleman's research had begun, specifically, at a Toronto symposium on lead in 1981. As Lydia Denworth describes the scene in *Toxic Truth*, after Needleman and several other lead researchers and industry spokespeople made their presentations, "Claire Ernhart, a psychologist in the psychiatry department at the Cleveland Metropolitan General Hospital, got up from the audience.... She said she was about to publish a paper in which she followed up on the children from her study with Perino [on lead levels and school performance] and no longer found a neuropsychological effect from lead." Needleman recalled being "puzzled" by Ernhart's comment, according to Denworth, because "her '74 paper was the best one on the subject at the time."[29] In the forthcoming paper, Ernhart not only reevaluated her own study but criticized Needleman's 1979 article because it did not account for some confounding factors. When Ernhart and her colleagues retested the children five years after their original study, the researchers said, and once parents' IQs were taken into account, there was reason to suspect that lead was *not* the factor that accounted for the children's lowered functioning on various psychological and educational tests.[30]

It was at this time that Ernhart began to receive grants from the lead industry for her work.[31] In 1981, as the controversy over Needleman's research was heating up, Ernhart went to ILZRO to seek funding for a study of asymptomatic lead levels in children and the effects on cognitive and behavioral "sequelae." ILZRO's Lead Environmental Health Committee noted that while Ernhart's study "was very well designed and complete ... it should not be funded" because it did not address the issue of how, over time, lead absorption correlated with behavioral problems. The committee noted that a recent article she had published in *Pediatrics* had established her "expertise" in this area, and they suggested that she "be asked to become a member of the Steering Committee" on another project. For this she would receive $8,000 as a "Special Consultant."[32] It was the beginning of a fruitful relationship: From 1983 through 1989, Ernhart received funding for several projects, as a special consultant and as a researcher. In addition, industry documents reveal that ILZRO was grateful to her for "other pertinent activities, such as chairing symposia on various aspects of low level lead exposure," writing "state of the art" reviews, "preparation of a letter to the editor" that she shared with ILZRO before publication "concerning the Needleman et al paper in the *New England Journal of Medicine*" in 1990, as well as sharing with ILZRO two manuscripts that were "now in press."[33] Such "sharing" of drafts became routine between Ernhart and ILZRO, as she made clear in her progress report to the group in 1986: "As usual, manuscripts will be sent to ILZRO as they are completed."[34] She received at least $376,347 (about $700,000 in 2012 dollars) from 1983 through 1990.[35]

From the industry's point of view, Ernhart's efforts shifted attention away from the culpability of the industry in creating the lead hazard, focusing it instead on parents, landlords, and regulators.[36] Donald Lyman of the Ethyl Corporation summed up Ernhart's importance to the industry when he remarked to Jerome Cole that she was "mainly responsible for Needleman's work being discredited," or at least questioned.[37] Whatever doubt or confusion Ernhart could interject into the emerging consensus about the dangers of low-level lead exposure was, as one would expect, highly valued by the lead industry.

Ernhart's and the industry's attacks on Needleman led to a dramatic confrontation in 1983, a year before CASAC's meeting, at an EPA workshop held at Research Triangle Park in preparation for revising the NAAQS criteria document.[38] According to Denworth, "The sides were clearly drawn. The meeting room was set up with a large rectangular table. On one side, Needleman sat among allies such as Ellen Silbergeld, who marshaled the evidence from animal studies, and Phil Landrigan, who describes his role as 'tactician.' Ernhart sat opposite them with Julian Chisolm, Jerome Cole, and other industry representatives. [Lester] Grant [the head of the EPA's Criteria Document Office] and his EPA staff tried to keep order from the middle." Almost immediately, Denworth notes, "sparks flew. Needleman and Ernhart accused each other of duplicity. She said he had not been fully accurate or honest. He questioned her motives. . . . When Needleman pointed out errors in her own study, Ernhart began to cry. But she was unbowed." Philip Landrigan told Denworth that at the meeting "Claire Ernhart informed us that a little lead poisoning in poor children didn't matter because their life was of little value anyway." According to Denworth, "That was too much for Julian Chisolm. Although he was conservative by nature and agreed with industry on the risks of 'overinterpreting' the data, he had also treated thousands of lead-poisoned children in Baltimore throughout his career." Landrigan told Denworth that "Chisolm got up from the industry side and said, 'every child's life is of value.' . . . Then he came around the table and sat with us."[39]

Julian Chisolm had in fact received numerous grants from ILZRO, but not because he was particularly "probusiness." Chisolm's point of convergence with the lead industry, Paul Mushak later commented, was that "as far as he was concerned, lead paint was the problem," not lead in gasoline, and "anything that deflected attention from lead paint was wrong."[40]

When the workshop adjourned, the bitterness of the session "spilled out of the meeting room," Denworth writes. "Workshop participants were staying at the Governor's Inn. After a long day of hearings, they returned to the inn for dinner. When two of Needleman's friends and allies, Jane Lin-Fu and Carol Angle, a professor of pediatrics from Nebraska, went into the ladies room, they found Ernhart brushing her teeth. 'You should wash your mouth out with soap,' said Angle."[41]

Shortly thereafter, the Science Advisory Board appointed a six-member Expert Committee to attempt to resolve the dispute over the Ernhart and Needleman results. The Lead Industries Association claimed credit for sowing the seeds of doubt that prompted the creation of this Expert Committee and hoped that it would provide a forum for undermining Needleman's contributions.[42] The committee was composed of Lawrence Kupper, a biostatistician at the University of North Carolina School of Public Health who had done work on lung cancer and tobacco; Sandra Scarr, a Yale University child development psychologist; Lyle Jones, a psychologist from the University of North Carolina; Lloyd Humphreys, a professor of psychology and educational psychology at the University of Illinois; Richard Weinberg, from the University of Minnesota's Department of Psychology; and Paul Mushak. They met with Ernhart on March 17 and 18, 1983, at Research Triangle Park and then with Needleman in Pittsburgh on March 30 and 31.[43] The committee's preliminary report found methodological problems in both the Needleman and Ernhart studies, which made it impossible to resolve the dispute without further work. The draft report criticized Ernhart's study on a number of grounds, including the lack of proper controls for factors other than lead in children's performance, and they wanted a closer reanalysis. The report questioned several methodological issues in Needleman's work, for his research was not, according to the committee, supported by others and was new in its conclusions. For Needleman's studies to be accepted, the committee asked for a reworking of the data and what it considered better controls of confounding variables. "The Committee recommends that the entire Needleman data set be reanalyzed, correcting for errors in data collection and entry, using better Pb exposure classification, and appropriately adjusting for confounding factors."[44] This preliminary report was sent to Needleman on November 28, 1983, and elicited a dramatic and angry response.[45]

Mushak said the committee did not have enough time to evaluate Needleman's data properly, and he can now understand why Needleman was so infuriated at not having been given an opportunity to review the draft report, which contained errors of its own.[46] In any case, as Lydia Denworth recounts, Hill & Knowlton, the public relations firm that had represented the lead industry for decades, took advantage of access to the committee's draft report to initiate a new stage of its public relations campaign against Needleman and his research. The PR firm, writes Denworth, "copied the Expert Committee's draft report . . . [but] removed the stamp REVIEW DRAFT: DO NOT QUOTE OR CITE and the admonition that it should 'not be considered to represent Agency policy.'"[47]

Hill & Knowlton sent a letter to *Newsweek* and to science writers across the country enclosing a copy of the "edited" Expert Committee draft, with a cover letter calling Needleman's work "worthless as a peg for government policy." The public relations firm stoked the fires of doubt in the media: "As you are probably aware," the cover letter began, "there is a continuing debate on the environmental effects of lead going on around the world as the United States, Canada and Europe consider the new restrictions on the use of the metal." James D. Callaghan, senior vice president of Hill & Knowlton, laid out why Needleman himself was so important: "At the heart of this debate in recent years has been the work of Dr. Herbert Needleman, which purports to show that exposure to low levels of lead can reduce children's learning abilities." Callaghan went on to cite the draft report, which had raised questions about the methodologies and analyses of both Needleman and Ernhart, and he sought to portray this critique as the government's official position.[48] Hill & Knowlton was clear that it was seeking to undermine the impact on federal policy of Needleman's recent research findings: "All of this is of importance because the Needleman study has served as the emotional underpinnings for efforts here and in Canada, England and Europe for ever more stringent regulations of lead. The idea that children's minds are being damaged by lead is very powerful stuff when it comes to rallying public or governmental support for regulations."[49]

By 1983, the lead industry clearly realized that public relations efforts had become integral to its cause. As Donald Vornberg, the environmental health manager for the St. Joseph Lead Company, a mainstay of the LIA and the leading lead producer in the country, explained: a public relations campaign was critical "to try and raise lead's pitiful image." In addition to the assaults from the lead research community, Vornberg saw that "multi-million dollar community lawsuits are mushrooming [and] anti-lead regulations are epidemic." The message that the LIA's environmental health meeting in 1983 sent back to its members was "go home—spread the word—and budget."[50]

SCIENCE AND SELF-INTEREST

While the EPA Science Advisory Board's Expert Committee was grappling with the science and politics of lead, CASAC members were also facing the broader public policy implications of the new research that emerged following Needleman's 1979 paper. At the next CASAC session, held on April 26–27, 1984, once again most of the scientific community experts on lead found themselves at odds with the lead industry. The intensity of the discussion was highlighted in the public comment session following presentation of the scientific data. As a prominent lead researcher in the country, Sergio Piomelli, alert to the modern politics of science and the ability of a determined interest group to manufacture doubt about the meaning of scientific research, opened the session by relating his fear that the lead industry had unduly influenced government decision making by falsely emphasizing uncertainty in science where there was none. The EPA's attempt to produce a statement summarizing the state of scientific knowledge regarding a specific substance—a Criteria Document for Lead in this case—was not the way science should be pursued, he said. It was, unfortunately, the result of an adversarial procedure, "on one side the lead producers, on the other side the health and medical community."[51]

Piomelli pointed out the dangers in giving the industry and independent scientists equal status in the deliberations: "As a result of this, the document ends up being often an anthology with equal emphasis on good and bad sides. This degrades the value of scientific studies and dignifies foolish ones which are reviewed and criticized as a group. In my opinion, the EPA fails to fulfill its role of protector of the environment by assuming a role of arbiter of conflicting views."[52] Piomelli specifically took on the industry position that claimed that "medically, small increases in EP [erythrocyte protoporphyrin, the marker for lead in the body using the pinprick method] have not been viewed generally as of great concern." He argued that the participants at the CASAC meeting could not accept the lead industry's position that a raised EP level was not of clinical importance. Far from EP being insignificant, as the industry claimed, "it's clear," Piomelli argued, that lead's interference in the production of blood was "an indicator of dam-age to the neuro tissue."[53] His conclusion was that "henceforth, we cannot, in my opinion, accept anymore a blood lead level of 30 micrograms as being safe, we have to aim at a lower blood lead level as the maximum permissi-ble."[54] To protect the health of America's children, Piomelli concluded, the scientific evidence clearly indicated that "atmospheric lead should be totally removed."[55]

Piomelli was followed by the LIA's director of environmental health, Robert Putnam, who, not surprisingly, opposed lowering the blood lead level considered unsafe for children. In contrast to Piomelli, Putnam argued that the issue of what was a dangerous blood lead level was far from certain; other scientists had provided "a one-sided view of the issues," he claimed.[56] Putnam cited the Expert Committee's preliminary report, which, he said, "concluded [that Needleman's and Ernhart's studies] provide no basis for definitive conclusions on the subject. . . . We cannot see how EPA can now conclude otherwise."[57] The industry had expended a great deal of effort and money promoting the importance of the draft report, and Putnam was not about to abandon the attempt to represent it as the final word.

After Putnam came Ralph Bradley of the University of Georgia, a repre-sentative of the Ethyl Corporation, whose interests were most threatened by proposed changes in the air quality lead standard. Bradley told CASAC that "variables other than gasoline lead use, and not unreasonable variables, can explain blood-lead decreases in NHANES II."[58] He reverted to the industry's fallback position whenever faced by adverse evidence: nothing can be said (or done) without "further research." "The U.S. public," Bradley declared, "expects. . . any proposed government regulation to be based on sound, thorough, scientific investigation."[59] The "sound science" gambit as a means of delaying regulation and obscuring danger—first used by the lead industry early in the century and soon to become a right-leaning political mantra—was being perfected.

John Rosen, a professor of pediatrics at New York's Albert Einstein College of Medicine and Montefiore Medical Center, took on industry's claim that the jury was still out on the "soundness" of the latest science. It was not only lead poisoning that had been dramatically redefined in the preceding few years as a result of "recent advances in cell biology and in medical and biomedical techniques," he said, but other diseases as well. Lead poisoning was unlike diseases of the past that were characterized simply by their "overt clinical symptoms." Rosen observed that "toxic effects of lead are characterized today by highly sensitive biochemical indices."[60] Cell biology and medical techniques had demonstrated that lead impaired "the metabolism of red cell nucleotides, erythrocyte protoporphyrin, hemoglobin synthesis and the hormonal form of vitamin D, namely, 1,25-dihydrooxyvitamin D. All these pervasive effects of lead have been demonstrated at blood lead concentrations well below the so-called 'maximum safe' level of 30 micrograms per deciliter."[61] Rosen, who devoted his life to protecting children from the scourge of lead poisoning, argued that a new awareness of environmental danger had developed over the course of the previous two decades as new technologies and new attitudes regarding acceptable risk had redefined medicine broadly and lead toxicology more specifically.

The two-part question that dominated the CASAC's discussion was, what constituted disease (and more broadly, what constituted harm)? And at what point was it the responsibility of society to protect the vulnerable from harm? The meeting had brought together some of the nation's medical and intellectual leaders, and the discussion that ensued often pitted older notions of disease against newer views of environmental danger and risk. Hans Grunwald, chief of the Division of Hematology at Queens Hospital Center and associate professor of medicine at the State University of New York–Stony Brook, made the most precise critique of the emerging paradigm in addressing whether biological change resulting from lead exposure was in itself a reason for concern. He argued against regulations based on biological changes that did not have demonstrable clinical effects. He asserted that there was a "lack of scientific evidence that these effects are adverse to health." In his view, the threshold level for lead should not be lowered based on information that was not directly linked to observed disease.[62]

Grunwald's argument stirred up a flurry of questions from the psychologists, lead toxicologists, and public health officials who saw in it a flawed logic and lack of awareness of recent research but that, if given credibility, could doom any attempt to lower acceptable blood lead levels. Harvard professor Jerome Kagan, among the nation's preeminent developmental psychologists, began the probe by critiquing the underlying framework of Grunwald's argument, stating that "implicit in your comments is the notion that if it doesn't affect the mean, we don't care about it." Kagan argued that if there was harm to the most vulnerable, that was a population that deserved to be protected, despite its small number.[63]

Although Kagan and some others in the audience assumed that the number of those affected was small, the lead researchers who were following the unfolding debate closely knew that it was anything but. In fact, Paul Mushak and other key coauthors of the EPA Criteria Document for Lead accepted the lead researchers' underlying position: that a huge number of children was potentially at risk and perhaps many, many thousands were poisoned without a clear diagnosis.

The CASAC members fundamentally rejected Grunwald's arcane view, arguing that virtually any clinician would "treat" patients with abnormal yet subclinical conditions, even in situations much less serious than in lead exposure, with its potential for irreversible neurological damage to children. Ben Ewing, the director of the Institute of Environmental Studies at the University of Illinois, asked Grunwald what he would do if he were "confronted with a child who did not have lead poisoning but had changes in [biochemical] parameters . . . indicative of iron deficiency, but he was [clinically] well. . . . Would you treat him for iron deficiency?" Grunwald answered simply, "Yes," which closed the discussion.[64]

HERBERT NEEDLEMAN'S VINDICATION

The second day of the April 1984 meeting of CASAC returned to the most contentious issue, the integrity of Herbert Needleman's research, because the thrust of the analyses and recommendations for the Criteria Document for Lead were based on his studies. Joel Schwartz, an environmental epidemiologist at the EPA Office of Policy Analysis, and a young economist, Hugh Pitcher, had been assigned the task of evaluating Needleman's research and had traveled to Pittsburgh to meet with him and review primary data.

Before CASAC considered Schwartz and Pitcher's report, Needleman was given an opportunity to respond to the criticisms that had originally been made of his work. Needleman addressed the fundamental flaw in the Expert Committee's critique that had led it to question his results in the first place: The attacks on him had posited that epidemiological proof could be attained through rigorous statistical analyses and that anything less than a finding of statistical significance disproved a relationship between exposure and damage. Needleman argued that there were numerous misconceptions in this view and they reflected a profound lack of understanding of epidemiology and what it could and could not do. "The first [misconception] is how you prove a relationship." This was the wrong question, he said. "Epidemiologists are not in the business of demonstrating [or] proving causality. We try to pile up incremental coherent pieces of evidence that lead to some kind of acceptable picture of relationships."[65] "No study is perfect," he acknowledged. But even if a study were perfect, the nature of epidemiological studies was such that they "could not prove causal relationships. There's always another co-variate out there in multi-varied space."[66]

Needleman was also concerned by the statistical turn epidemiologists had taken over the years and the rigidity with which they sometimes used the concept of significance. He asked the committee to consider "the meaning of the word significance" because it had come to lose any common-sense connotation. "We have heard today that studies are not significant. They may have P values of .07, or .08," referring to the probability that the effects were real: traditionally, the results of scientific and social science experiments were considered "real" when the probability that they occurred by chance was 5 or fewer times in a hundred trials. Where the probability of the event occurring by chance was P = .05 or less, the result was termed "statistically significant." Needleman recalled Sir Ronald Fisher, the father of modern statistics, and wondered what he would have thought about such a narrow understanding of statistical significance. "Does Fisher really mean that [.07 or .08] is to be ignored, . . . evident of no relationship? Of course, he didn't mean that. But yet we have heard that and subconsciously that does get into decision making."[67]

In his remarks, Needleman was reflecting an ongoing debate within the field of epidemiology on whether statistical convention should be the determinant of "truth." As early as the mid-1960s, Bradford Hill, the British epidemiologist and statistician widely considered one of the fathers of modern statistical epidemiology and author of the "Bradford Hill" criteria for establishing causal associations, had warned of the dangers of a slavish dependence on the very tools he helped create. In his "criteria" he worried that "the pendulum" may have "swung too far," valuing statistical significance over common sense. Like Needleman, Hill warned that when the stakes are high and a population (in his case, industrial workers) is threatened by an environmental toxin, "crossing every single 't' and swords with every critic" is not necessary "before we act."[68]

After Needleman was finished, Pitcher reported to the committee next, on his and Schwartz's findings about Needleman's research, focusing on three methodological and substantive issues: "One was sets of confounding problems. The second had to do with exclusion of observations; and the third had to do with errors in variables. And our analysis, or our reaction to the results of Needleman's reanalysis, is essentially that the results that we found are robust to all of the checks, the empirical checks that were made on these issues."[69] Pitcher and Schwartz's formal report was even more definitive in its defense of Needleman's research: "We believe the additional work done by Dr. Needleman resolves, insofar as empirical work can, the specific issues with respect to confounding, exclusion of observations, and errors in variables that have been raised in either the committee's or our own examination of Needleman's work."[70]

Throughout the two-day meeting there had been references to the controversial nature of Needleman's work and there lurked the real possibility of division among the scientists and federal officials who made up the committee charged with making a final judgment. Yet in the end, the decision making seemed a bit anticlimactic. When Morton Lippmann, the chair, asked whether Needleman had been "responsive to the requests of the committee," Lloyd Humphreys, a prominent professor of psychology at the University of Illinois, simply answered, "Yeah, he has." The chair then said, "If there's a consensus on that issue, let's move on."[71] All twenty-three members of CASAC, including those on the smaller Expert Committee, vindicated Needleman.[72] The committee included Paul Hammond and Julian Chisolm, both of whom were then receiving grants from ILZRO, so the unanimity of the board was even more impressive. In a final repudiation of the lead industry, CASAC used the data that Needleman and others had accumulated to revise the Criteria Document for Lead.[73]

But the lead industry had not given up. Researchers supported by the LIA continued attacks on Herbert Needleman and defended Claire Ernhart for "courageously revers[ing] her position" about lead's low-level effects.[74] ILZRO even contacted individual members of the Expert Committee after the CASAC meeting in an attempt to revisit the committee's conclusions.[75] ILZRO president Jerome Cole, for example, wrote directly to Paul Mushak trying to resurrect the original complaints that had appeared in the preliminary report of the Expert Committee. Cole said he was concerned that the committee had cleared Needleman and was especially chagrined that Lester Grant, the committee chair, had presented the "lack of dissent from the Committee" to mean that Needleman "adequately address[ed] the concerns of the panel and should be accepted." Cole acknowledged having had "discussions with some of your Committee's members" and wanted Mushak to look at the data again in the hope that he would "change your overall conclusions with regard to the relationship between low level lead exposure and neurobehavioral effects in children."[76] Mushak was outraged by this industry attempt to bypass the normal scientific procedure and undermine the scientific evaluation of the evidence. "I have to tell you," Mushak wrote to Lester Grant, "that I find this letter and its intent not only offensive and highly irregular, but there is a question in my mind as to the legality of this action." Mushak suggested that the EPA might investigate whether Cole's actions violated "the obligations of the Committee of which I am a member to preserve the integrity of its actions from outside interference or influence."[77]

THE INDUSTRY COUNTERATTACK

Having lost on the scientific issues underpinning the EPA's Criteria Document for Lead, the industry worked assiduously to block implementation of the EPA's phasedown of lead in gasoline. It continued to fight on two fronts: on one, the lead industry sought to maintain its market for lead in gasoline by continuing to contest the consensus that relatively low-level blood lead levels were damaging to children; on the other front, it denied that there was a relationship between the decreasing use of lead in gasoline and the declining blood lead levels in children. The industry was particularly worried that existing studies might give legitimacy to lowering the ambient air lead standard below the 1.5 micrograms per cubic meter adopted in 1978, which would have meant eliminating virtually all lead from gasoline. Donald Vornberg, environmental health manager for the St. Joseph Lead Company and a member of the LIA's Environmental Health Committee, in 1982 had blamed "environmental forces" for mounting pressure on the EPA. They "are well organized, armed with new data, and not to be taken lightly." While he had taken solace in what he described as environmentalists who "apparently made unobjective asses of themselves in pushing their points of view," Vornberg had recognized that "the most difficult data to deal with will be a study which has been represented to show that children's blood leads are dropping in strict correspondence to air lead decrease and gasoline phase down."[78] He would say at an LIA Environmental Health Committee meeting the following year that the NHANES data—which showed "a one to one drop in blood lead with gasoline lead reduction"—was "devastating to lead interests."[79]

What would the economic benefits be of removing lead in gasoline? Joel Schwartz created an econometric model that incorporated the biological effects of lead and the cost to society of the deficits likely to result. Coming at a moment in history when industry was pressing regulatory agencies to take account of the financial costs of environmental regulations, his analysis projected that "there would be a savings of three quarters of a billion dollars [by] 1988 if there was a marked decrease in lead in gasoline."[80]

In May 1984 the LIA challenged these estimates, charging that its own economic analysis indicated "that the Environmental Protection Agency overestimated the benefits and underestimated the costs of banning leaded gasoline or requiring a drastic reduction in its lead content by a factor of three." The LIA also hired Jim J. Tozzi, a former official in the White House Office of Management and Budget, to challenge yet again both the relationship between blood lead levels and lead in gasoline and the science indicating that "cognitive and behavioral 'deficits' occurred in children with more than 30 micrograms per deciliter." Such "deficits," the LIA claimed, could not be verified "after proper control for confounding variables."[81]

In testimony before the Senate Environment and Public Works Committee in June 1984, Jerome Cole even made the astounding claim that "there is simply no evidence that anyone in the general public has been harmed" from lead's use as a gasoline additive. The "government has been shooting from the hip" in its attempt to demean lead, he charged, and pleaded for a more beneficent understanding of lead in the human environment. Recycling Robert Kehoe's arguments of previous decades, Cole argued that "lead is not some alien substance created in some chemical laboratory. . . . Lead is an element. . . . Man has always lived with it and adapted to it." Far from being a major environmental pollutant or human toxin, lead produced some "minor biochemical changes" that were "sometimes correlated" with lead exposure. But much more research was needed, he claimed, to determine the effects of these "changes." In response, Vernon Houk, director of the CDC's Center for Environmental Health, noted that "the position the Lead Industries Association has taken on the health effects of lead is reminiscent of the position the tobacco industry has taken on the health effects of cigarette smoking."[82] This was not surprising, given that both the tobacco and lead industries used the same consultants—Hill & Knowlton—to defend their toxic products.[83]

As the lead industry began to face the inevitable that lead in gasoline would one day be eliminated, its focus shifted to maintaining the demand for lead where it could and to limiting the damage to lead's image and market more broadly. It was none too soon. In March 1985 the EPA announced it would lower the allowable limit of lead in gasoline from 1.1 grams to 0.1 gram per gallon as of January 1, 1986, based on the harm being done to children.[84]

The recent history of lead regulation was troubling for the industry. Up through the 1950s and even the 1960s, the industry had played a major role in defining the problem of childhood lead poisoning as one of landlords who did not maintain properties, city health agencies that did not enforce existing lead paint regulations, and parents who did not supervise their children properly. The danger now was that the public could hold the industry itself responsible for the lead dispersed from leaded gasoline and its effect on blood lead levels. There was a further danger too: that industry's culpability would be seen to extend beyond leaded gasoline to other sources of lead in children's environment. As the LIA's and St. Joe's Vornberg would succinctly put it: "As the lead in gasoline issues fades, lead in water and house lead in urban street dusts will take the forefront. We need to be responsive or we will lose image again."[85]

STORM OVER WASHINGTON

The lead industry was under pressure not only from the EPA but also from other federal agencies that were being forced to deal with the new science of lead and its implications for public policy. As lead exposures at lower and lower levels were identified as problems, and the National Health and Nutrition Examination Survey detailed the unsettling percentage of American children who were affected, public health advocates sought to redefine the debate, arguing that lead poisoning was a broad social problem affecting all classes and races. As long as it was defined as a problem of the "slums," there was no political constituency for major reform. If it was defined more broadly, there was a real possibility of action. While NHANES had shown that elevated blood levels were concentrated in poor neighborhoods, when the CDC lowered the danger level from 30 to 25 micrograms per deciliter of blood in 1985—based on Needleman's, Piomelli's, and Rosen's work that had been the subject of so much debate at CASAC—it increased the pool of children who could be considered at risk, including more children who lived in the suburbs.

As scientists and others grappled with the public health implications of recent lead research, they met continued political resistance from the Reagan administration and an industry fighting to maintain the older definitions of disease and vulnerability. In the mid-1980s Paul Mushak and Annemarie Crocetti were at the center of this controversy, as political actors sought to tamper with their work and to alter its meaning. The new epidemiological evidence of the broad prevalence of lead poisoning among American children had clearly sent shivers up the spine of the lead industry.

The Superfund Amendments and Reauthorization Act of 1986 required the Agency for Toxic Substances and Disease Registry (ATSDR) to submit a report to Congress on the nature and extent of lead poisoning in children from environmental sources. In November of that year, the ATSDR hired Mushak and Crocetti to write the report.[86] Over the next six months, the two researchers composed and submitted a detailed three-hundred-page draft that documented the possible effects of lead at levels at and below the CDC's definition of poisoning, 25 µg/dl.[87]

In a June 4, 1987, telephone call Frank Mitchell, the project officer at the ATSDR, informed Mushak "that the decision has been made 'at the highest levels of CDC' . . . to submit to Congress a shortened, drastically revised and potentially very diluted version of only the Summary Chapter from the Draft Report plus EPA's separate chapter on childhood lead exposure at Superfund sites as the total agency response to Section 118(F) of the 1986" Superfund legislation.[88] The next day Mushak and Crocetti resigned in protest because, as the *Washington Post* reported, the "condensed version . . . fails to present the national scope of an environmental problem once thought to be confined to poor, inner city dwellers, and to detail the health consequences." Mushak told the *Post*, "No way in hell you can comprehend the complexity of this problem in a boiled down, very misleading, essentially neutral document."[89] Mushak and Crocetti, in the words of the *Post* reporter, were especially "angered by the short shrift given to lead's dangers at the level of 15 micrograms per deciliter of blood absorbed by the estimated 17 percent of pre-school children in 1984, approximately 3.4 million children. Their draft described in great detail such ill effects as IQ and hearing loss, growth retardation and impaired hemoglobin formation."[90] The *Post* then quoted the chief medical officer of the ATSDR, saying that "the 330-page draft had been cut to 46 pages to create a 'readable, usable' document for Congress" and that "the socioeconomic scope of the problem 'isn't missed at all' in the June 5 [46-page] version." But the *Post* reporter observed that this was not the case: "None of the draft's broad socioeconomic judgments appear in a copy of the June 5 text obtained by The *Washington Post*."[91]

Missing from the summary version was their report's "most important finding," Mushak and Crocetti told the *Post:* "'there are no strata' of children who are 'exempt from the risk of lead levels high enough to represent a potential adverse health impact.'"[92] The political implications of this finding were not lost on the *Post* reporter: "A large number of white, suburban, affluent youngsters are as vulnerable to dangers of lead as traditional victims in the inner city."[93]

On the same day the *Post* was preparing its story, Representative John Dingell (D-MI), chairman of the House Subcommittee on Oversight and Investigations, wrote to James Mason, the director of the CDC, demanding an explanation regarding "allegations that a Congressionally-mandated scientific report on an important public health issue has been substantially modified to weaken the report."[94] Mason responded that the ATSDR had acted appropriately, because it "thought that a less lengthy and more readable/understandable document would better serve the interests of Congress and others interested in the report," but that he was also planning to provide the full Mushak and Crocetti draft of May 19.[95] After Dingell expressed concern that there be appropriate peer review of the two versions, the ATSDR caved in to congressional pressure and asked Crocetti and Mushak to withdraw their resignations and continue to participate in the report to Congress.[96]

But even a year later, in the spring of 1988, neither report had been officially submitted. A watchdog newsletter, *Inside EPA Weekly Report*, charged that the U.S. Department of Health and Human Services was "deliberately delaying the report in an attempt to soften the impact the study is expected to have on [environmental] legislation to be introduced by the House Energy and Commerce Subcommittee on Health and the Environment Chairman, Henry Waxman."[97] By June the same periodical aired accusations that the White House Office of Management and Budget (OMB) had attempted "to tamper with the full report to minimize its conclusions." Leading scientists called "the move 'outrageous,'" it said. Representative Dingell, who also chaired the House Energy and Commerce Committee, now began to probe "allegations that OMB had become personally involved to downplay the report's recommendations" because of the potential costs associated with those recommendations.[98]

Scientists were particularly upset that the OMB was controlling the fate of the now fourteen-month-old report. According to *Inside EPA*, "Scientists familiar with the report say that OMB wants to alter the report's results" because "the problems addressed in the report will be difficult and expensive to mitigate." Congressional sources told the weekly that "OMB is pressuring HHS [the Department of Health and Human Services] to make 'unnecessary' changes to the report and spearheading efforts to 'deliberately' delay its release . . . in order to thwart the impact the report may have on upcoming lead legislation."[99] Over the next couple of months, the pressure from members of Congress as well as from scientists from around the country grew, finally leading HHS on July 15, 1988, to release Mushak and Crocetti's original report to Congress and the broader public.[100]

Although the report received little popular attention, it reached deeply into the public health and medical communities. When the report's release was announced in the *Journal of the American Medical Association* in September 1988, the journal attached an "editorial note" from the CDC. What had become clear over the preceding two decades was that "long term effects (particularly neurobehavioral, cognitive, and developmental) are increasingly being observed in studies of children with lead levels much lower than previously believed harmful." Even more alarming, "several million" children were now at risk. How to prevent children from being damaged was not so clear, the CDC said, because "the remaining important sources of lead in the environment (primarily lead paint in older housing

and lead in dust and soil from past deposition and from deteriorating housing) will be difficult and expensive to remedy." Nevertheless, the CDC
embraced the report and forthrightly identified the solution as well as the
problem inherent in that solution: "Childhood lead poisoning is one of the
most common environmental diseases of children in the United States. In
concept, it is a totally preventable disease—remove the lead from the child's
environment and the disease will disappear. In practice, eliminating childhood lead poisoning will require substantial commitment."[101] Implicit in
the CDC statement was the question of whether there was the political will
to do what was necessary and right.

The EPA's lead regulations had both national impacts through the
National Ambient Air Quality Standards and specific local impacts in communities affected by emissions from "point sources," such as lead smelters.
One factor affecting the intensity of the controversy, little noticed by the
press or by congressional staffers, was the lead industry's concern that
the EPA would use Mushak and Crocetti's report as the basis for lowering
the ambient air lead standard even further, from 1.5 to 0.5 micrograms per
cubic meter, a change that would dramatically affect lead smelters—the
factories that converted lead ore from the nation's mines into pig lead
ingots that were then distributed to the battery, auto, and other industries
and fabricated into consumer products. That may seem a minor source of
pressure. But the premier lead smelter in the United States at the time was
run by the St. Joseph Lead Company, a major financial contributor to the
LIA, with a long history of leadership in the organization.[102] The St. Joe
smelter in Herculaneum, Missouri, together with another Missouri smelter,
Homestake, by the mid-1980s produced 94 percent of the primary lead in
the country.[103] One reason the LIA in general and St. Joe's specifically were
so concerned was that children who lived less than a half mile from St. Joe's
smelter were already known to have elevated blood lead levels. In 1986,
St. Joe's, which was not meeting even the existing emissions standard of
1.5 $\mu g/m^3$, estimated the cost of complying with a lower standard of
0.5 $\mu g/m^3$ relative to compensating communities located near the nation's
smelters.[104] The company concluded that prevention of exposures through
engineering controls at its plant alone would cost over $287 million, while
medical treatment—for a condition that could lead to permanent brain
damage—would be less expensive, coming to only $163 million.[105]

The continued inability of the St. Joe smelter to meet the existing ambient air quality standard for lead was an ongoing cause of additional concern
for the company, as the potential liability for damages increased over
time. As ambient air lead standards were lowered, the company's financial

liability for childhood lead poisoning increased. One consultant was surprised at St. Joe's continual violations of the standard over a three-year period in the mid- to late 1980s. He discussed with company officials the option of "buying up all the property in Herculaneum" for an average price of $38,000 per house, thereby sending the families and children out of harm's way. But St. Joe's rejected this attempt at preventing future damage as "too hazardous and simplistic." The consultant succinctly described the company's rationale: "An all-out program to . . . relocate families, raze the buildings and return [the land] to its pristine state would very likely precipitate a massive class action suit" as families became aware that they were living in a toxic environment created by the smelter next door. Instead, St. Joe's continued to buy individual properties as they became available and rented them "under a lease which has a clause stipulating that no children may live in the home."[106] This slow process would protect the company from suits, it was thought, but would leave families who remained in the area unaware of the dangers and their children at risk of brain damage.

On January 28, 1987, some months before Mushak and Crocetti turned in their draft report, the LIA had a meeting with the EPA aimed at convincing the agency not to push for downward revision of the air lead standard. In the group's notes for the meeting, the LIA proposed to tell the EPA that "our motives are not masked" and the 0.5 standard "petrifies us." The LIA planned to pressure the EPA to question the science behind the proposed revision "to ensure that it is good science."[107] The industry, intent on winning this round, also paid a visit to the elected representatives of Missouri, home to the nation's main smelters. In a meeting with Republican senators Christopher (Kit) Bond and John Danforth to elicit their help with the EPA, the Jefferson Group, ILZRO's public relations and lobbying firm, made the case that the $60 million cost of meeting a lowered air quality standard for the primary smelter in Herculaneum, south of St. Louis, was prohibitive "and would render the smelter not economically viable."[108] This ambient air lead standard was in fact not lowered until 2008, when it was reduced to 0.15 $\mu g/m^3$, ten times lower than the 1978 standard of 1.5 $\mu g/m^3$.[109]

"WE CAUGHT HOLD OF THE TAIL OF THE TIGER. BUT NOW WE'RE STARTING TO SEE THE REST OF THE BEAST"

In late 1989, many of the top lead researchers gathered in Research Triangle Park, North Carolina, to attend a three-day conference sponsored by the National Institute of Environmental Health Sciences and the National Institute of Child Health and Human Development. The meeting sought to bring participants up to date on the latest data and address the "implications for environmental health" of the outpouring of lead research in the last decade. The organizer of the conference, Kathryn Mahaffey of the NIEHS, introduced the meeting by stating the disturbing implications for public health in general and children's health in particular that the findings of clinical and basic research now presented. "Recognition of the nature and extent of the adverse effects of lead and current exposures indicates an alarming situation," she said, in stark contrast to the industry view. It was especially upsetting that so many children lived with blood lead levels just below the 25 microgram per deciliter standard and thus with no "margin of safety between lead exposures associated with adverse health effects and lead exposures typical in the recent past of the general population."[110]

Ellen Silbergeld, by then a prominent researcher at the University of Maryland in Baltimore, set out the agenda she saw emerging from the previous decade of research. On the one hand, she said, "it can be claimed that of the major environmental factors in human disease, more has been done worldwide to reduce sources of lead exposure than for any other single toxicant." On the other hand, because toxic effects had been found at lower and lower blood lead levels, "the overall prevalence of lead [poisoning] has not been reduced." She identified one major reason for this contradiction: "the lack of effective action to remediate known sources of lead in the environment," especially, old housing, but also including lead smelters. Silbergeld produced a chart showing that there were more than 41 million lead-painted houses with more than 12 million children living in them.[111] This presented a horrendous prospect for timely and effective remediation, especially since recent research had shown "demonstrably adverse [biological] effects" at blood lead levels far below the CDC's recently reduced recommended level of 25 µg/dl.[112] She called for a major effort to remedy this tragedy of the public's health: "Although the past decade has seen substantial success in controlling certain lead sources, the advances in our knowledge of lead toxicity have outstripped our ability to identify and control lead exposure overall. The only way out of this treadmill is to develop an integrated public health and environmental policy based upon a goal of reducing lead in all persons below 10mcg/dL by substantially reducing all controllable sources of lead."[113]

From 1986 to 1989, Silbergeld served on the EPA's Clean Air Scientific Advisory Committee that was charged with reevaluating the health impact of low levels of lead. At the end of her term, in a major statement on the changing understanding of risks that relatively small amounts of lead posed to children, CASAC recommended a substantial lowering of the danger level for blood lead from 25 to 10 µg/dl, based on a variety of studies by Richard Lansdown, Mary Fulton, Kim Dietrich, David Fergusson, and others, all of which indicated that the existing threshold was inadequate.[114] "It is the consensus of CASAC that blood lead levels above 10 µg/dl clearly warrant avoidance, especially for development of adverse health effects in sensitive populations," particularly young children. The potential dangers of low-level lead to the fetuses of working women had become especially contentious as companies sought to protect themselves from potential lawsuits.[115] In order to avoid ambiguity about what was dangerous, the committee said that "the value of 10 µg/dl refers to the maximum blood-lead level permissible for all members of these sensitive groups, and not mean or median values." The committee concluded "that the [Environmental Protection] Agency should seek to establish an air quality standard which minimizes the number of children with blood lead levels above a target value of 10 µg/dl." The report was revolutionary in not only questioning but in fact rejecting the very concept of the threshold, the basis of much of the fields of toxicology and risk assessment: "In reaching this conclusion, the Committee recognizes that there is no discernible threshold for several lead effects and that biological changes can occur at lower levels." CASAC rejected industry arguments, in other words, that the damage caused by lead was so small as to be insignificant.[116]

The committee was also forthright about the importance of small changes in IQ. It countered the then-common (and ever since) argument that a loss of a few IQ points was not a meaningful enough effect to justify dramatic outlays of resources. But the CASAC report illustrated that a small shift in the IQ of an entire population could have an enormous impact: "a seemingly modest decrease in the mean or median value for IQ . . . [would mean a] reduction in the number of bright children (IQ >125) and [an] increase in the number of children with IQ < 80."[117] Julian Chisolm, citing another investigator, had some years earlier commented on the "practical implications of a 3–5 point reduction in IQ": statistics showed that a 5-point drop in mean IQ would "result in more than a two-fold increase in the percentage of individuals [with an IQ] below 70, i.e., a *doubling* of mentally retarded children!"[118] At the other end of the spectrum, a similar shift of 5 points would result in a decrease in the number of "gifted" children, those children with IQs above 130, from 6 million to 2.4 million, based on the nation's population at the time.[119]

The variety of studies the CASAC members reviewed had a profound impact on their thinking with regard to an appropriate air lead standard. Even what an expectant mother inhaled of lead-laden air was now

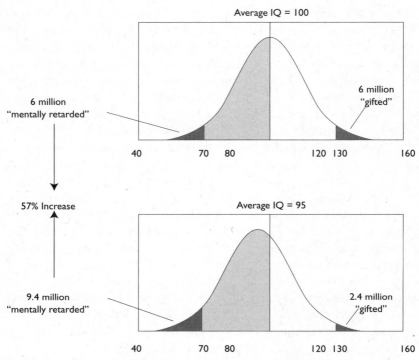

FIGURE 7.   Impact of small change in IQ on populations. Systematic lowering of
IQ due to childhood lead exposure can have major effects on a population scale. A
five-point decline in IQ for a large population increases the number of individuals
considered "mentally retarded" by more than 50 percent. Source: Mount Sinai
Children's Environmental Health Center, available at www.worstpolluted.org/
projects_reports/display/66.

understood to constitute a potential threat to the fetus. David Bellinger,
Kim Dietrich, and others had published groundbreaking articles in 1987
that documented the impact on children's early cognitive development
following exposures that resulted in blood lead levels of less than 25 μg/dl
while still in utero. Dietrich and his colleagues found similar results in a
group of children of "305 lower socioeconomic status women" who had
been exposed to low levels of lead during pregnancy.[120] It was thus essential
that the air lead standard be reduced: "The Committee believes that you
[the EPA] should consider a revised standard with a wide margin of safety,
because of the risks posed by lead exposure, particularly to the very young
whose developing nervous system may be compromised by even low level
exposures."[121]

Industry representatives were livid as they watched the federal government move toward adopting the positions of some of its most avid critics. Jerome Cole, president of ILZRO, appeared before Congress and wrote to Senator Harry Reid (D-NV) objecting to the potential lowering of the action level for blood lead. Cole argued that there was "no evidence that blood lead levels below today's guidelines (below 25µg/dl) result in any harm to health."[122] In fact, the LIA held that the whole nomenclature of the lead debate should be changed. In its view, not only was it misguided to believe that there was no limit below which lead was safe but the idea that children were poisoned by low lead levels should also be abandoned. "We urge CDC not to adopt the proposed new definition under which a blood lead level of 10 µg/dl is considered 'lead poisoning'" because, the LIA asserted, "the studies on which it is based remain subject to considerable scientific uncertainty."[123] Cole was particularly outraged that Herbert Needleman had been named by Joseph Lieberman (D-CT) as the preeminent scientist in the field. Cole maintained that the work of Julian Chisolm, Paul Hammond, and Claire Ernhart "have contributed at least as much as Dr. Needleman to the understanding of lead's effects on health." Without identifying these scientists as having received industry support, Cole "objected to Dr. Needleman's assertion that lead industry–sponsored research is somehow suspect."[124]

For thirteen years Herbert Needleman and his work had been the focal point of the lead industry's attempt to undermine the growing attention being paid to the devastating effects of its product. The attacks on Needleman's research and on his scientific integrity culminated in 1991 when Claire Ernhart and Sandra Scarr filed charges with the Office of Scientific Integrity at the National Institutes of Health, alleging that Needleman had engaged in scientific misconduct.[125] Using the same arguments Ernhart had used in 1983 to challenge his methodology, they demanded, and received, another inquiry, which led Needleman's own university, the University of Pittsburgh, to begin another investigation of his research. It was a "horrible" period in his life, Needleman recalls. The university refused to allow him to bring in outside experts, though it called on others who had previous professional relationships with his accusers. The university initially refused to open the hearings to the public; it took a petition campaign from scientists around the country to persuade the campus officials otherwise. He was shunned by colleagues who worried about being associated with him. But in 1992 despite some methodological criticisms, Needleman was vindicated of wrongdoing by the university and, similarly, three years later by the Office of Research Integrity of the

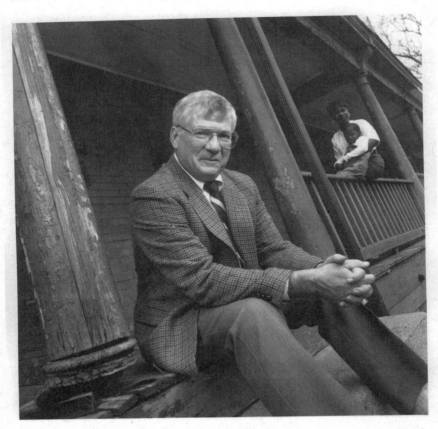

FIGURE 8. Herbert Needleman, ca. 1995. Needleman's research on low-level lead exposure and its effect on children transformed the nature of lead research, which along with his advocacy for removing lead from children's environments earned him the ire of the lead industry. Source: Heinz Family Foundation; Jim Harrison, photographer; reprinted with permission.

Department of Health and Human Services, the federal agency of which the NIH is a part. And in 1996 Needleman won the prestigious Heinz Award.[126]

In this effort to discredit Needleman, Ernhart had served industry's interests once again. But the question of scientists disclosing associations and conflicts of interest had not yet emerged as the major issue it would become in the next decade, as scholars uncovered the extent and effects of industry involvement in pharmaceutical and tobacco research.[127] Nevertheless, the lead industry already felt that its power to affect the scientific community had eroded.

By the early 1990s, the industry had lost the battle with scientists over the definition of what constituted dangerous blood lead levels in children. But the public health community, as well as other concerned citizens knowledgeable about the issue, were frustrated by the persistence of a broader problem whose source was documented, identified, and obvious: the issue of remediation extended beyond resistance from the lead industry to whether state and federal government, and society at large, had the political will to keep children from preventable harm. Lead, ultimately, had to be contained or even removed from the children's environment, but doing so was proving to be a political, economic, and technological nightmare. The science had progressed to the point where tiny amounts of lead could be detected in children's blood and its effects documented, but the public health community, as Julian Chisolm put it, had "not been able to develop programs in which more than one-half to two-thirds of the children at high risk [were] reached."[128]

Scientists had come a long way in their effort to understand the scope of the problem and the implications of their findings for what would be needed to protect children from harm. But they and their public health colleagues were also taken aback by exactly how far needed to be traveled to truly protect America's children. Local ordinances demanding warnings on the sides of paint cans, chelation therapy, surveillance and identification of poisoned children, dramatic reduction of lead in gasoline and its elimination in paint, programs to remove the obvious lead hazards in older homes—these were landmarks in the long struggle against this pervasive threat. But every victory had seemed to reveal a new challenge and another battle to be fought. Ellen Silbergeld captured the sense of the moment when she observed: "We caught hold of the tail of the tiger. But now we're starting to see the rest of the beast. And it's bigger than we thought."[129]

A central issue for lead researchers and public health workers in general in the 1980s, as we have seen, was identifying the main sources, other than paint chips, of the low-level lead exposures that were occurring—specifically, dust from crumbling paint and auto exhausts and smelters in some areas—and then figuring out a means of eliminating or at least controlling them. With the amount of lead in gasoline declining, researchers began to focus increasingly on lead dust on windowsills, walls, floors, and other objects around the home as the most important sources. The dangers of dust had been recognized at least since the beginning of the twentieth century but generally ignored as an important source of lead pollution.[130] A host of local studies from Rochester, Boston, New York City, Hartford, El Paso, and Baltimore, as well as cities in Belgium and Great Britain, identified the danger from paint dust.[131]

As the CDC and numerous researchers elsewhere were revealing that lower and lower amounts of lead posed a serious threat to children, the dust from the millions of pounds of lead that had been laid at children's fingertips continued to poison and destroy. In new and dramatic ways, the truth of John Ruddock's 1924 observation that a "child lives in a lead world" continued to haunt scientists, advocates, and public policy makers alike three-quarters of a century later. Julian Chisolm, by now elder statesman of the lead research community, had watched as literally thousands of children had come into Johns Hopkins's lead clinic only to be sent to the hospital for chelation therapy because their cases were so severe. These children, he knew, had then been sent back to their homes only to be exposed once more, returning again to his care. More than three decades of experience in the field had left him troubled by a purely clinical approach to the problem. "In the overall long-term management of lead poisoning, chelation therapy can have short-term benefits," he observed. "However, these benefits must be accompanied by drastic reduction in environmental exposure to lead if therapy is to have any long-term benefit."[132]

The public health community was faced with knowing the long-term answer to a century-old problem—the removal of lead from children's environment—yet lacking the power or means to effect this change. The story of leaded gasoline, which had been largely removed from the market by the late 1980s, had demonstrated the extraordinary power of primary prevention as an effective means of lowering overall blood lead levels. In this, the public health community's historical principle of working to actually prevent disease was seen to be operative. Yet, such a principle had not been applied to the continuing problem of lead-based paint. Paul Mushak and Annemarie Crocetti summarized the situation to date in 1990: "Certain primary lead prevention measures, i.e., the phase down of lead in gasoline, the promulgation of ambient air standards ... and phase-out of lead-soldered food cans have been effective in reducing overall childhood lead exposure." But this was not the case with the nation's housing stock. "By contrast, other lead sources and pathways, i.e., leaded paint in older U.S. housing and public buildings and lead in dusts and soils, remain as significant contributors to U.S. childhood lead exposure and intoxication. To date, little in the way of nationwide abatement efforts have been implemented for these routes and those that have been attempted have generally failed."[133]

In the first half of the 1980s, scientists and public health advocates had to confront and defeat a fierce attempt by the lead industry to stymie a reduction in and the final removal of lead from gasoline. Yet as it became obvious that lead at lower and lower levels still caused major learning and behavioral problems for children, and as lead was removed from gasoline, researchers began to understand that lead dust was not just coming from gasoline exhaust but was present in dangerous amounts even in homes in which the most obvious lead hazards had been removed. Though lead could no longer be an ingredient in household paint starting in 1978, dust from old paint continued to haunt scientists and public health officials and to destroy the lives of young children. To truly protect children from the ravages of lead, homes needed to be detoxified to a degree never before attempted. How could this be done? In a nation where millions of children lived in housing built before lead was banned from paint, the potential danger was mind-boggling to public health advocates. Was it necessary to remove all lead paint from the nation's housing? Was there a way of addressing this national disaster short of rebuilding entire cities?[134]

5   The Rise of Public Health Pragmatism

> Childhood lead poisoning has already affected millions of
> children . . . it damages their brains and limits their abilities.
> Deciding to develop a strategic plan for the elimination of childhood
> lead poisoning is a bold step, and achieving the goal would be a great
> advance.
>
> CENTERS FOR DISEASE CONTROL, 1991

As concerns about lead contamination spread from the dangers of paint chips to leaded gasoline and lead-tainted soil and house dust, the problem of addressing the threat began to extend beyond the traditional limits of public health activity. In the 1960s, local public health departments headed the effort to address lead paint poisoning, and the medical care system treated acute lead-induced conditions. At the same time, local and federal housing authorities detoxified and remediated the often dreadful conditions that exposed children to peeling and flaking paint in both public housing projects and privately owned tenements neglected by absentee landlords. It was not until the 1980s, though, that federal and local housing agencies, among other advocates, began to focus on what to do about the dust from lead paint that still covered much of the nation's walls, the disturbing results of some early remediation efforts, and the reluctance of state and federal governments to finance an effective campaign to protect children from lead's increasingly evident harms.

THE SHIFTING GROUND OF THE LEAD PROBLEM

What had been considered a narrow concern of local public health officials by the 1980s had become of national interest to more than sixteen federal agencies, among them the Department of Health and Human Services (which provided grants to local health departments), the Department of Housing and Urban Development (responsible for controlling lead poisoning in federal public housing), the Centers for Disease Control (which documented lead poisoning and established unsafe blood lead levels for children), the Food and Drug Administration (which regulated the lead content of food), the Consumer Product Safety Commission (which regulated the content of new paint), the Environmental Protection Agency (which regulated lead in gasoline, air, and drinking water), and the Occupational Safety and Health Administration (which regulated workers' exposure to lead on the job).[1] The federal effort to control the lead problem was thus multifaceted, but it was also fragmented and, according to the General Accounting Office, "operating under at least eight separate statutes."[2]

As the enormous scope of the problem of detoxifying a nation became apparent, and as political leaders in the age of Reagan retreated from commitments to large federal programs, many of these agencies sought to limit their responsibility and define the problem so that other agencies would assume their burden. The Children's Bureau in the Department of Health and Human Services, for example, at times argued that lead poisoning was primarily a housing issue and that responsibility for protecting children from household paint demanded a housing rehabilitation program. When the dangers of leaded gasoline came to the fore, to take another example, Department of Housing and Urban Development officials argued that the EPA had the primary responsibility to address the crisis. It was only in the 1990s, J. Julian Chisolm noted, that HUD "set up an office of prevention of lead paint poisoning in children, under Congressional mandate."[3]

By the 1980s lead poisoning was recognized by many as affecting millions of the nation's children, requiring a remedy of legislative and administrative action in areas as diverse as housing, public health, and environmental protection. The very definition of public health was then in flux: some still saw it as defined by bacteriology and the laboratory, while others had refocused on environmental factors ranging from pollution to urban poverty. Some believed that the tools of science—epidemiology, laboratory analysis, statistics, empirical data—along with new and better research, were the motors that drove health-related public policy; public health departments, they felt, needed increasing amounts of evidence in order to convince lawmakers to act. Others believed that a healthy nation overall would result only if public health aligned itself with social movements to demand a radical restructuring of society. This latter group pressed the public health profession to return to its roots in the nineteenth and early twentieth centuries, when it had addressed crises of epidemic diseases by lambasting urban conditions that fed the problem and proposing a wide array of reforms. The leading public health departments in cities such as New York, Boston, Providence, and Chicago formed alliances with social movements of the time—from labor to housing and urban reform—to improve living conditions and thereby thwart the spread of cholera, typhoid, tuberculosis, and other diseases. Huge investments were made in the aqueducts and tunnels—sometimes a hundred miles long or more—that brought pure water to the slums and suburbs to control waterborne diseases. Housing codes and construction standards were developed to allow fresh air into the crowded apartments and tenements of the growing cities.

Likewise, such activist-oriented advocates argued in the 1980s, in order to confront the myriad environmental issues arising from the dumping of dioxin and PCBs on the streets of Times Beach, Missouri, or the chemicals leaching into the soil at Love Canal, public health officials needed to build strong bridges to environmental and political movements and the organizations, both public and private, that formed the political and professional base for reform. An example of such an alliance would come in the late 1980s with the coalition of public health officials and groups like ACT-UP, which joined to confront the AIDS crisis by marshaling a powerful combination of scientific and political support. AIDS activists would be instrumental in getting the federal government to allocate money for research and treatment. But they would also be critical in efforts to destigmatize AIDS and put it on the agenda of policy makers and the public alike. Many of those concerned with childhood lead poisoning were also recognizing that medical research alone was inadequate to address a broad social problem; solutions to the lead poisoning epidemic required confronting, at the very least, the problem of contaminated housing.

By 1980 the solution to childhood lead poisoning was very clear: get lead permanently out of the child's environment—abatement—and stop new uses of lead from polluting it in the future. But practical and political limitations would compromise both the field and its practitioners. Public health as a field had defined itself historically as a preventive science, concerned with identifying problems and, when possible, addressing them before a crisis developed. But with lead poisoning, prevention required a significant financial investment as well as regulation of—which typically meant confrontation with—powerful industries that had a stake in the continuing use of lead. It also required a clearly thought out set of social policies—and the political will to implement them. However good the intentions for reform among health and housing officials generally, though, the American reality of the 1980s was characterized by profound political and economic retrenchment and growing skepticism inside and outside Washington about the ability of government to take bold action on crucial issues of the day. In this context, many public health advocates believed that the field needed to rethink its historical mission of prevention. Sights should be lowered, they thought: the best that public health could do was to ameliorate health problems by *reducing* the level of harm where possible, rather than *eliminating* it.

DIVERGENT VISIONS AND RISING TENSIONS

These divergent visions of public health, as prevention or harm reduction, played out in the lead arena mainly through positions taken on lead in urban housing. To some, the implications of work by Herbert Needleman and others in reconceiving low-level exposures meant that the necessary goal was complete elimination of the major sources of lead—whether in paint, air, or soil—from children's environment. Others saw this as unrealistic and utopian. To public health advocates of this latter persuasion, less extensive—and less expensive—means had to be found to lower exposures to a level that would limit lead's impact on children. These visions were not necessarily incompatible, at least in the short run—partial removal of lead could be part of a long-term national strategy to remove all of it from the nation's housing stock. But in the 1970s and 1980s there was no long-term strategy, and partial abatement of lead came to substitute for its complete removal.

In fact, one critical federal agency, HUD, seemed resistant even to taking on responsibility for partial abatement.[4] In 1980, the GAO issued a harsh and unrelenting report on HUD's abatement activities in its own properties, which ranged from huge public housing projects in New York, Chicago, St. Louis, and other major cities to subsidized housing units in communities throughout the country. Nearly a decade earlier, HUD had been mandated to detoxify federally owned housing, a small if significant percentage of the total housing stock in the country. The vast majority of housing was private and therefore under local control, which generally meant lax or nonexistent lead regulations. But since passage of the Lead-Based Paint Poisoning Prevention Act of 1971, HUD had not even developed effective means for evaluating the extent of its own problem or a methodology for correcting it. "Nine years and $9 million of HUD-sponsored research have [resulted in] innovative lead paint abatement products and techniques," the GAO reported. "But their high cost has prevented any from having a practical use."[5]

The GAO indicted HUD's conception of lead abatement and its use of existing, inadequate removal and abatement techniques. Considering that lead research in the 1970s, culminating in Needleman's pathbreaking article a year before the GAO report, had documented the extraordinary prevalence and danger of low-level lead exposure, HUD's response was feeble. "HUD limits its regulations to correcting only peeling or chipping paint," reported the GAO, "yet children can be and are exposed to hazards by chewing on 'intact' paint on accessible surfaces. HUD's own lawyers have determined that 'intact' surfaces containing lead paint should not be ignored." The GAO also criticized the agency for only inspecting and elim- inating lead paint "when dwelling units change occupancy" and for paying scant attention to preventing exposure in HUD-sponsored apartments. In addition, even though "lead paint was commonly used in the 1950s and 1960s," HUD notified "tenants of lead paint hazards only in pre-1950 dwelling units." Even worse, HUD did not even follow its own inadequate regulations. Of the twelve local housing authorities under HUD's jurisdic- tion that the GAO contacted, "several of which are among the Nation's largest," "none were complying with the requirement to notify those residing in pre-1950 dwelling units about the dangers of lead-based paint."[6]

THE ECONOMICS OF LEAD ABATEMENT

The enormity of the task and the huge cost of abatement even for its own properties, among other considerations, discouraged HUD from taking decisive action. In what would turn out to be underestimates, a National Bureau of Standards report quoted by the GAO indicated at the time that of the country's nearly 60 million housing units—both public and private—"28 million dwelling units likely to contain lead" and "the cost of total abatement" (removing all the lead paint) would be "between $28 and $35 billion in 1976 dollars" (between $111 and $139 billion in 2012 dollars). "The cost of correcting only defective paint"—peeling or deteriorating paint—was estimated at $2.1 billion in 1976 dollars ($8.36 billion in 2012 dollars),[7] while "the cost [per unit] of abating pre-1940 interiors range[d] from $370 to $2,886 in 1976 dollars" ($1,473 to $11,410 in 2012 dollars).[8]

But it was not only costs that made HUD officials wary of complete abatement as a policy. Could full abatement, whether in public housing or private, be conducted without increasing the risk that children would be poisoned? During the 1980s, recalls Dave Jacobs, director of HUD's Office of Healthy Homes and Lead Hazard Control between 1995 and 2004, "dust measurements and control of the dust was not done very well" and could result in the creation of new and potentially more dangerous health hazards. "The abatement jobs did result in reduced exposure probably for the vast majority of children," but "for a significant percentage, the early abatement jobs resulted in children's increased exposure, because we did not have the scientific understanding of the importance of dust.... I sus- pect a lot of these jobs in the early days were done while kids were present in the home and getting exposed in the course of the work or to the dust and debris left behind after the work." New research in the early 1980s showed two of the most commonly used methods to remove lead paint were especially dangerous when dust was not adequately controlled and debris not thoroughly cleaned up: burning off the paint with a blowtorch and power sanding, Jacobs said.[9]

Saul Kerpelman, a Baltimore lawyer representing lead-poisoned children in lawsuits against landlords, recalls that in the 1980s "we saw literally dozens of Kennedy Krieger records" where children had been lead poisoned during abatement. "Dr. Chisolm would say, 'This child needs to be hospitalized because the workers came in with blow torches, removing the lead yesterday morning and the child was in the house.' Now he had a lead level of 90 [micrograms per deciliter of blood] so he was hospitalized for chelation therapy." The Baltimore code from the 1970s simply required lead be removed using any means necessary. As Kerpelman recalls, "They would come in with blowtorches and no safety equipment and just melt the paint off and scrape it off, and they'd throw particle lead all over the place."[10]

GETTING THE LEAD OUT

For all these reasons—the costs, the enormity of the task, and the inadequate methods of full abatement—researchers began to search for less ambitious approaches: some form of partial abatement. In Baltimore in 1983, Evan Charney and Barry Kessler, along with two young graduate students at Johns Hopkins, Mark Farfel and David Jackson, published a study they hoped would point the way to a practical means for limiting the damage to children exposed to lead dust;[11] by this time, even in poor neighborhoods, peeling and chipping paint were largely taken care of by the local public health department. Could children's blood lead levels be reduced if there was "a reduction" of the amount of lead in the child's home? Charney and his colleagues acknowledged that "it would be optimal to move all such [exposed] children to a guaranteed lead-free environment, and there is evidence to suggest that their blood lead levels would then fall." But, the researchers said, "the limited availability of [lead-free] low-cost new housing in urban areas" made that option for protecting children impossible.[12]

To reduce exposure to lead dust, Charney and his colleagues tested the practical effects of wet mopping areas of homes that showed high levels of lead dust, together with frequent washing of children's hands. From the lead-poisoning clinic at the John F. Kennedy Institute at Johns Hopkins, they selected forty-nine children between the ages of fifteen months and six years with blood lead levels between 30 and 49 micrograms per deciliter. The homes of fourteen of these children—the experimental group—received a series of treatments aimed at controlling lead dust emanating from "hot spots" (deteriorating paints in different areas of the house). The other thirty-five homes were controls and did not receive the dust treatment. In both the experimental and control homes, however, the sources of obvious lead exposure—specifically "all peeling or deteriorated lead-containing interior and exterior surfaces within the child's home"—were "treated" by the removal of peeling paint and/or the covering or removal of lead paint below four feet "if they presented an accessible surface from which paint might be chewed (windowsills, stairs, porches, and the like)."[13] "A 'dust-control team' of two research assistants visited each experimental home twice monthly, and all rooms (including windowsills) in the home that contained > 100µg . . . of lead per sample were wet mopped."[14]

The researchers hoped that changing the practical behavior of parents—training them to clean the "hot spots" with Spic and Span and keeping children's hands washed before bedtime and meals—could lower the exposure of these children and, thus, their blood lead levels to a point where the children would no longer be at risk, at least by the threshold standard of the time. After one year, the investigators found that the experimental group's blood lead levels had fallen on average ten times more than the controls' (a decline of 6.9µg/dl compared with 0.7 µg/dl).[15]

In the published paper, the abstract focused attention on the success of the lead dust reduction strategy. But the body of the paper showed how difficult it was to achieve positive results in the treated group, especially compared to the lead levels of new housing where lead paint had never been introduced. While cleaning was effective in reducing lead immediately after the cleaning, "in most homes the initially high levels were again present within two weeks after the first visit." It took many weeks "before all homes [in the experimental group] had a reduction in the lead-containing dust that persisted between visits." Children thus would have been exposed to dust during these interim periods. Perhaps even more disturbing, the authors found that "even though all homes [in the experimental group] eventually showed a marked improvement, only 5 of 14 had continuing values below" the highest levels of lead found in new homes in Baltimore. "The provision of completely lead-free housing for all children remains an important goal," the authors agreed, but in its absence they recommended including the techniques they had studied in future abatement strategies.[16]

Further questions about the effectiveness of dust control (which meant wet mopping and vacuuming to keep dust down throughout the house) were raised the following year.[17] In a 1984 article published in the *Journal of Pediatrics*, Julian Chisolm, along with Sergio Piomelli, John Rosen, and John Graef, wrote, "*It must be understood that dust control is not a substitute for abatement.*" They acknowledged that where air was polluted by car exhaust, industrial emissions (e.g., from smelters), and by lead paint contaminated homes, "it may be helpful to institute a regular program in and about the home to control lead-bearing dust." Scrubbing floors and woodwork with Spic and Span and Tide, washing children's hands, and vacuuming might provide some short-term benefits, but "the definitive way to prevent recurrences is for affected children and their families to move into housing free of lead paint hazards."[18] Despite this research, through the 1990s public health authorities continued to promote dust control as an accepted means to reduce children's lead exposure.

Meanwhile, Chisolm and others continued to search for additional ways to lower children's exposure.[19] In 1985 Chisolm and his colleagues published a study testing the effects of different types of housing exposures on the blood lead levels of preschool children in Baltimore. The researchers studied 184 preschool-aged children who were diagnosed with high blood lead levels (above 50 µg/dl) and who had received chelation treatment.[20] This was a "prospective study"—it followed these children for a year after they returned to their homes. The researchers studied children in five groups: (1) those living in pre–World War II homes that had been "partially abated according to local ordinances"; (2) those in newer, lead-free public housing where lead paint had never been used; (2a) those in lead-free public housing who did not visit lead-contaminated homes; (3) those in "completely gutted and renovated" old houses believed to be free of lead-based paints; and (4) those in old, unrenovated pre–World War II houses "incompletely abated according to local ordinances."[21] Even though homes in the first group (those abated according to local ordinance) were believed to have been detoxified, almost 40 percent of the children returning to these homes had to be chelated a second time because their blood lead levels rose to dangerous levels once again. More than half of these children even had to be chelated a third time, as they came back still again with blood lead levels at 50 µg/dl or above.[22] The conclusion of Chisolm's study was telling: "Children's PbB [blood lead] reequilibrated with their new level of environmental lead exposure [the type of housing they lived in] after approximately three months and . . . the levels of exposure differed significantly according to housing group."[23] Only the children who lived in newer "lead-free" public housing or in completely gutted and renovated private housing—and did not visit lead-infested housing—had no need for chelation again.

"The data from this study raise serious questions about the adequacy of current methods of detection and classification of lead-in-paint hazards as well as [about] *traditional* policies and practices for the abatement of lead-in-paint hazards in old housing," wrote Chisolm and his colleagues.[24] In short, the partial abatement methods being used in the mid-1980s were typically unsafe. Further, the methods used were not standardized and often were performed by workers who were untrained and unaware that the dust produced by sanding, blowtorching, scraping, and other techniques was in itself hazardous. Often the children still lived in the home while abatement was underway, and the dust remained on windowsills, floors, and furniture that children came in contact with again and again. While these methods of abatement removed the chips, peeling paint, and other of the most obvious lead dangers—and in themselves led to a reduction in acute, life-threatening poisonings—it was still common for many children to appear in clinics with highly elevated blood lead levels and suspected neurological damage. Thus, in the mid-1980s, the choice for public health advocates and officials in Baltimore and elsewhere was to either find more effective means of abatement—whether partial or complete—or, quixotically (at least so it seemed to most people at the time), to advocate rebuilding America's poor neighborhoods. The same year that Chisolm's study was published, 1985, Mark Farfel (at this point a researcher in the Johns Hopkins School of Public Health), signaled his rise to prominence in the lead-poisoning research community with an article in the *Annual Reviews of Public Health* that outlined current thinking about this long-standing problem. There was a dramatic contrast, he said, between the extraordinary impact that restrictions on lead in gasoline had had on children's blood lead levels and the lack of progress in reducing children's exposure to low levels of lead in their homes. Chisolm's recent study, Farfel wrote of his mentor's work, demonstrated "that practices used to delead homes often do not prevent asymptomatic lead poisoning."[25]

Farfel presented a damning indictment of abatement practices around the country, practices that often put the very children they were meant to protect at further risk. Although many public health officials used the term *abatement*, Farfel argued that there was little agreement as to what the word meant, and the actions done in its name had vastly different effects on the blood lead levels and lives of children. Variation was to be expected because public health depended on the actions and interests of many local authorities and differing municipal requirements for lead abatement. Baltimore landlords, among many others, used techniques—"open flame torching and scraping"—that created greater dust, and therefore danger, than existed before. New York City used half measures, including "wall coverings of canvas or hard barrier materials to prevent exposure to deteriorating paint," while other cities required "the removal of only deteriorating paint." Some cities specified that lead paint be removed from "surfaces within four or five feet of the floor" (i.e., the height of a small child), whereas others more generally required remediation on "surfaces with lead paint accessible to children." The "incomplete clean-up of paint chips and dust after abatement" was particularly worrisome, noted Farfel, as it "subjects children to new sources of readily ingestible lead, yet post-abatement assessment is not keyed to dust monitoring."[26] Farfel reported that when "intact paint . . . is not removed [it] is subject to deterioration, sometimes within weeks, which leaves occupants at risk for further exposure." In fact, "one study found that 75% of a group of homes reduced of lead paint hazards had new areas shedding paint one year later." He concluded that "studies show that partial abatements of lead paint hazards as currently practiced in various communities are inadequate to reduce or sustain PbBs within the currently acceptable range," then defined as a blood lead level of less than 25 µg/dl.[27]

Baltimore was a specific, tragic example of the failures of abatement, Farfel's analysis indicated, since "studies show no reductions in mean blood lead levels" in children "one year after their homes were deleaded by current practices." Indeed, in "the vast majority" of cases, children's blood lead levels remained constant "for several years unless they move to housing completely free of lead paint."[28] Whether called partial or full abatement, both approaches as then practiced ended up poisoning children.

This dismal record meant, Farfel wrote, that there was an urgent "need for research on improved abatement methods." But the Reagan administration had undermined efforts even to identify and evaluate lead-removal methods. Since 1981, "appropriations for HUD's Division of Environmental Hazards Research were discontinued," and, as a result, "little has been done to identify and evaluate improved abatement techniques."[29] Lead abatement funded by HUD was only occurring in a small proportion of existing housing: some federal public housing projects and some private housing where rents for low- or middle-income families were subsidized by the government.[30]

Farfel identified some problems that stifled lead-abatement programs: they were costly; they generated political opposition from landlords and property owners; they met ideological resistance from those who argued that abatement was unnecessary because the fault of lead contamination lay with parents who did not supervise their children properly. These points of resistance, in turn, diverted attention away "from the environmental aspects of lead poisoning."[31] In short, children were not being protected.

Public health practitioners needed to find cost-effective means of partial abatement that would protect children as well as full abatement, Farfel emphasized. Such an approach had to control lead dust in a way that would not endanger the workers doing the abatement and that would "achieve long-lasting effects similar to those of lead-free housing on children's PbBs."[32] The next year, in 1986, Chisolm called for "fresh approaches to adequate removal of lead-based paints from old housing . . . so that new soundly based public health policies and procedures can be developed which will result in adequate reduction in this environmental hazard to children."[33]

If the long history of frustration with partial and inadequate abatement techniques was by the mid-1980s leading some, such as Farfel and Chisholm, to see reducing harm rather than eliminating it as a "new approach" suited to the political realities of the time, others were drawing quite different conclusions. They called on public health leaders to abandon the half measures that had dominated regulatory efforts and public health activities since the 1960s. In 1987, as the toll of low-level exposures continued to be revealed, the American Academy of Pediatrics published a report based on work led by Philip Landrigan and Joseph Greensher that called for "all hazardous lead based paint (exterior and interior) [to] be removed from all housing."[34] The report reflected pediatricians' frustration that children were continuing to suffer the effects of a completely preventable condition.[35]

Despite some important improvements, one horrible fact remained: "children are used as biologic monitors for environmental lead," said the American Academy of Pediatrics.[36] As long as it was "accepted" that lead would remain in children's environment, testing children's blood lead levels was the primary way to identify a particularly dangerous condition. This was, in their view, unacceptable—and implicitly unethical. If the goal was "to prevent lead exposure in children," didn't using children as research subjects to signal places of the greatest danger from lead contradict it? It was the responsibility of "public agencies to develop safe and effective methods for the removal and proper disposal of all lead-based paint from public and private housing."[37] The Centers for Disease Control weighed in later that same year, in 1987, and called for complete abatement of the lead hazard, a position, the agency said, that reflected a growing consensus among leading clinicians and government officials.[38]

HOUSING, LEAD POISONING, AND HUD

In the meantime, parents were becoming increasingly frustrated with HUD's lack of action. In 1983 Claudia Ashton, the mother of a lead-poisoned child living in public housing in Washington, D.C., decided to press the issue by suing Samuel Pierce, the secretary of HUD, alleging that the public housing authority had failed to protect her daughter and other children who had been lead poisoned. The federal district court found in favor of Ashton and her daughter, faulting HUD for failing to eliminate the hazards that had caused this child's poisoning. HUD appealed the case to the U.S. Court of Appeals for the District of Columbia before Justices Edward Allen Tamm, Ruth Bader Ginsburg, and Robert Bork, who upheld the decision of the lower court on August 26, 1983.[39] In the process, the court outlined the dangers for children in a new and potentially important way. As Dave Jacobs, the former director of HUD's Office of Healthy Homes and Lead Hazard Control, succinctly put it, "The court defined a lead paint hazard to be the presence of lead paint."[40] As long as lead was present on the walls or woodwork of a house, children were endangered. Further, the court held HUD accountable because it had failed to meet the legal requirements to remedy the "immediate hazard" that lead paint posed to children.[41]

The court decision had profound implications for publicly supported housing, Jacobs points out: "The result was that all that lead paint . . . would have to be removed" from the walls of all public housing.[42] This was a frightening prospect for a department that was already strapped for cash and under siege from an unfriendly Congress and a president who were ideologically opposed to a substantial federal presence in the nation's housing market.

At least on the surface, the ruling highlighted primary prevention as the way to deal with lead poisoning. What came out of the decision as well was passage of the 1987 Housing Act, which for the first time recognized officially that the primary hazard to children was the lead paint and lead dust that were on the nation's walls. The legislation directed HUD to perform a "lead inspection" in all public housing developments and provided limited funding for the complete rehabilitation and modernization of public housing, which included the complete abatement of lead paint.

The breadth of the problem left HUD and public health officials aghast. While all agreed that children should be protected, there was little agreement on what protection meant or what the best means of achieving protection were. The simple problem of removing the lead safely was daunting enough, though no one had yet established safe levels for the lead dust that remained after abatement. It would take congressional action to define what a national program to end lead poisoning should look like, even if just for federal housing. HUD did estimate how much deleading the nation's housing stock would cost, as Jacobs explains: "We had an estimate back in

1990 of about 64 million [public and private] housing units with lead paint. The cost of removing all the lead paint on average was $10,000 per housing unit." "The price was just astronomical," Jacobs continues. "It gave Congress sticker shock." In his view, it "produced policy paralysis" in HUD and in the broader public health community,[43] though in that age of Reagan it could be argued that a kind of paralysis was all-too-evident already at the national level.

The ground had shifted. Removing lead from paint and gasoline had already succeeded in dramatically lowering average blood lead levels for children. The next steps, however, were proving more difficult. How did one remove all lead from the walls and backyards of the nation's housing? It was no longer an issue of stopping lead from being *introduced* into consumer products in a factory or refinery. Now it was a matter of removing the century-long accumulation of lead. Federal housing and public health officials in HUD and the Department of Health and Human Services, along with some lead researchers and sympathetic allies in community organizations, began to formulate new goals for a lead-control effort. If removing the lead from walls was too costly, especially in the prevailing political climate, what methods could be used to at least limit, if not eliminate, the lead hazards that children faced?

The *Ashton v. Pierce* decision did, however, force public housing authorities to confront the immediate prospect of additional lawsuits from tenants. Because HUD had begun to collect data documenting the lead hazard in public housing, this now left them more vulnerable to potential lawsuits: the data HUD was collecting documented the department's own knowledge of the dangers, while its inaction in removing the lead was proof of its failure to fulfill that responsibility to protect tenants from danger.

In the absence of a comprehensive program to detoxify the public housing stock safely, a variety of interim solutions were sought. According to Jacobs, in 1987 "a group of housing authorities [at the state and local levels] banded together and created the Housing Authority Risk Retention Group," a private organization tasked with providing insurance to public and low-income housing agencies. The idea was "to set up a procedure by which these housing authorities could insure themselves against lead poisoning cases. So they asked me to help devise some risk management procedures between the time they could do the abatement, which may be years down the road, and right away." Jacobs turned to the research "that Mark Farfel and many others [including himself] had done," which, Jacobs believed, provided "a sound scientific basis to establish such procedures," in part because customary abatement practices by the late 1980s had not proven effective in preventing lead poisoning in children. With such an interim program, the Housing Authority Risk Retention Group (later called the Housing Authority Insurance Group) would provide HUD and local housing authorities with insurance, but the group still needed to measure actual lead exposures to assess the risk. The group identified the three common pathways that put children at risk: deteriorated paint, lead in soil, and lead in dust. "The theory was," Jacobs continued, "that if you control those three pathways of exposure, then your risk will be managed and you're unlikely to get sued, because no children would be poisoned."[44]

But the realities on the ground were very different than the theory. The housing authorities had limited budgets with which to address lead poisoning and control those pathways. Whatever was done to abate the lead problem "were thought at the time to be sort of temporary fixes," Jacobs said. The working assumption was that this was "sort of a stopgap measure" because most people expected that "within twenty years all the public housing would get abated."[45] In Jacobs's view, it was neither necessary nor practical to remove all lead paint from the walls of the nation's homes. He advocated a more layered approach, dealing with the worst conditions more aggressively and triaging the rest.[46]

If Jacobs and many others believed the only option to be an incremental approach, Herbert Needleman took a more radical position. In a 1990 article on lead toxicity and housing, he did not mince words. Whether federally financed or private, leaded homes were "the twentieth century equivalent of pest houses or open sewers," putting kids at risk for brain damage, with black children at particular risk because so many lived in housing that was deteriorating and neglected by landlords. "Fifty-five percent of poor black children have elevated blood lead levels," then defined as more than 25 micrograms per deciliter. This was more than an injustice. This was "one of the greatest single threats to the polity," to civil society.[47]

And Needleman came forward with a specific plan to right that wrong. "Why not train unemployed persons," Needleman asked, "in safe (and inexpensive) deleading [skills]." Why not, he asked, "pay them, and allow them to purchase equity in these [abandoned] houses?" To Needleman this seemed a rational and reasonable means of addressing the lead crisis, the housing shortage, and the unemployment problem that were chronic issues in Reagan-era America. "Current estimates are that a home costs $5,000 to delead," wrote Needleman, taking issue with the HUD estimate of at least $10,000.[48] "To delead 2 million homes would cost $10 billion. If 30,000 individuals were employed at $20,000 per year, with a 5% annual increase, this would cost $7.8 billion and leave $2.2 billion for training, materials and insurance." Needleman argued that this was not "utopian," when one remembered that no one objected to Congress's plan to spend $11.6 billion "for new prison construction." In any case, HUD's own estimates were dramatically higher.[49] By the 1990s, building new public housing for low-income residents, a "realistic" objective in the 1960s, had become "utopian," even for the most avid advocates for children's health. By this time the Reagan-era attacks on the Great Society government programs of the 1960s had virtually halted new government housing, which was replaced instead by federal cash subsidies for rents in privately owned housing.

Yet public health leaders, housing officials, and lead researchers had still not solved the disjuncture between the *ideal* of abatement and the *reality* of how to carry it out. Researchers Paul Mushak and Annemarie Crocetti identified the paradox at the time: neither full nor partial abatement as then executed would protect children. Unless the flaws in abatement practices could be resolved, children would continue to have repeated encounters with lead. Mushak and Crocetti asserted that the evidence clearly showed "that conventional methods often result in incomplete removal and often carry associated exposure roots." Mushak and Crocetti reminded readers of Julian Chisolm's observation that "when lead-poisoned children are returned to 'lead abated' structures, their PbB levels invariably increase to unacceptable levels."[50] The "major difficulty," they said, was "the relatively high mobility of old, powdering (chalking) lead paint, which enters cracks and crevices, settles on contact surfaces, and readily sticks to children's hands." They criticized the public health community for ignoring the "hidden assumption [that] underlies efforts to remove leaded paint from the homes of children found to have lead poisoning: that the child will remain in the lead-abated home [either while the abatement was taking place or would return shortly after]."[51] Mushak and Crocetti's assessment was a damning indictment of prevailing practices in stemming the lead-poisoning epidemic.[52]

But Needleman continued to believe that ways could be found around these obstacles. Public health prevention, he believed, meant exactly that: making sure that there was no toxin in the child's environment. For a brief moment in the George H. W. Bush administration, Needleman thought that true prevention was about to become public policy. He was invited in 1991 to a meeting with Assistant Secretary of Health James Mason, Vernon Houk of the CDC, and others for what seemed a fruitful discussion of the lead issue. "On the wall," journalist Lydia Denworth tells us, "Needleman noticed a plaque commemorating the end of smallpox in the United States. 'There's room for another plaque,' he told Mason. At the end of the meeting, Mason was unequivocal. 'I want a plan to eliminate childhood lead poisoning, and I want it on my desk in six months,' he told the group. Needleman's mouth dropped. 'It's happened!' he thought and floated out of the room."[53]

The moment of hope was dashed almost immediately, however. Needleman, fellow lead researcher John Rosen, and others would soon face growing opposition that would derail the possibility of ending lead poisoning in America anytime soon. Conservatives were well aware of the implications of defining lead poisoning as a housing problem. Citing the experience of Baltimore, where recent legislation required that "landlords pay for thorough renovation of inner-city buildings if sufficient quantities of lead paint are found," the *Wall Street Journal*, for example, in June 1991 argued that the state's "lead-paint abatement program [would develop into] an environmentally mandated public housing program." Like other environmental regulations that, in the paper's eyes, were forms of social engineering, "Maryland's lead poisoning rules are just another set of environmental regulations crafted to impose social policies under false pretenses." The "Lead Scare" was little more than "Leftist Politics by Other Means," the *Wall Street Journal* headline read.[54]

Despite such opposition, the Senior Advisor to the National Center for Healthy Housing as of 2012, Don Ryan, when he was a congressional staffer on the powerful House Appropriations Committee in the late 1980s, was determined not to let the issue die or fall into a bureaucratic vacuum between various agencies. He, along with Nick Farr, Director, and Dave Jacobs, Deputy Director, of the National Center and others, pressed the EPA and HUD to decide which of them would take responsibility for developing a national program to detoxify the country of lead. But each resisted taking the primary role, Ryan recalls, just as they had in the 1970s and early 1980s. When it came to lead, the EPA wanted to narrow its focus to "lead in air, lead in water, lead in soil, lead in Superfund sites." But "the elephant in the room was [lead paint]," and that was casually dismissed. The EPA simply avoided it by saying, "oh-well, that's a HUD problem."[55]

In the end it was neither HUD nor the EPA that took the initiative to develop a full-fledged lead paint abatement plan. It was the CDC, in February 1991.[56] The plan was written by Susan Binder and Henry Falk of the CDC, with assistance from Jane Lin-Fu, Joel Schwartz, Richard Jackson, Don Ryan, John Rosen, Sergio Piomelli, Herbert Needleman, and Lynn Goldman, along with consultants David Bellinger, Julian Chisolm, and Philip Landrigan, all of whom had long been associated with the struggle to control lead. Ultimately, the plan sought to reconcile complete and partial abatement strategies. The goals of the committee were to increase public awareness; improve prevention programs; abate lead paint and paint-contaminated dust in high-risk housing; reduce lead exposure from water, food, air, and soil; and establish a national surveillance system for children with elevated blood lead levels. "The public health benefits and cost effectiveness of lead-based paint and dust abatement are greatest in the housing most likely to contribute to lead poisoning," the authors noted. They therefore recommended that "in the early years the emphasis should be on abating the housing units of affected children and the units likely to poison children in the near future." The committee acknowledged the paradox of public health: if the goal was "to eliminate completely this disease," it was necessary "that all housing with lead-based paint eventually be addressed." But limited resources and the need to prioritize demanded that "high risk housing be abated first."[57] Nonetheless, the CDC insisted, "a concerted societal effort could virtually eliminate this disease in twenty years"[58]—that is, by 2011, a goal that has clearly not been met.

Even at the time, the CDC was willing to compromise the long-term possibility of ending lead poisoning. "In general the most thorough abatements are believed to be the most effective in reducing blood lead levels and residual lead in the environment," the CDC said. But "given the limited resources for abatement, a balance must be struck between doing the best possible abatements in fewer units and using reasonably good, less expensive methods in more units." The CDC, interestingly, called for precisely the kind of evaluations of the "cost effectiveness of alternative paint abatement methods" that the Farfel and Chisolm Kennedy Krieger Institute study eventually would attempt to evaluate.[59]

ANTILEAD ACTIVISM IN THE 1990S

Six months after the CDC's report was released, a conference held at the Omni Shoreham Hotel in Washington, D.C., brought together hundreds of public health officials, community activists, educators, union leaders, realtors, parents, researchers and policy makers—all of whom were deeply concerned about the unfolding tragedy caused by both low and high levels of lead. The inspiration for the conference came from Don Ryan, whose commitment to ending childhood lead poisoning had begun two years earlier.

At the very end of 1989, Ryan, then a congressional staffer who held a "job in Washington that no one had ever left," actually left to help establish the Alliance to End Childhood Lead Poisoning, the sponsor of the October 1991 conference. Ryan remembers vividly what led him to leave the House. In December, when he took over the staff position at the Transportation

Subcommittee of the House Appropriations Committee, he recalls, "I found it deadly boring. I recall getting a briefing on time delays and cost overruns in FAA's new air traffic computer system and thinking, 'I don't want to do this.' Meanwhile, I was literally dreaming night after night about how to unravel the policy snarl related to lead-based paint. Lead poisoning had grabbed me and simply wouldn't let go." He remembers when he told his wife that he wanted to leave his job and begin a new career, one with no security, no guaranteed paycheck, and no benefits of any kind. Despite the uncertainty, his wife and friends supported his decision and on the first workday of 1990, Ryan submitted his resignation "to go and work in the public interest."[60] Within months, Ryan had established with Herbert Needleman and others the Alliance to End Childhood Lead Poisoning, a public interest advocacy organization that sought to focus the nation on primary prevention and to create a national campaign to "end childhood lead poisoning."[61] Among those who served on the Alliance's original Board were Needleman, Ellen Silbergeld, Philip Landrigan, Richard Jackson, David Rall and Teresa Heinz. The Alliance was instrumental in bringing together scores of community groups, especially those in areas most affected by poverty and lead poisoning.

The welcome address at the inaugural alliance conference set the tone for the seriousness of the effort. It featured Louis Sullivan, secretary of the Department of Health and Human Services, who identified lead poisoning as "the *number one* environmental threat to the *health* of children in the United States." He told the packed conference-center audience that "President Bush and I are committed to ending this senseless, totally-preventable tragedy." These were not insignificant statements, coming as they did for the first time from policy makers at the highest levels of the U.S. government. In his address, Sullivan announced the CDC decision to lower the threshold for blood lead levels from 25 to 10 micrograms per deciliter and proposed a four-part strategy to address the lead problem. It included (1) screening of children; (2) reduction in exposure to a variety of lead sources, including lead in water, food, soil, and air; and, perhaps most significantly, (3) an ongoing program of national surveillance of blood lead levels in children. Critical to the long-term effort to eliminate childhood lead poisoning, of course, was (4) the development of effective methods of abatement in housing, but Sullivan hedged on what that would mean. Rather than call for complete abatement of the country's existing leaded housing stock, Sullivan asked for "cost-effective and safe lead-based paint abatement."[62]

The conference was a landmark in joining divergent strands of thought and action that existed primarily at the local level all across the country. In the words of the conference's final report, it "ushered in and gave legitimacy to a new emphasis in fighting lead poisoning: primary prevention."[63] The Alliance to End Childhood Lead Poisoning recognized that the CDC's lowering of the level of concern from 25 to 10 µg/dl had vastly increased the scope of the problem, because so many children once defined as "safe" were now seen as "at risk."[64] The CDC had estimated that in 1984, the last year for which it had estimates of the number of children affected, between three and four million children had blood lead levels above 15 µg/dl. It was not unlikely that several millions of children still, in 1990, had blood lead levels above 10 µg/dl.[65] The alliance argued that it was necessary to develop "new approaches emphasizing prevention through source identification and elimination rather than sole reliance on belated identification and 'tracking' of already lead-poisoned children." Regarding abatement practices, this meant "correcting lead hazards in housing before the child gets lead poisoning."[66]

Within the lead advocacy coalition there were divergent meanings of abatement. For Herbert Needleman, abatement aimed at primary prevention meant detoxifying all housing so that no child—whether residing in the home now or in the future—could come in contact with lead paint or lead dust. But for most in the alliance, primary prevention meant something different: the conference's final report said that, given the financial and political realities of the time, "resources should be directed to the most serious problems and used cost-effectively to produce the greatest benefit." To do this, the alliance proposed a set of "lead hazard reduction principles."[67] These principles included the goal of providing "a lead safe house, not necessarily a lead free one," "interim measures" that could be "short of [complete] abatement [but that] could effectively control or stabilize the situation to reduce lead exposures to acceptable levels in the short to midterm." The title of the report's appendix, "Lead Hazard Reduction," captured the fundamental approach and the essential difference in interpreting *primary prevention* between those who advocated removal of all lead paint from all of America's housing stock and those who proposed pragmatically, in their view, to at least *reduce* the hazard by eliminating worst cases through a "hierarchy of response."[68]

The CDC and the alliance were responding to exactly the conundrum that many researchers and policy makers confronted in the late 1980s and early 1990s, Dave Jacobs recalls. In principle, he agreed with Needleman that the goal should be "to remove all the lead paint in all the housing," but in practice he advocated what he saw as the more achievable and effective goal of partial lead abatement. There were both practical and financial impediments to removing all lead from the nation's walls, Jacobs said. In fact, without careful controls, full remediation was "dangerous because it increased exposures in some cases," though that could be true of partial abatement.[69] Jacobs believes that the enormous success of the effort in the 1970s and 1980s to eliminate lead in gasoline had created an unattainable model for proponents of complete removal of lead paint. "They were mired in the gasoline lead experience in the 1980s," he says, "which was resolved by changing a centralized source—change the gasoline refineries so that lead was not added. And of course that did work."

"Housing was entirely different," Jacobs argues. There were no companies that could be ordered to remove lead from the nation's walls. There was no "centralized source" because lead was "dispersed throughout millions of housing units."[70] Lead—like other environmental pollutants such as PCBs, mercury, and a host of chlorinated hydrocarbons—had become ubiquitous throughout the land. Looking back from the perspective of two decades, Jacobs acknowledges the logic and power of Needleman's approach: "Now Herb is right and others are right to point out if . . . the lead paint is still there [it] could deteriorate further and [cause] problems down the road." But, Jacobs argues, "that's true with every disease. You know if you don't pay attention to preventing a disease, some of them start coming back again, like TB." It was a classic argument between those advocating radical change and those who sought—or felt compelled to settle for—incremental reform. "In an ideal world I'd love to have all houses have all lead paint removed," Jacobs went on. "I mean, that would be ideal. But that just was not working, so I helped to craft an exposure-control approach that I thought might break the impasse."[71]

By 1991, the CDC, the EPA, scientists, and Congress all agreed in principle that something dramatic had to be done to protect the nation's children from lead exposures. The EPA's administrator at the time, William K. Reilly, in Senate testimony on February 21 of that year, summarized the long struggle to find an answer for this persistent public health problem. Reilly reminded Congress of the enormous strides that had been made over the previous two decades. The society had "banned the use of lead in house paint and in the solder and pipes used in public drinking water systems. It has encouraged the phase-out of solder in food cans." Most significantly, the EPA had made a "major contribution" through its "aggressive action to virtually remove lead from gasoline." Despite these efforts, lead continued to haunt the country and demanded coordinated action from many federal agencies. But the agencies so far had failed "to develop a federal plan of action that would be both comprehensive and cost effective" to remove lead from the children's homes. Congress had recently given the EPA four million dollars to develop a program with HUD that would assess various abatement techniques. Over time, Reilly told Congress, they would be able to evaluate "how abatement methods hold up . . . in reducing exposures."[72]

Concerned officials in the federal government were seeking practical ways to prevent, or at least limit, further exposure of children to lead paint and dust. They were not the only ones. In the 1990s community groups such as the Arkansas People Participating in Lead Education (APPLE) and United Parents Against Lead formed alliances with public health workers to press for legislative, technical, and pragmatic programs to address the lead problem. One major result of these efforts was passage of Title X of the 1992 Housing and Community Development Act, an attempt to shift national policy and to develop both long-term strategies to end childhood lead poisoning and interim measures to reduce children's contact with lead. And within HUD, the Guidelines for the Evaluation and Control of Lead Based Paint were drawn up in 1995 to standardize method for risk assessment, abatement, and the like.

By the opening years of the twentieth century's final decade, then, recognition of the harm that low-level lead exposures could cause millions of children had prompted a spirited debate over what should be done—and what, it was imagined, could be done. Thus began, among other efforts, the Johns Hopkins "Repair and Maintenance" studies.

6 Controlled Poison

"It's patronizing, they say, or worse, it's racially motivated. We're white, middle class people saying to black, lower income families, that's good enough for you."

Harvard Kennedy School of
Government Case Program, 1990

During the 1980s in Baltimore, J. Julian Chisolm and his young colleague Mark Farfel had been at the center of research on, treatment for, and implementation of policies regarding low-level lead poisoning. The two researchers had shown that existing abatement practices advocated by public health officials and instituted in Baltimore and elsewhere were inadequate, if not dangerous, for young children exposed to lead. Children were being used as "canaries in the mines," their blood lead levels and their deficits revealing—after the fact—which homes were "leaded" and which were not. State-of-the-art public health practice by 1990 typically identified children after they had developed lead poisoning and, if their lead levels were above 40 micrograms per deciliter, admitted them to hospitals for chelation treatments—the intrusive, extensive, and often debilitating procedure designed to chemically leach lead from their bodies—after which they were generally returned to the very same houses whose lead had made them ill in the first place. A close look at Farfel and Chisolm's research on the shortcomings of both partial and even full abatement practices at the time indicates, however, that children were also being used as canaries in a second way: in defining what were and what were not safe abatement practices. Whatever the intentions of deploying the existing abatement methods, those methods were failing to protect children.

Although Maryland's regulations called for abatement of the lead hazard in the apartments where young children resided, this work was often inadequate or improperly done, if done at all. As early as 1951, Baltimore had pioneered banning the use of new lead paint on walls, but that was only one aspect of the multifaceted lead problem. While there was some detection of lead in homes before children living in them were identified with high blood lead levels, the main way that lead-contaminated houses were discovered was for a child saturated in lead to show up at a lead clinic or a hospital. This was still the norm in Baltimore, and in most other cities, when the Johns Hopkins Kennedy Krieger Institute research study was initiated in 1991.

According to the Baltimore Health Department at that time, a child identified in a clinic with a blood lead level above 20 micrograms per deciliter should trigger an "environmental investigation of sources and environmental remediation." Specifically, someone from the public health department would "inspect the child's primary residence" and, based on visual and x-ray analysis, develop a plan with the property owner to abate the problem.[1] This is still largely the practice today all across the country. For Chisolm, who saw the suffering of children and their families firsthand and saw these same children being exposed to more lead dust when they returned home, this "treatment" protocol was unacceptable. If a way could be found of doing abatement cheaply, Chisolm and others believed that governments at various levels, or even some landlords themselves, might cough up the money to save children from the most dangerous exposure levels before damage occurred.

Mark Farfel had far less personal experience in the poor neighborhood surrounding KKI, but he shared Chisolm's deeply felt social values. Farfel's father, a pediatrician in Baltimore in the 1950s, had, in the words of the *Baltimore Sun*, "upset the city's racial conventions when he admitted the first black baby to Sinai Hospital while a resident there." Farfel himself was deeply involved in the community. After graduating from McGill University in Montreal, he went into public health because, he told the *Sun*, "it seemed like a great way to wed science and socially meaningful work." At Johns Hopkins "he was struck by the contrast between the wealthy institution and the impoverished neighborhood that surrounded it." He also "reached the central epiphany of his career." Johns Hopkins and KKI were providing "world-class" care for lead-poisoned youngsters. "But who was 'treating' the inner-city row houses that were sickening kids in the first place?" He lamented the predicament of those in public health and medicine in the 1980s, for "all we were doing was waiting for children to be poisoned."[2] Ellen Silbergeld, the prominent lead researcher, Johns Hopkins professor, and student of Chisolm, notes the humane motives that led Chisolm (and also Farfel) to seek means to improve the lives of Baltimore's children. "He [Chisolm] really *saw* his patients as people. It wasn't just lead vs. children. He knew how they lived. He knew what their circumstances were."[3]

The public health community had been faced by a stark reality in the conservative 1980s: severely limited resources and relatively weak political support. AIDS had emerged as a problem for cities, many of which were already overwhelmed by a crack epidemic, deindustrialization, and the debasement of their tax bases and educational systems. In this context, public health workers lacked political support for attaining the legislation and appropriations needed to end childhood poisoning. Yet the paint problem was enormous. The country's homes at the time were covered with an estimated three million tons of lead paint spread over the walls of 14 million housing units, of which, the Centers for Disease Control estimated, 3.8 million had deteriorating lead paint and were occupied by young children at risk for a host of neurological and behavioral problems related to low-level lead exposures.

Short of completely removing lead from housing or developing a program to replace inner-city housing—two options deemed unacceptable given the politics of the time—what could be done to limit, if not eliminate, the danger to children? The challenge, even if not acknowledged at the time, had changed. Most public health workers no longer saw elimination of lead from the child's environment as feasible and hence had subtly shifted their goals toward identifying "acceptable" exposures to this toxin. Building on his work in the 1980s to find effective means of reducing childhood lead exposure, Mark Farfel began in the spring of 1990, with the aid of a $65,000 EPA grant, to design a study for what was called the "Lead-Based Paint Abatement and Repair Maintenance Study (R&M)." The Johns Hopkins Kennedy Krieger Institute, research home of both Chisolm and Farfel, and the premier lead research unit in the country, housed the study, with Farfel and Chisolm serving as the joint project managers from its inception.[4] To understand the KKI case, and why it provoked such outrage from some and a strong defense from others, it is important to look with some care at the nature of the research that Farfel and Chisolm conducted. This can illustrate for us on a small scale how the issues of political will, social concern (and lack thereof), and economic interest were at play in the 1980s and 1990s and how many of the local forces at work mirrored national debates.

From the first, Farfel and Chisolm's aim was to use Baltimore, with its extensive lead problem, as the site for a national demonstration project. "Lead has been identified as a significant cause of neurobehavioral and learning deficits in young children which are long lasting, if not indeed permanent," the contract for the initial study funding began. "The recent report to Congress by the Agency for Toxic Substances and Disease Registry (July, 1988) points out that lead in existing residential paint, household dust and soil now constitute the major sources of high lead exposure in U.S. children." If children were going to be protected, "new policies and practices" would have to be developed. "This study," the contract continued, would "evaluate the effectiveness of alternative methods of reducing residential sources of lead in paint and dust."[5] The advantages of siting the study in Baltimore were many. In addition to its legendary lead program and stellar researchers, Baltimore's Department of Health was well aware of the problem's dimensions, and Maryland was already giving the city one million dollars a year for abatement activities. In addition, Baltimore was the site of a HUD Lead-Paint Abatement Demonstration Project that could provide funding for the renovations and abatement necessary for the KKI study. The pieces for what the study contract called a "natural experiment" seemed to be in place. All the EPA would need to fund was the "evaluation of the abatement, not the abatement itself."[6]

Baltimore itself in the 1930s through 1950s, inspired by the efforts of city health commissioner Huntington Williams, had led the nation in identifying the depths of the lead-poisoning crisis and engaging in innovative and, for its time, radical attempts to publicize and prevent lead paint poisoning among children. But, in recent decades, Baltimore had fallen behind other major cities in a host of regulatory, surveillance, and prevention efforts. By the 1980s, other cities had developed more extensive childhood screening and testing programs; and some cities, such as New York, and states, such as Rhode Island and Massachusetts, were screening nearly half of all children below the age of six years. In comparison, Maryland as late as 2001 had screened fewer than 18 percent of the state's children.[7] And as late as 2002, the estimated number of housing units in Baltimore that remained a hazard was still staggering. According to one Baltimore foundation, approximately 57,000 of the city's housing units had been built before 1950, when lead paint was commonly used. Of these especially dangerous apartments, more than half, at least 32,000, "remained untouched by Maryland's lead law and City abatement efforts" because of lack of enforcement.[8] These somber statistics, which represented a vast improvement over the situation in 1990, are indicative of the environment the Johns Hopkins researchers faced.

Serious planning for the Farfel and Chisolm abatement study began in the summer of 1990, with consultations with housing experts, property owners, state and local health and housing officials, biostatisticians, community leaders and organizations, and construction contractors. Questionnaires about the demographics and housing characteristics of the neighborhoods were designed; informed consent forms and questionnaires were written; equipment and supplies were ordered; detailed technical and financial plans were composed; the application for the Johns Hopkins Joint Committee on Clinical Investigation, the university's institutional review board that had to approve the plans for protection of human subjects in the research, was drafted; a plan for training outreach workers and laboratory assistants was developed; letters of commitment and written waivers from regulatory agencies were solicited.[9]

The researchers also explored what became the most controversial aspect of the proposal but was then considered state of the art for lead researchers: "determination of the relationship between lead in house dust and children's blood lead levels." The goal was to find the methods of abatement that would reduce the most amount of dust and therefore, presumably, the absorption of this toxin by children. Since traditional abatement methods had been shown to be inadequate and sometimes even harmful, Farfel and Chisolm proposed to use methods that they believed would do a superior job of limiting the production, spread, and residue of lead dust during the abatement process.[10] To the two researchers, demonstrating the comparative effectiveness of such methods seemed to demand an objective biological measure—children's blood lead levels measured over a span of years.[11]

A tremendous amount of the conceptual and organizational preparation for the KKI study had been done in advance. For the previous five years, Farfel and Chisolm had been conducting pilot projects that explored the very questions their larger study now aimed at finally answering. In 1985 both Farfel and Chisolm had concluded in separate publications, for example, that abatement as it was practiced in Baltimore and elsewhere did not protect children from levels of lead that could result in neurological damage.[12] And just before beginning the KKI study, Farfel and Chisolm published an article comparing what they characterized as traditional and modified forms of abatement.[13]

Traditional abatement in 1990 entailed either removal or "encasement"—the use of wallboard or plastic covering of lead-painted walls—up to four feet, the estimated maximum height a young child could reach or suck on. The paint was often removed using a blowtorch or sanding machine, with little attention paid to repainting, cleaning up, or disposing of the lead-containing debris. Typically, those doing abatement would at most "dry-sweep" the area.[14] Little thought was given to protecting either the inhabitants or the workers doing the abatement.

The "modified abatement" methods Chisolm and Farfel looked at as an alternative were increasingly being used in Baltimore and elsewhere. Although the extent of abatement was still the first four feet up from the floor, in modified abatement the lead paint on interior window frames was also totally removed. Instead of using a torch or a sander, which generally produced a lot of respirable dust, a heat gun was used; cleanup was more thorough and included "wet cleaning with high phosphate detergent together with dry vacuuming using standard shop vacuums." Further, the abated surfaces were repainted and the debris disposed of more carefully. Perhaps most significantly, the crews that did the work were given specific training and "were more likely to warn parents of hazards and provide instructions on dust control," though even children in these homes "had some contact with the home during abatement."[15] Chisolm and Farfel considered this comparison in methods a "natural experiment" because they "had no control over the implementation of either form of abatement."[16] Rather, they were documenting the results of activities of city workers and others employed by landlords to meet city requirements.

Traditional abatement procedures, Farfel and Chisolm found in their 1990 study, often actually substantially increased the lead hazard: in "nearly half the occupant children," blood lead levels rose, contrary to the objectives of the law and public health reformers. The modified abatement practices were not much better: they "represented modest short term improvement compared with traditional practices but were also inadequate." Further, "by six months, it was clear that neither form of abatement resulted in long-term reductions of PbB or house dust lead levels." It seemed that the best of intentions, then, had actually left children "at continued risk of excessive exposure to lead and permanent adverse neurobehavioral effects." The challenge for public health officials, Farfel and Chisolm argued, was thus "to identify abatement strategies that will be practical and well suited to the current understanding of low-level lead toxicity."[17]

From this failure of then-current practices came the seed for the new, more extensive KKI study that Chisolm and Farfel hoped would protect children but that would ultimately hold KKI up to the opprobrium of a skeptical and outraged public. The researchers argued that "a new approach" was needed, one that would require "more extensive, if not complete, abatement of lead paint on interior and exterior surfaces using replacement, paint removal and encapsulation methods which prove to be safe, practical and effective in the long-term." It would also include "more effective clean-up measures which may well require the use of vacuums equipped with high efficiency particle air [high-efficiency particulate air] (HEPA) filters." Farfel and Chisolm called for testing the amount of lead dust that remained on interior surfaces of the dwelling before the child returned home and an "evaluation of costs and health and environmental outcomes of alternative abatement methodologies."[18]

To make these "evaluations," Farfel and Chisolm's view of what constituted convincing science demanded something else, as already noted: the ultimate test of their hypothesis required *measuring* the blood lead levels of children who would reoccupy the houses. It also demanded a more controlled experiment than the earlier "natural" one had been, with a calibration of the environments to which the children were returned and the introduction of "control" groups for purposes of comparison—families living in roughly similar circumstances but whose homes were not subject to the abatement methods of the "experimental" groups. New means of protecting the children themselves during these renovations would also have to be found. If done properly, the researchers decided, either the children would have to be recruited after the homes had been renovated or be relocated while the abatement work was in progress.[19] Overall, the critical question that Farfel and Chisolm sought to address was, how much—or how little—"repair and maintenance" had to be done to gain what level of protection for the children?

In May 1991, Johns Hopkins's institutional review board approved the first, planning, phase of the "Lead-Based Paint Abatement and Repair Maintenance Study in Baltimore."[20] As the researchers finalized planning for the study early that summer, one last hurdle remained: how would Johns Hopkins find the housing and the tenants that were essential for the research? Here, they had to confront the heritage of racism and housing in Baltimore.

BALTIMORE AND THE LEGACY OF RACE

A growing port city, Baltimore in the nineteenth century had, up until the 1870s when it was overtaken by Washington, D.C. in this respect, the largest African American population of any city in the country.[21] Located below the Mason-Dixon Line, Maryland was a slave state, but nevertheless home to a large free black population, the vast majority of whom lived in Baltimore. On the eve of the Civil War (Maryland remained in the Union), less than 10 percent of Baltimore's African Americans were slaves.[22] As Samuel K. Roberts relates in his impressive history of tuberculosis in Baltimore, in the decades between the Civil War and World War II the population of "Afro-Baltimoreans" increased from 53,000 to 166,000, while this group's proportion of the city's total population remained relatively constant, fluctuating between 15 and 20 percent.[23]

The history of housing in Baltimore was shaped by the evolving class and racial relationships that marked what Roberts calls "a distinctly southern feature," segregation in virtually every aspect of peoples' lives and poverty for the vast majority of African Americans. The Druid Hill neighborhood of northwest Baltimore, for example, had two very different kinds of housing, segregated by class and race. Along the avenues were large, three-story single-family houses "occupied by working class whites (often German) and middle class blacks." In the "alleys" between the avenues, "poorer blacks . . . resided in one- or two-story houses."[24] The vast majority of both the avenue and alley housing were rentals. According to a 1913 survey, Roberts notes, Baltimore, despite its large black middle-class population, ranked next to last of seventy-three cities in percentage of black home ownership.[25] By the 1950s, the vast majority of the black population was segregated in the poor, largely neglected neighborhoods of Druid Hill and an area of northeast Baltimore just north of Johns Hopkins University and hospital, where the housing stock was old, run-down, and covered with decades of lead paint.[26] These were the two neighborhoods from which virtually all the families and children would be drawn into the KKI study.

While the study was being planned, Baltimore was confronting its most serious housing crisis in decades. Nationally, there had been a profound decline in federal support for the construction of new public housing. After World War II, Washington had committed itself to providing housing to millions of returning veterans and their families. It had also provided monies to many cities to build public projects as part of a massive program to rebuild cities whose poor populations still lived in nineteenth-century tenements. The lack of investment in new housing during the Depression and World War II years had created tremendous housing shortages for the working and middle classes. New York, among other cities, took advantage of the new federal funds to "clear its slums," replacing them with high-rise public housing projects. However problematic these "urban renewal projects" were—as populations were sometimes displaced and communities destroyed, forcing poor residents into overcrowded conditions in other areas of cities, producing new urban decay, and encouraging white flight to the suburbs—this investment represented a significant social commitment on both national and municipal scales.

By the 1970s and early 1980s, however, the construction of new public housing had come to a virtual standstill as the War on Poverty waned and a new conservative culture equated publicly supported housing with socialism. By the 1990s, not only had construction stopped, but all forms of housing subsidies also had succumbed to this antigovernment onslaught. At the same time that major cities in the Northeast and Midwest were experiencing a disinvestment by the federal government in housing and social services, they were also experiencing a dramatic decline in overall population, caused primarily by the flight of middle-class whites to the suburbs and the flight of factories to the South and West, and later overseas, to reduce wage costs. In 1950, Baltimore had been the sixth-largest city in the country, with a population of about 950,000. But by 1980 it had fallen to tenth place, with a population of 786,000, a decline of more than 17 percent. By 2000, Baltimore's population had dropped to 631,000, a decline of 33.44 percent over the course of a half century. This loss of population, coupled with an increase in the percentage of people living below the poverty line and a decline in the tax base, led to the abandonment of thousands of homes and row houses.[27] Not only had the tax base eroded, but the economics of urban housing had shifted as well. In the early 1980s, real estate speculators had begun buying up many of the housing units with an eye to making a huge profit. According to the Baltimore Department of Housing, this process had led to an excess of 70,000 substandard homes, "800 of which were lost yearly to abandonment." The "city targeted these abandoned properties, rehabilitating as many as possible."[28]

Initially the city spent between $60,000 to $90,000 per building, providing new floors, modern plumbing, new heating systems, and new kitchens.[29] But this practice soon ran up against the realities of tight state budgets and restrictive federal funds. In the mid-1980s a new nonprofit group, one that would become central in the KKI case, City Homes, was established with the goal of buying up large numbers of abandoned or dilapidated housing and doing "selective rehabilitation" to avoid high renovation costs.[30] In 1986, City Homes promised to buy 101 occupied houses from private landlords who were on the verge of abandoning their properties for the staggeringly low cost of $11,000 each and to rehab them for $10,500 apiece.[31]

Whatever the economic appeal of City Homes, its attempts to bring dilapidated housing up to at least minimally acceptable standards were soon challenged by city and state inspectors and administrators. Nancy Rase, director of Maryland's Community Development Agency, for example, commented on City Home's "frugal rehabilitation standards" and feared that such minimal rehabilitation efforts would not provide adequate housing for the city's poor population. And a state inspector, Jim Brown, found the City Home units he visited to be "in worse shape than others." He was, he said, "very uncomfortable going into a unit where the walls are obviously destroyed and [City Homes's] idea of fixing them is to put a little patch here and there and throw some wall paper up."[32] By 1990, estimates for "full lead abatement" of a two-story, three-bedroom house ran about $15,000, "much more than many of these houses are even worth," according to an independent evaluation by the Harvard Kennedy School of Government. But City Homes expected to spend only $10,500 to renovate an entire building and thus could only do cursory abatement at best. The

Harvard case study of City Homes, done while these housing units were being bought, argues that the group's policy was "to paint or wall paper over chipping surfaces and use a high-powered particle vacuum cleaner after rehab to pick up any stray dust or paint chips," a practice that the public health community had already documented as inadequate.[33] Rase and other government officials were worried: "We were fully aware that there was a 99% chance that [these units] had lead paint, and yet [City Homes] was doing almost nothing to address it."[34] One official acknowledged how awkward it was for upper-middle-class reformers to advocate for solutions they would not accept for themselves or their own children: "It's patronizing, they say, or worse, it's racially motivated. We're white, middle class people saying to black, lower income families, that's good enough for you."[35]

This history of abandonment set the context for the decisions to implement the KKI study. As Ellen Silbergeld recalls, Farfel and Chisolm "certainly were seeing that landlords were abandoning housing. It was a tremendous wave of abandonment at that time in Baltimore," and the prospect of having to invest in deleading homes may have contributed to this wave.[36] Farfel and Chisolm hoped that finding inexpensive ways to detoxify children's homes would keep landlords from abandoning housing.

To find appropriate housing for its study subjects, Farfel and Chisolm needed both apartments that could be renovated with minimal disruption to tenants who lived in them and apartments that needed extensive work and had to be vacant during renovation. Farfel wrote to Thomas Hendrix, the chair of the Johns Hopkins Joint Committee on Clinical Investigation, the medical center's institutional review board (IRB), that he and Chisolm were looking into "the feasibility of collaborating with a local housing organization, City Homes, on the main study." City Homes, it seemed, was seeking a way to rehabilitate its image; it had, Farfel explained, "adopted a new lead poisoning prevention program and would like to collaborate with the Kennedy Institute."[37] City Homes was an attractive partner for KKI because it "owns and manages 200 low-income rental units [and] has agreed to be the primary source of study dwellings which will receive the Repair and Maintenance interventions."[38]

City Homes planned to visit each apartment "to provide the educational component of their prevention program." This would entail informing "tenants of the upcoming study" and assessing which residents were amenable to participating in the KKI research effort. Then, according to Farfel, City Homes would give KKI "a list of families who would be willing to speak to us further."[39] The initial screening of those who would participate in the study was not done by the researchers themselves but by others outside their immediate control.

In addition to City Homes, other owners of low-income housing "stepped forward" to make their properties available, Farfel recalled. To qualify, the homes "had to be approximately 800 to 1200 square feet . . . two story, six-room row house[s] in Baltimore City with 8 to 10 windows in a structurally sound condition" built before 1941. Such relatively small dwellings were required, Farfel explained, because "we had a certain amount of resources to do the experiment, and we didn't want to use large houses." Most importantly the house "had to have what we called elevated levels of lead in dust in at least two sites in the house."[40] In practice this meant that Johns Hopkins had to establish relationships with landlords who potentially violated existing lead ordinances. For example, one landlord, Lawrence Polakoff, who would become the focus of lawsuits brought by tenants whose children were lead poisoned, had been cited by the Baltimore Department of Health at least ten times between "1977 and 1984 for extensive lead content."[41]

City Homes agreed to "give priority to families with young children when re-renting the vacant units following R&M interventions,"[42] because, Farfel recalled, "we were looking for families that had at least one child under the age of 48 months and older than five months at the start of the study."[43] The children "were not to be mentally retarded or severely handicapped in any way that would limit their physical movement," and the researchers needed to feel sure that the family would not move from the dwelling "because we were interested in following the family over a period of years."[44] KKI personnel would then obtain informed consent forms from the tenants after they had moved in.[45]

KKI provided a script that City Homes personnel used to evaluate whether or not residents with young children in the group's housing would be willing to participate in the KKI study. "As you can see," a City Homes representative was told to begin, "City Homes is committed to finding a practical and responsible way to address the lead poisoning problem." The representative would then describe the City Homes program as "new and unlike any other program that we know about in the U.S." The representative would tell parents that "we want to find out how well it works so that more children can benefit." At this point the City Homes representative would explain the role of KKI, emphasizing that Johns Hopkins, "a leader in lead poisoning prevention," would be leading the study. City Homes would then ask if the family was "interested in being part of this effort." If the tenant was interested, the City Homes representative would say that

KKI staff would periodically visit "your home during the next two years . . . to take samples of the dust, water, and soil." Johns Hopkins would test these samples "at no charge" and would inform the tenant "of the results." City Homes emphasized that one of the benefits of the program was that residents would be told how their "own house cleaning efforts [could] reduce lead exposure." Additionally, KKI would provide blood lead testing "at no charge to you."[46]

In 1992, Chisolm and Farfel laid out to the EPA the prevailing dilemma of public health as they saw it. The "public health goal" was "to maintain PbBs [blood lead levels] of children and fetuses below levels associated with adverse health effects (i.e. PbB below 10–15 µg/dL)." But here was the rub: there were practical realities that researchers and officials had to face. An estimated "57 million privately owned and occupied U.S. housing units contain[ed] some lead-containing paint," of which some 10 million were homes to children under the age of seven. "The extent and potential costs of the problem," said the researchers, made it "imperative that we investigate low-cost and practical . . . forms of lead-paint abatement." Accepting the premise that "future generations of children . . . will continue to occupy older housing which cannot be fully abated or rehabilitated without substantial subsidy," the KKI study aimed at providing "a practical means of reducing lead exposure."[47] In short, said the researchers, "the public health challenge is to obtain the maximal reduction in children's body lead burdens with a finite set of resources."[48]

Farfel and Chisolm's report to the EPA acknowledged that, as public health researchers, they had their feet planted in two worlds. In one, the discipline of public health strove to be a basic science, discovering the way the world worked and letting the political chips fall where they may. The responsibility of the public health scientist in this sense was to provide scientifically sound research that could pass muster with scholars from a variety of scientific disciplines. By the 1980s, sophisticated epidemiological methods and statistical analyses were essential tools in establishing an academic researcher's legitimacy and authority. The relative prestige of publishing in an epidemiological journal and the rigor associated with tests of statistical significance could determine whether or not the broader scholarly community would accept a given set of research findings. In the second world, public health science was judged by its relevance to practical application, amenable to translation into policies that could improve people's health.[49] Thus the KKI study was developed to employ a scientific, epidemiologically and statistically valid method for comparing the results of expensive, comprehensive lead abatement with "less costly and potentially more cost-effective Repair and Maintenance interventions." A prospective, well-controlled study was the coin of the realm for epidemiologists and public health scientists because the variables that might affect the findings could be isolated. By establishing separate groups of research subjects (cohorts) that had similar socioeconomic and other characteristics, and varying their experience systematically, researchers could assess the effect of the factors that were being tested. The researchers would evaluate the effectiveness of these interventions by following children over time and periodically testing their blood for lead, hypothesizing that all of these interventions would result in at least "interim" declines in children's blood lead levels, but in some cases more than others.[50]

Evaluation of the various methods of abatement was essential to the development of good public health practice, and KKI developed a multi-tiered methodology for this purpose. The core of the study was to compare the effects on blood lead measures of three different levels of abatement.

I. Level I abatements were minimal renovations in which loose and peeling paint were removed and painted over, "to [the] limit of [the] budget," in occupied and unoccupied dwellings. Floors were left untouched except for the placement of a "textured walk-off mat at the main entrance." Stairways remained untreated and windows had "well caps" (coverings for the windowsills) installed, with exterior and interior window trim repainted. Doors had peeling paint removed as well, again only "to limit of budget"—$1,650 for the entire operation.[51]

II. Level II abatement was somewhat more extensive, also performed in homes that were occupied and to which the same family would return. A "textured walk-off mat" was placed at each front and rear entrance and if lead based paint was present, a floor covering was provided to make the floor smoother and thereby ostensibly easier to clean. All lead-based paint was removed from the trim of exterior and interior surfaces and repainted "to limit of budget," which was capped at $3,500 for this level.[52] If stairways were found painted with lead-based paint, the treads and risers were encapsulated. And if lead-based paint was found on windows, attempts were made to reduce friction, install well caps, stabilize exterior trim, and repaint interior sills with a nonflat paint. Doors were also planed to "reduce friction," and peeling paint was removed and the area repainted. Finally, a more extensive renovation was reserved for damaged walls. If lead-based paint was found on the walls, and more than 25 percent of the wall was damaged, the wall was repaired and treated with a "flexible encapsulate or rigid enclosure," probably wallboard.[53]

III. Level III abatement was the most extensive, with spending capped at $7,000. It was only done in unoccupied homes. Floor, stairway, wall, and door treatments were essentially the same as level 2. But unlike level 2, all trim was sealed, encapsulated, and enclosed and all windows were replaced.[54] Unlike a control group of fully abated homes built before 1978, not all of the lead was removed from the walls and ceilings. Lead on these surfaces was only patched and encapsulated if 25 percent or more of that surface was damaged.

The blood lead levels of children aged six months to four years would be periodically tested, as would the amount of lead in house dust, soil, and drinking water, measured in "three groups of 25 dwellings (total of 75 dwellings), each receiving one of three levels of Repair & Maintenance interventions." Homes that were occupied would "be randomly assigned to receive either R&M Level I or R&M Level II intervention in a ratio of 2:1 respectively." Homes that were not occupied would "be randomly assigned to receive R&M Level III or Level II interventions, in a ratio of 2:1 respectively." Thus each of the levels would have approximately 25 homes assigned.[55]

In addition, the blood lead levels of children aged six months to four years would be periodically tested and the lead in house dust, soil, and drinking water measured in 50 other homes, 25 of "which received comprehensive lead-paint abatement performed by pilot abatement projects in Baltimore between May of 1988 and February of 1991,"[56] and "25 [of which were] modern urban dwellings built after 1980 . . . as negative controls (i.e. dwellings which are not likely to contain lead-based paint)."[57]

Families in each of the five groups of the study would be asked to complete questionnaires at the time of enrollment and every six months thereafter, providing demographic information and "covariates which could influence lead exposure in the home (e.g. hobbies, child behavior, diet and occupation)."[58] KKI hoped to measure the efficacy of the test abatement techniques for up to four to six years. "These types of long-term follow-up data currently do not exist, yet they are essential for developing scientifically sound prevention and remediation policies," the researchers said. In the end, 108 housing units, rather than the 125 originally envisioned were included in the study.[59]

As required by law for all research involving human subjects, Farfel and Chisolm submitted their research protocol to the Johns Hopkins medical center's institutional review board for approval. This process, created by federal mandate in the 1980s in response to revelations about Tuskegee research and other human rights abuses, was meant to protect people who agreed to participate in research efforts. In response to the researchers' application, Thomas Hendrix, the board's head, replied with just two questions. One had to do with how the researchers would deal with a situation where there was more than one eligible child in a study household. The second raised an issue of ethics: how to deal with federal guidelines "regarding using children as controls in projects in which there is no potential benefit" to the children, in this case those in the two control groups, in homes that had received comprehensive abatement and in homes built after 1978. Federal guidelines limited the use of children and other vulnerable populations as controls under these circumstances, but Hendrix suggested that there were ways to illustrate potential benefit, thereby avoiding the government restrictions. He pointed out that the children were likely exposed to lead from numerous sources beyond the home, such as their schools, daycare centers, and playgrounds, and said the value of this study lay in finding out "whether [lead] safe housing alone is sufficient to keep the blood-lead levels in acceptable bounds."[60] Curiously, the IRB did not raise any issue about potential harm that children in the *partially* abated homes might face from living there. In his response to the two questions Hendrix posed, Farfel said that the study would have a separate consent form for each child and would include a section in the protocol that incorporated Hendrix's suggestions, redefining the potential benefits to children in the control groups.[61] The proposal was formally approved by the IRB on May 18, 1992.[62]

Farfel included in his letter to Hendrix a copy of the proposed consent form that parents would be required to sign in order to participate in the study. "As you may know," the form began, "lead poisoning in children is a problem in Baltimore City and other communities across the country." Alluding to the repairs that were done in conjunction with City Homes, the form went on to explain, "We understand that your house had special repairs done in order to reduce exposure to lead and dust. We are interested in finding out how well the repairs worked." The explanation that the parents were given reinforced the view that this was a passive, observational study. "We are now doing a study to learn how well different practices work for reducing exposure to lead in paint and dust. We are asking you and over a hundred other families to allow us to test for lead in and around your homes seven to eight times over the next two years." The form went on to say, "We are also doing free blood lead testing of children aged six months to seven years, seven to eight times over the next two years."

1991

CLINICAL INVESTIGATION CONSENT FORM

The Johns Hopkins Medical Institutions
(The Johns Hopkins Hospital
The Francis Scott Key Medical Center, etc.)

Title of Research Project:
Lead-Paint Abatement and Repair & Maintenance Study
(Older dwellings which have received R & M)

Patient I.D. Plate

Explanation of Research Project to Subject:

PURPOSE OF STUDY:
As you may know, lead poisoning in children is a problem in Baltimore City and other communities across the country. Lead in paint, house dust and outside soil are major sources of lead exposure for children. Children can also be exposed to lead in drinking water and other sources. We understand that your house had special repairs done in order to reduce exposure to lead in paint and dust. We are interested in finding out how well the repairs worked.

1993

CLINICAL INVESTIGATION CONSENT FORM

The Johns Hopkins Medical Institutions
(The Johns Hopkins Hospital
The Francis Scott Key Medical Center, etc.)
The Kennedy Krieger Institute

Title of Research Project:
Lead-Paint Abatement and Repair & Maintenance Study
(Older dwellings which have received R & M)

Patient I.D. Plate

Explanation of Research Project to Subject:

PURPOSE OF STUDY:
As you may know, lead poisoning in children is a problem in Baltimore City and other communities across the country. Lead in paint, house dust and outside soil are major sources of lead exposure for children. Children can also be exposed to lead in drinking water and other sources. We understand that your house is going to have special repairs done in order to reduce exposure to lead in paint and dust. On a random basis, homes will receive one of two levels of repair. We are interested in finding out how well the two levels of repair work. The repairs are not intended, or expected, to completely remove exposure to lead.

FIGURE 9.   Kennedy Krieger Institute consent forms, 1991 and 1993. These consent forms were intended to explain potential risks and benefits to parents of the children enrolled in the KKI study. The 1991 form did not clearly state that lead was still present in the home and children could be endangered. The 1993 form added simply, "The repairs are not intended, or expected, to completely remove exposure to lead." Source: Ericka Grimes v. Kennedy Krieger Institute Inc., No. 128, and Myron Higgins et al. v. Kennedy Krieger Institute Inc., No. 129, 366 Md. 29, 782 A.2d 807, 2001 Md. LEXIS 496 (2001).

KKI personnel would collect "samples of outside soil, house dust, and drinking water." They would also collect "dust from bare floors, carpets, windows, and upholstered furnishings." The researchers assured the parents that "these procedures would [not] damage surfaces," and they explained what the blood sampling would involve: "free transportation will be provided to and from the clinic"; about "one third of a teaspoon of blood" would be taken from the child's arm each visit; and for the child, "there may be some discomfort but no danger is involved in this procedure." Families were also asked to complete a questionnaire "about other potential sources of lead exposure in your home."[63]

Potential benefits were also explained on the form. The Kennedy Krieger Institute promised the families compensation of fifteen dollars "each time the questionnaire is completed." In addition, coupons and T-shirts would be given to the families.[64] Further, the dust, soil, water, and blood samples would be tested for lead at KKI "at no charge to you," and the institute "would contact you to discuss the test results and steps that you can take to reduce any risks of exposure." The information collected "would be considered confidential and will not be shared with landlords or anyone else without your express permission." If parents had questions or wanted further information, they could "contact your physician or the Baltimore City Health Department's Lead Poisoning Prevention Program."[65]

By January 1993, "following EPA's final approval of our study plan," the researchers were ready to begin data collection. One hundred and eight low-income African American households were selected as subjects in the study.[66] But almost immediately the study faced financial limitations: the EPA wanted the researchers to "reduce the scope of work to match available resources."[67]

Other problems began accruing too. In a September 9, 1993, letter Farfel informed the Baltimore Health Department that though there was still lead dust in the homes, the vast majority of study houses tested had lead levels below the legal standard—called "clearance levels" in Maryland—following the renovations.[68] However, lead readings in a few apartments were above the legal standard, probably because the floors did not "receive floor treatments to make them smooth and cleanable." While "in all cases," Farfel reported, dust lead levels appeared to have been reduced, he reminded the department that "floor treatments, other than cleanings, are not an element of R & M Level 1 and cannot be done in all rooms in occupied R & M Level II dwellings due to logistical problems." He informed the Department of Health that "for these and other reasons, the Maryland Department of the Environment (MDE) is not holding us to the Maryland Clearance levels in the latter two types of units."[69]

The following spring, Farfel applied to the Joint Committee on Clinical Investigation (JCCI), Johns Hopkins's IRB, for a renewal of the project's approval.[70] He extolled what the researchers considered the success of the project to date: "The blood-lead results are monitored on a regular basis. To date, only one child out of over 130 study children has had a blood-lead increase during follow-up that has required chelation therapy. This child lives in a previously abated house [one of the study's controls]. The child's provider and the Health Department were immediately notified. The child received chelation therapy and remains in the study. Based on the most recent follow-up blood lead values none of the other study children have had an increase in blood lead above baseline that triggers case management (i.e., ≥20 µg/dL)."[71] Farfel also reported having increased the incentives for families and children to participate. Now, not only T-shirts, $10 coupons, and $15 payments for filling out questionnaires were given, but also "hats, gloves, and toys for the children and certificates of appreciation." KKI also sponsored a "roller-skating party" for all study families.[72] In May 1994, the JCCI approved the project through 1995 with a new, revised consent form. It included a new line stating explicitly that "the repairs are not intended, or expected, to completely remove exposure to lead."[73]

In 1997 the EPA's Office of Pollution Protection and Toxics reported its findings for the first two years of the KKI study, 1993 through 1995, the only evaluation of the study that has been issued. The report noted the "growing interest in the use of interim measures to temporarily control the problem of extensive residential lead-based paint hazards . . . in a cost-effective manner." And it noted certain measures of "success" in the Baltimore study: "all three levels of R & M intervention were associated with statistically significant reductions in house dust lead loadings and total dust loadings that were sustained below pre-intervention levels during two years of follow-up."[74] One of the two "control" groups—the one consisting of houses built after 1978 and therefore considered lead free—"had significantly lower dust lead loading and concentrations across time" than did any of the partially abated houses, as one would expect.[75] After two years, the study's Level III houses, which had had the most extensive partial abatement, had dust lead levels "generally similar to" "the [group of] previously abated control houses four years to six years post abatement."[76]

The Johns Hopkins researchers, the EPA evaluation noted, concluded that there was a direct correlation between house dust levels and blood lead levels in the children, a finding that confirmed the 1990 study that Farfel and Chisolm had already conducted and published in the *American Journal of Public Health*. Those children who lived in homes built after 1978 "had significantly lower blood lead concentrations than children in each of the other four groups," and their "blood lead concentrations were <10 µg/dL, the Center [sic] for Disease Control's level of concern."[77] Overall, the EPA authors concluded, the interventions were a success: "Children with baseline blood lead concentrations ≥15/dL in each of the

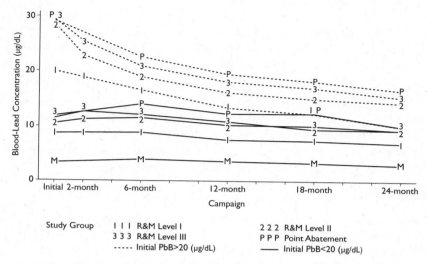

FIGURE 10. Kennedy Krieger Institute Repair and Maintenance (R&M) Study, effect of abatement strategy on children's blood lead levels at designated intervals ("Campaign"). While children with very elevated blood lead levels appear to have benefited from all forms of abatement, no levels were reduced to the then-accepted level of concern, 10 μg/dl. Children in "modern-urban" (M) (i.e., lead-free) housing had the lowest blood lead levels at the beginning and end of the study. Source: U.S. EPA, Office of Prevention, Pesticides, and Toxic Substances, "Executive Summary," in *Lead-Based Paint Abatement and Repair and Maintenance Study in Baltimore: Findings Based on Two Years of Follow-Up*, EPA 747-R-97-005 (Washington, D.C.: U.S. EPA, December 1997).

three R&M groups and the previously abated group had statistically significant reductions in blood lead concentrations during follow-up, after controlling for age, gender and season."[78] For children whose blood lead levels had been below 15 μg/dl at the start of the study, however, there was virtually no change (see figure 10).[79] The summary did not draw conclusions about the efficacy of partial abatement as a substitute for complete removal of the lead hazard. But it did show (as illustrated in figure 10) that, in contrast to previous efforts at partial abatement, both lead dust levels in the home and the blood lead levels in children could be reduced for a significant period of time.

But, the "success" of the KKI effort was undermined by at least two significant factors: first, between the time the study was conceived and the time the results were being gathered, the scientific community had dramatically reassessed the conception of what level of lead in a child's blood constituted a threat. In the mid-1980s that level was 25 µg/dl. In 1991 the Centers for Disease Control had lowered the level of concern to 10 µg/dl, and many suspected that there was simply no level below which lead could be considered "safe" for children. By the time Farfel and Chisolm actually started collecting data, January 1993, the CDC threshold had been reduced to the 10 µg/dl level for two years, below the level (>15 µg/dl) at which the KKI study had determined that abatement techniques were most effective. Second, the statistical success of the KKI study was undermined by the fact that a few of the children's blood lead levels actually rose, and the blood lead levels of many children were found to fluctuate greatly over the two-year study period.[80]

The level of abatement in the KKI study was determined by the elimination of specific hazards—for example, windowsills were to be scraped clean of lead or floors smoothed and sealed. But the renovations in all categories were capped by specific dollar amounts, thereby limiting their efficacy. The effect of such a dollar limitation could be problematic, as it was, for example, in one home on Durham Street that was scheduled to have a Level II renovation. The field report and spectrum analysis for the home listed a wide range of paint hazards throughout the house. But when Environmental Restorations Inc. (ERI), the contracting company employed by City Homes to prepare houses for the KKI study, put in its proposal for renovating the home, only about half of the lead hazards were addressed. Specifically, of the 58 sites in the house that were identified in the "Lead Paint Field Report" as containing lead, only 28 were cleaned up by ERI.[81]

In December 1993, to take another example, Lawrence Polakoff made the property at 1906 Federal Street, just eight blocks north of KKI, available to the institute, and it was assigned a Level II lead intervention, meaning that $3,500 would be invested in renovations.[82] The house sat "smack in the middle of a string of fading row houses, a Baptist church and an old corner store."[83] ERI undertook the restoration in which Kathy H., a 21-year-old single mother, and her son, Michael H. (3-1/2 years old), and Joan M., a 20-year-old single mother, and her two daughters, Abby M. (age 5) and her sister Annabel M. (age 2), would live for a monthly rent of $315.[84] From the start, ERI president Jean Eddy was concerned about possible danger to the families and the company's liability for possible lead poisoning. Eddy wrote to Polakoff to make clear that the partial abatement could leave the incoming residents endangered. "This scope of work does not provide for the complete removal or enclosure of existing lead based paint surfaces," he reminded the landlord. "It is hereby understood and agreed that Owner's contract specifications governing the abatement of lead-containing materials by ERI from the subject premises, do not include provisions for the complete removal of all lead containing materials from said premises." But more than that, Eddy insisted on making clear that his company had been "expressly" told not to "remove [some of the] lead-containing materials from said premises" and could not be held liable for having followed those instructions.[85]

PARTIAL ABATEMENT: THE STATE OF THE SCIENCE

By 1998, a series of studies conducted in other cities had begun to document that the new methods of partial abatement, while successful in lowering lead exposures and blood lead levels of children, could not protect all children down to the new action level of 10 µg/dl. The EPA, in conjunction with the Ohio-based research and development firm Battelle, evaluated nineteen of at least thirty-five lead-remediation projects, including the KKI study, that had been completed between 1981 and 1998 to determine what had been learned about the efficacy of different lead-abatement techniques. The studies, principally carried out in the United States but also in Canada, France, and New Zealand, showed the limited success of partial abatement methods in protecting children. The goals and methodologies of the studies varied, with differing sample sizes, statistical measurements, and objectives. The Baltimore KKI study stood out, however, as the only one in which the researchers directed the nature of the partial abatements that were to be evaluated and placed children into these environments. In all but one other case the children were observed in the homes they already lived in.[86]

Battelle provided a mixed review of the efficacy of partial abatement. There was "a growing body of evidence that lead hazard interventions can reduce exposed children's blood-lead concentrations and dust-lead levels in homes." But Battelle went on to point out that, based on the limited data available, "none of the intervention strategies studied to date have consistently brought blood-lead concentrations below the level of concern [10µg/dl]." While the various partial techniques did have an observed impact on children with high blood lead concentrations, these partial solutions "may not be as successful among children with lower blood-lead concentrations." Furthermore, the firm was critical of the limited goals of the abatement studies. They were designed to evaluate techniques of lowering the blood lead levels of already exposed children and hence represented merely "secondary prevention." The goal of public health interventions, Battelle suggested, should not be "secondary prevention" but rather "to prevent childhood lead exposure before it occurs."[87]

The Battelle and EPA summary provides a window into the broader crisis that public health (and society) faced as it confronted the insidious nature of damage to children caused by low-level lead exposure. The KKI study was clearly part of much broader and somewhat desperate search for reasonable ways to address a century of lead pollution. Underlying all of the evaluated studies was the hope that more research could provide the catalyst for effective policy. After literally thousands of studies of lead and its pernicious effects, the EPA noted in 1998 that "a number of data gaps" existed and specifically asked for more research to determine whether "primary prevention" was more effective than "secondary." For researchers and policy makers interested in scientific exactitude, this issue might be important. But for a parent of a child whose permanent brain damage was the result of secondary rather than primary prevention, this research might seem a nicety. Hence, the EPA came back to the common-sense conclusion that "primary prevention can be assumed to be at least as effective as secondary prevention and may be considerably more effective."[88]

Around the same time the EPA released its evaluation of the partial abatement strategies, Herbert Needleman challenged the public health community to confront the limitations of its own activities and commitment to preventing lead poisoning. In an article in the *American Journal of Public Health*, Needleman told the story of "the promise and abandonment of primary prevention," the approach that he believed responsible public health practitioners should have pursued. He recounted the hope embodied in the CDC's 1991 pathbreaking *Strategic Plan for the Elimination of Childhood Lead Poisoning*. An entire decade had been lost to ineffectual action since then, Needleman charged, and "the drive to eliminate childhood lead poisoning is stalled." Two critical components of that strategic plan "had been abandoned," he said: universal screening of children between the ages of one and five years and "comprehensive lead abatement."[89] He criticized the entire public health, medical, and political establishments whose responsibility it was to protect children: the CDC, faced with a hostile Republican congress, had backed off its earlier commitment to universal screening; HUD had allowed the real estate and insurance interests to become the predominant voice in its task force "to make recommendations on lead-based paint reduction and financing."[90] Even the Alliance to End Childhood Lead Poisoning, founded with Needleman's participation in 1990, and its sister organization, the National Center for Lead-Safe Housing, did not escape his critique. The two groups, Needleman argued, had both become dependent on HUD and EPA grants and had lost their ability to advocate for full abatement and, therefore, for primary prevention.[91] He blamed these groups and the more potent conservative atmosphere in Washington for undermining the momentum for change that had seemed to be building in the late 1980s and early 1990s: "It derailed an undertaking that promised to wipe out childhood lead poisoning forever, that would have lifted the disease out of the pediatric textbooks and entered it into the histories of medicine and disease controls."[92]

Needleman traced the relationship between the history of the country and the sad history of lead poisoning. In this, "one important factor is racism," he pointed out, which he believed had played an important role in stifling the efforts to protect children. Twice as many African American children had elevated blood lead levels as non-Hispanic whites, he noted, and this had "resulted in a widely held belief that lead poisoning is a problem exclusively affecting African American children. As the current attitude of indifference of the poor and minorities developed, the attack on lead exposure lost its urgency."[93]

This critique, coming from a person who had contributed so much to the discovery of the devastating effects of low-level lead exposure on children and who had felt the full brunt of the lead industry's power and wrath, sparked a huge controversy among advocates, government officials, and researchers. The *American Journal of Public Health* editors noted that "the Journal received an unusual number of responses" to the article and printed six of them in July 1999. Don Ryan, who had founded the Alliance to End Childhood Lead Poisoning to force lead's dangers onto the national agenda, protested that "a rigid national program of full abatement would squander resources on homes with minimal or no hazards and fail to provide near-term protection to the children who are at highest risk."[94] Dave Jacobs, then at the Office of Healthy Homes and Lead Hazard Control at HUD, countered Needleman's assertions of failure with the view that "primary prevention is now a reality across the country" and argued that "we have moved beyond the simple (and, I submit, potentially dangerous) notion that total removal must be the only hazard control option." If total abatement was not politically or fiscally possible, then holding out for it meant hundreds of thousands more children would not receive potentially helpful partial abatement, he argued. The National Center for Lead-Safe Housing replied to Needleman's critique by arguing that "making housing lead-safe is a more effective approach to preventing childhood lead poisoning than requiring complete abatement of all lead-based paint."[95] While some critiqued Needleman, others did support him. Paul Mushak and John Rosen, both of whom had gone through the lead wars of the 1980s, argued that

Needleman was on target with his critique of a retreat in the commitment to eliminate childhood lead poisoning.

Needleman responded to the criticisms by reiterating that in 1991, in the midst of a nationwide recession, there had been an opportunity to employ the jobless "in safe deleading and housing rehabilitation," which would have provided them income. In the process it would have wiped "out lead poisoning forever." But by temporizing and compromising, the country had only achieved a "limited 'interim' (i.e. temporary)" goal that amounted to little more than "scraping, patching, and painting, and an attempt to insulate landlords from lawsuits by parents of poisoned children." Needleman pointed out an obvious but frequently overlooked fact: "If true de-leading had been done, every child who moves into [a given] house will be protected." And if this had been done years previous, many children would have been saved from lead poisoning. The abatement approach was threatening the very foundations of public health. "Shortly after I began to study lead toxicity," he said, "I became puzzled by the persistence of the problem in the face of so much information." It was "easy to see" the "role of the lead industry" then. But "I came painfully to understand," he went on, "that bureaucratic caution, lack of imagination, and unwillingness to engage and fight essentially evil forces—slum landlords and their political and economic allies—were just as damaging to any real solution."[96]

The debate over abatement was emblematic of a much larger social debate that was then overtaking the public health and public policy communities over what the nation could "afford" to provide its citizens and which citizens "deserved" support. The Clintons' proposal for national health insurance, for example, foundered in large part on the "ability" of society to "afford" health insurance for all of its citizens; state governors argued that welfare reform was needed in part so that states could balance their budgets. Many of the oldest ideological battles over the role of the state in providing services to the needy were fought using the rhetoric of efficiency and scarcity.

Within public health, the effort to control AIDS ironically fed the broader ideological movement away from prevention and toward "harm reduction." In the late 1980s, public health practitioners, faced with the prospect of an uncontrolled epidemic that could literally wipe out millions of people—if not tens of millions—sought to slow the spread of the virus that caused AIDS (HIV) by establishing programs that promoted clean needle use among intravenous drug users and safe sex practices. By the mid-1990s, antiretroviral (ARV) drug therapy changed the landscape of AIDS in North America and western Europe as treatment transformed

AIDS from a deadly, acute disease to a chronic condition. By the late 1990s, best practices to treat AIDS included providing clean needles and promoting safe sex among "at risk" populations and treating HIV-positive patients with ARV drugs. But for much of the world, HIV infection remained a death sentence. In Africa, the cost of ARV drug therapy was out of reach for the victims and their governments. Many public health and policy makers as a consequence began searching for less expensive and, admittedly, less effective protocols for treatment.

An enormous controversy ensued over the ethics of providing people only partial protection against a disease because of cost. One especially heated debate involved international health campaigns. On one side were those who noted the injustice of treating the poor, often voiceless African population with less effective treatments than their European and American counterparts. On the other side were those who saw the inequalities between nations and peoples as insurmountable and who therefore argued for doing *something* to help people who were suffering, even if it was not ideal. The debate raged in leading medical, public health, and policy journals as well as in publications for the broader intellectual and academic community, carried out by some of the nation's leading scholars.[97] Harm reduction, rather than full prevention, was a controversial topic at the center of discussions over tobacco use as well. Public health advocates were divided over whether or not low-tar and low-nicotine "safe" cigarettes were preferable to smoking bans and heavy taxation to discourage smoking among the young. Once again, around the major public health issues in the late twentieth century, harm reduction contended with the prevention of disease for the attention of public health practitioners, policy makers, and concerned citizens more generally.[98] But at heart, a larger issue lurked: was there the political will and economic support to cope seriously with these issues? This question was central to what would ultimately become the firestorm over the Johns Hopkins lead research studies.

7 Research on Trial

In most cases of research involving human subjects, respect for persons demands that subjects enter into the research voluntarily and with adequate information.

BELMONT REPORT, 1978

Social indifference . . . has let generations of children suffer the insidious menace of lead poisoning.

ELLEN SILBERGELD, 2010

Young Enid G. lived on North Monroe Street in the northwestern district of Baltimore, one of the two major African American neighborhoods that were part of the Kennedy Krieger Institute lead study.[1] She was born May 30, 1992, to a single parent who had lived at the North Monroe Street address since the summer of 1990 in a house that ostensibly had been completely abated in the late 1980s, and therefore was supposedly "lead free."[2] In March 1993 the family was recruited to participate in the KKI Repair and Maintenance study, and Enid's mother signed a consent form that would play an important role in the lawsuit she would later bring on behalf of her daughter against Johns Hopkins. Her home was designated as one of about twenty in the "pre-1978" control group that would be used to compare the efficacy of the various partial abatement efforts (described in chapter 6).[3]

The day before Enid's mother signed the consent form, the home was tested for lead exposures and found, despite its lead-free designation, to have a number of "hot spots" in the first-floor window wells and the exterior entrance, where lead paint could pose a danger to Enid. (An additional dust test done five months later, in August 1993, showed no remaining hot spots.) Enid was found to have a blood lead reading of 9 micrograms per deciliter in April 1993, when she was approximately eleven months old. But by the time she began to walk in September, her level had risen to 32 µg/dl.[4] Not until three months later, in mid-December (and nine months after the initial dust test had been completed),[5] was her mother told about hot spots of lead in the apartment that might have accounted for Enid's lead poisoning. In a handwritten addendum at the bottom of the letter informing Enid's mother of the results of the various tests, the project's outreach coordinator told the mother how to protect her children: "You might want

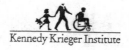

Kennedy Krieger Institute

A comprehensive resource for children with disabilities

3/28/94

Dear Ms. [name deleted]

This is to inform you that your child [name deleted] has a high blood lead elevation based on test results of the blood which was taken from the arm at the Kennedy Krieger Lead Clinic on 3/25/94. His/her blood lead test result is 22 micrograms/deciliter. This places your child in CDC Class III. We have already informed the Baltimore City Health Department of this result. <u>You should provide the test result to your child's primary health care provider</u> right away. As you know, the test was performed as part of the special project sponsored by the U.S. Environmental Protection Agency.

<u>If you have any questions please contact me at 550-9241</u> or the clinic nurse at 550-9035.

In September 1993, [name deleted] Sincerely,
blood lead was 32 ug/DL.
So, this shows some improvement! [name deleted]
Try to keep her hands away from [name deleted]
her mouth! Outreach Coordinator
cc: [name deleted]
KKI Medical Records 046377 121-01-12

707 North Broadway Baltimore, Maryland 11205 (410) 550-9000/Telephone (410) 550-9344/Facsimile (410) 550-980 E. 36

FIGURE 11. Kennedy Krieger Institute letter notifying parent of her child's elevated blood lead level, 1994. The form letter says that the child's blood lead level is at least twice the CDC level of concern. The mother is told to take her daughter to "the child's primary health care provider right away." The handwritten note reassures the mother that this blood lead level is an improvement over the previous level of 32 µg/dl and that she should "try to keep [the child's] hands away from her mouth!" Source: [name deleted] v. Kennedy Krieger Institute Inc., No. 128, and Myron Higgins et al. v. Kennedy Krieger Institute Inc., No. 129, 366 Md. 29, 782 A.2d 807, 2001 Md. LEXIS 496 (2001).

to wash your front step more often to keep dust from being tracked in. Happy Holidays!—Ruth."[6]

But the story did not end there. Three and a half months later, in March 1994, Enid's blood lead level was measured at 22 µg/dl, somewhat lower than the September reading but still more than twice the level of concern that the Centers for Disease Control had established three years earlier. KKI sent a form letter giving these results, with a handwritten note at the bottom: "In September 1993 [Enid]'s blood lead was 32 µg/dl. So, this shows some improvement! Try to keep her hands away from her mouth!" The letter told Enid's mother that her child was in the CDC's Class III, "highly elevated," category and that she should consult the family's physician.[7] In the KKI study, families such as Enid's were thus receiving conflicting messages from Johns Hopkins. On the one hand, KKI was there to help improve their situations with renovated apartments that research scientists believed would reduce children's exposure to lead. On the other hand, when the renovations were shown to be inadequate the burden fell to the parents to protect their children through half measures that shifted responsibility away from Kennedy Krieger and to the parent, who was told to "mop up."

The KKI study had modestly benefited the majority of the 130 children who lived in the houses that were being evaluated. The amount of dust to which they were exposed declined and their blood lead levels fell as well. But Enid was certainly not in that majority. For her and a few other children, the housing proved to be particularly contaminated and their blood leads had risen dramatically.

Another child in the study who did not fare well was Michael H., the five-year-old son of Kathy H.[8] Kathy filed suit on February 26, 1995, in the Circuit Court for Baltimore City against Lawrence Polakoff, their landlord, because she discovered that Michael's blood lead levels were rising and that he was being poisoned. Throughout the 1980s, childhood lead poisonings had prompted numerous lawsuits against Baltimore landlords, many of which were brought to court by Saul Kerpelman, a Baltimore attorney. Kerpelman and his young associate, Suzanne Shapiro, had visited the family's home after the KKI abatement study had begun and had seen conditions that Shapiro knew represented a real hazard (the house had been assigned as Level II, the medium partial abatement). They initiated the suit against just the landlord and did not add Kennedy Krieger until 1999, when the attorneys realized that Johns Hopkins had sponsored the home's renovation as part of a research study. Shapiro recalls that the law firm did not, at first, consider KKI to be culpable in any way. KKI was "usually involved in treating the firms' clients" and J. Julian Chisolm, one of the KKI researchers, had testified on behalf of hundreds of these poisoned children.[9] In fact, a close, informal relationship had developed since the early 1980s between the lawyers representing kids and KKI because Chisolm treated nearly all of these children at the institute. When the Baltimore Health Department discovered children with high blood lead levels in the course of routine screenings, they were likely to be referred to KKI for treatment.[10]

The lawsuits that emerged on behalf of Michael H. and Enid G. alleged that "the children [in the study] were poisoned, or at least exposed to the risk of being poisoned, by lead dust due to negligence on the part of KKI." Specifically, the lawsuit charged that KKI had "failed to warn" the families of the potential harm to the children from the lead remaining in their homes and had not made the families "fully informed of the risks of the research."[11] The lawsuits would reverberate throughout the lead research community and ultimately through the worlds of public health and bioethics because the questions raised were fundamental to the research of many scientists and the programs of many advocates. The internal debates among scientists and lead activists in the 1990s over thresholds of safety for lead and primary versus secondary prevention provided the fodder for what would ultimately become one of the most explosive issues in public health ethics in decades. But seen through the lens of history, this story is ultimately about something larger: the ethics of a society that treats the health of a portion of its citizenry with indifference.

THE OPENING SKIRMISH

The lawsuits of two children, Michael H. and Enid G., were initially filed separately in the lower court, the Circuit Court for Baltimore City.[12] On February 22, 2000, Johns Hopkins and KKI's attorney, Susan Boyce, asked that the charges be dismissed, on the grounds that "there is no contract or special relationship between KKI and Ms. [H.]" and that KKI was under no "duty to protect the plaintiff from harm." In its initial written defense, then, KKI denied responsibility for the lead poisoning that any children may have suffered in its lead study. KKI argued that its "role" was simply to conduct research and that it had no role inducing the family "to occupy the subject property." Furthermore, Boyce argued, KKI had not leased the apartment and had only "limited contacts" with Ms. H. "*after* she moved into" the apartment and "voluntarily consented to participate in the study." Boyce predicted dire consequences for science if the court held KKI responsible in this case, suggesting that it "would have a chilling effect on all research projects that are being conducted every day in hospitals and institutions all over the country . . . that are designed to try to *eliminate* hazards in the most efficacious way." To hold KKI responsible "would be a terrible tragedy for all citizens. And particularly for the children of Baltimore City who are being exposed to lead based paint in older homes every day."[13]

"If KKI is guilty of anything it is guilty of trying to help these children, not harm them," when you considered the social context within which the study was constructed, Boyce continued. Poor African American children in Baltimore had been at risk of lead poisoning before any had volunteered to be part of the study; the housing the children lived in already had a lead hazard and, therefore, "it was not the study that presented any risk of harm" to the children. "It was the circumstances in which [the children] found themselves completely independent of whether they participated in the study." For a century, lead poisoning had been a plague on the homes of Baltimore's children, and almost no one had "taken up the banner of children exposed to this hazard."[14]

In their argument, the lawyers for Johns Hopkins and KKI were returning to one of the fundamental rationales for the study's design in the early 1990s: it was utopian to "require that all lead paint will be removed from all houses." Hence, Hopkins supported research "to find out whether there are lesser treatments than full abatement which can be helpful in limiting exposure to lead dust." To test which of the "differing approaches to remediation of lead paint dust" was most effective, Hopkins maintained, any research had to "involve the presence of lead paint."[15] According to this argument, good research required that children be exposed to lead.

In oral arguments before Judge Allen L. Schwait, in early April 2000, Boyce amplified KKI's two basic arguments. First, KKI was merely "an observer" that "collect[ed] information about an existing and evolving condition which KKI neither created nor controlled." Because the danger from lead exposure already existed, "KKI did nothing to introduce appellants to any hazardous conditions." Second, KKI was carrying out a study that, in order to meet the requirements of epidemiological rigor, compared systematically the effects on children of differing levels of lead exposure in the home. If anything, Boyce argued, the plaintiffs in the case and all the study participants had benefited from being part of KKI's research study because "all flaking, chipping and peeling paint was removed and some degree of additional remediation was provided."[16]

Thus, according to KKI's attorneys, not only was the Mark Farfel and Julian Chisolm study unquestionably good in its intentions, it was purely observational and entailed no manipulation of variables or conditions. In making this initial case, KKI's attorneys employed a narrow, legalistic argument that they themselves subsequently recognized was untenable. With respect to the family in question, "all KKI [did] was to periodically enter the premises to collect dust samples and to obtain blood samples from [Michael H.]."[17] And because the study was merely observational, the KKI lawyers argued, it did not need to inform or warn parents or the children themselves about the potential danger that lurked in the dust in their homes. KKI's attorneys argued that the researchers were not involved in an experiment at all but were "passively" collecting data, rather than "actively doing something to the participants such as providing medical treatment or subjecting them to dangerous conditions such as a deep sea dive." Because "the law requires informed consent before an actor does something to a person," the legal team went on, KKI's "only duty to Appellants was to inform them of any risks in collecting the data." KKI did this by telling the study subjects of the very minimal "risks attendant to the collection of blood," and, therefore, KKI had met—even exceeded—the requirements of the law.[18]

The KKI lawyers were drawing a sharp distinction between active and passive research, medicine versus public health, a distinction that was rarely as clear in practice, and certainly not in this case. But the argument that KKI presented initially to the Baltimore City Circuit Court did capture many of the rationales behind observational public health research in the 1990s and why it differed from medical research. Medical research introduced new procedures, medicines, or technologies that were unavailable to the lay person. Public health research, by contrast, collected data useful in evaluating differing exposures and circumstances of persons in their everyday lives. Whatever the possible risks for individuals who lived in dangerous circumstances or engaged in unhealthful personal behaviors, the public health investigator was not actively subjecting the study participant to these dangerous circumstances or behaviors. Further, testing a proprietary drug or device by providing it to some individuals and not to others was fundamentally different from surveillance of individuals in their everyday habitat. The argument KKI developed was that the latter type of research could result in broad societal changes that could benefit entire populations and prevent illness, not simply treat it. Far from exploiting a vulnerable population, KKI saw its role as instead akin to being a "volunteer" in a neighborhood where children were at risk.

The lower court raised just this distinction at its hearing on KKI's motion for summary judgment on the merits of the case: Judge Schwait asked the attorney for the child "why KKI owed you [the plaintiff] anything at all? KKI is a volunteer here. What's the duty?" The attorney, Allen Mensh, responded, "My main argument really is the duty to warn, Judge." Schwait then asked, "Why do they have a duty to warn?" to which Mensh answered, "Because they know about the hazards; they know that there is lead paint dust here; that it's increasing; and they did actually have her sign a consent form."[19]

> The Court: "You consider this like a patient/doctor relationship where they have a duty to inform and other sorts of duties?"
>
> Mr. Mensh: "Well, there definitely is a relationship here. I mean, it's a medical institution coming in and doing a medical study. They're using these children as subjects to that study. I think there is a duty to warn."
>
> The Court: "I don't think it's medical. I think it's more like a public health, in this context."[20]

The lawyers for KKI gave a passionate defense of the institution and its public health mission, even arguing that far from being able to predict possible harm, the researchers could only anticipate positive outcomes for the children and their families. The only thing "foreseeable," as the lawyers and KKI saw it, was that the selected children from Baltimore's poor communities would have a lowered exposure to lead because Kennedy Krieger had been fixing up their houses and moving families into homes with lower lead dust levels. "If it hadn't been for this study, this house would not have been touched; this child would have been exposed to more lead," said KKI's attorneys.[21]

Furthermore, the KKI lawyers said, the H. family had already been warned by the landlord that lead was probably present in their apartment and was a danger. For example, shortly before Kathy H. and Joan M. (a roommate) and their children moved into the house on East Federal Street on May 17, 1994, they signed a "lease addendum" that Lawrence Polakoff had prepared to warn them about the lead dangers in the house: "Eating or chewing paint or plaster or household dust that contains lead, by children, especially under 6 years of age may cause severe illness. Areas in the property that are of particular concern for chipping, flaking, loose or peeling paint, plaster or wallpaper are doors, windows, woodwork and wood trim and molding." The lease addendum told the parents that if they found any of these conditions, "you must notify us within [sic] writing so that we can make the necessary repairs."[22] Although KKI would later say that by signing this lease addendum the parents "knew or should have known" the dangers that living in this apartment posed,[23] the addendum primarily addressed the traditional conception of lead poisoning and the danger to children of eating "flakes" and pieces of lead in plaster, and only in passing the peril for children of ingesting or breathing lead dust.

KKI also had warned study participants, Boyce said, "that lead poisoning in Baltimore City is a severe problem. That Kennedy Krieger was doing this study to determine whether they can find a cost-effective way to reduce a child's exposure to lead, that repairs and maintenance were done to this property and they wanted to do periodic dust sampling to find out whether the repairs and maintenance worked." Boyce concluded, "I mean, I don't know what more they could have told this woman."[24]

The Circuit Court for Baltimore City accepted KKI's argument and dismissed the case the same day, April 5, 2000, writing that "KKI was sort of an institutional volunteer in the community." KKI had come into the community with the best of intentions, the judge declared, and "the next thing you know they get sued."[25]

THE LAWSUIT APPEALED

There the matter stood legally for eight months, until January 2001, when the young attorney at Kerpelman and Associates, Suzanne Shapiro, filed an appeal with Maryland's Court of Special Appeals, which screened cases that might ultimately be brought to the state's highest court, the Court of Appeals. The appeal was specifically based on what Shapiro saw as a misinterpretation and misrepresentation of the KKI study. Far from merely being a surveillance of existing conditions, she said, the study was a research experiment with no therapeutic value to the children who were put at risk. These children were part of a vulnerable population because of their socioeconomic status and race as well as their age. As such, Kennedy Krieger had a special obligation to make it absolutely clear that the families were not benefiting from the research and that their homes were still dangerous environments for young children. Further, KKI could not claim that it was a passive "volunteer" helping a community in need when the institute itself was actively manipulating the conditions of the homes and the placement of families in these homes. In sum, the appeal was an indictment of the KKI lawyers' public health rationale for the study. KKI, working with poor children and young mothers, had a responsibility not only to document dangerous circumstances, Shapiro said, but also to inform the parents of all potential dangers and to protect the children from harm.[26]

After all, Shapiro argued, "Kennedy could reasonably foresee the danger to which the minor plaintiff was exposed." She pointed out that "Kennedy was well aware of the fact that the home contained unacceptable levels of lead in house dust," and that the children "could potentially ingest this leaded dust through normal hand to mouth activity, and that this ingestion could lead to permanent irreversible brain damage and neurobehavioral deficits."[27] While Kennedy Krieger may not have done the actual repairs or even paid for them, Shapiro argued, it was hardly a "passive" participant collecting data. It had designed the experiment, it had required that leaded homes be part of the study, it had contracted for limited repairs knowing that the danger of ingestion of lead dust by the children in residence was still a probability, it had received federal grants to carry out the research and the partial repairs on the houses, and, perhaps most damningly, KKI had "encouraged the landlord to lease the property to a family with a young child, and then waited for the minor plaintiff to move into the home in order to solicit the child's participation in the experiment."[28]

"Kennedy's intentions may have been benevolent," she conceded, as "it sought to advance scientific knowledge." But public health researchers had a greater obligation than to the limited goals of finding cost-effective means of reducing lead poisoning, or even to science. KKI "may have hoped that no child would be lead poisoned," but, Shapiro argued, there was every "expectation . . . that some children would develop lead poisoning." In essence, KKI was "sacrificing the health of the Study children" and was "utilizing them as guinea pigs to determine cost effective environmental treatment of lead-based paint."[29]

At the heart of the legal and ethical issues of the case, Shapiro suggested, was the disparity of knowledge and power between the researchers and the subjects of the study: "At a minimum, Kennedy owed a duty to warn of the specific hazards known to Kennedy and unknown to the participants." Whatever the minimal, technical requirements of the Johns Hopkins institutional review board's consent form, "every person has a right to freely choose what happens to his or her body and whether to participate in a research study that entails physical risks to his or her body." The rights of vulnerable children and young parents, and the obligation of IRBs, she argued, went beyond a specific legal form or a narrow definition of responsibility: "Consent to participate in research cannot be truly informed unless the researcher fully discloses to the subject all of the information necessary for the subject to freely choose whether to participate." Simply put, KKI understood that the lead and dust tests performed indicated that some areas "still contained high levels of lead in dust above the clearance criteria in Maryland for abated homes," but KKI did not inform Michael's mother for weeks, if not months later, that her child was at risk.[30] By this time, the child's blood lead levels had already risen.

The tension that marked the arguments of both the lawyers for Johns Hopkins and for Michael H. reflected a broader split in the lead research and advocacy communities that had erupted after the initial filing of the lawsuit. The fact that generations of children were struck down by lead paint on the walls of their homes made the study appear reasonable and even noble to some. The KKI research held out the promise of a methodology that could be repeatedly used for research in the service of protecting future generations while, at the same time, maintaining the housing stock that the poor lived in. Thus it came to be that the National Center for Lead-Safe Housing, a nonprofit corporation founded in 1992 and led by Nick Farr and Dave Jacobs, supported Kennedy Krieger in the lawsuit in an amicus brief for the appeal.[31] The center described the dangers of a victory for the plaintiffs in this case in stark terms: it would have "true potential to forestall the only type of research that can provide answers to the daunting problems faced by cities like Baltimore, with a substantial deteriorating housing stock, most of which contains old, deteriorated lead-based paint."[32] In the center's view, complete removal of lead was just not economically practical, given competing political agendas and the dilapidated condition of the nation's housing stock for poor people. "The dollar value of the houses involved may actually be less than the unit cost of such an extensive abatement process," the center suggested. That was why the KKI research was so important: the nation needed "a less extensive intervention methodology" that could "lead to successful lead-dust reduction."[33]

The National Center for Lead-Safe Housing specifically opposed the amicus brief of another advocacy organization, the Public Justice Center, which supported the suit. Founded in 1985, the Public Justice Center was, in its own words, a Maryland "non-profit, civil rights and anti-poverty legal service organization dedicated to preserving the rights of the underrepresented." The justice center recognized that "the development of scientific knowledge through research on human subjects is a valuable pursuit." But, it warned, "good intentions can have bad consequences, as exemplified by the misuse and abuse of humans, especially African Americans and children during many research studies." Contrary to the lead-safe housing group's argument that the suit against KKI would have a chilling effect on other research projects, the Public Justice Center argued that recognizing the duty of scientists and public health researchers to protect human research subjects from unreasonable harm "will improve scientific research by restoring and retaining the most critical element of all human research: the public trust."[34]

Kennedy Krieger's attorneys replied that lead poisoning as a result of the study's interventions was not foreseeable and, in fact, "the lives of each and every one of these children was improved." They cited the researchers' report to the Environmental Protection Agency in 1998 after completion of the project's second year. Those findings showed, they argued, that over time most children had reductions in blood lead levels, therefore proving the benefits of the research. Though KKI's lawyers did not dispute the results of Michael's blood tests, they refused to acknowledge that any harm might have been done to any of the children. In fact, KKI's attorneys said, "everything KKI did for the R&M Study benefitted the participants, from eliminating lead hazards in their homes to providing blood lead monitoring that they otherwise would not have had."[35]

The KKI lawyers also rejected comparisons made by the Public Justice Center and others linking Johns Hopkins research not only to Nazi medical experimentation but also to the infamous Tuskegee study in which the U.S. Public Health Service watched as more than one hundred African American men slowly succumbed to the effects of syphilis over the course of four decades, without offering them treatment.[36] The KKI defense said the accusations were absurd: "KKI concentrated its efforts in poor African American communities because that is where the need is greatest." Far from exploiting a vulnerable population, KKI had acted in their best interest. "One can hardly imagine a more noble cause than KKI's efforts to help the children of Baltimore fight against the scourge of lead paint poisoning."[37]

The positions of the plaintiffs and the university were starkly different: Suzanne Shapiro, the attorney for the children (the H. and G. cases were now consolidated in the appeal), argued that specific children had been injured and that KKI had had an obligation to protect them. Given their abrogation of responsibility, Johns Hopkins owed some form of restitution. The university attorneys insisted, however, that even those youngsters whose blood lead levels rose had not incurred any more injury than they would have had there been no experiment, given the terrible housing conditions that existed for low-income families in Baltimore. More broadly, the university's defense argued that the research conducted was both moral and necessary if children in Baltimore and other cities were to be protected in the long run from the scourge of lead poisoning. Essentially, the needs of the larger community demanded that the research be allowed to proceed.

Shapiro rejected the KKI argument by drawing a contrast between the needs of the researchers and the rights of the children and other vulnerable populations. "Affordable lead-safe housing may be scarce in Baltimore City," she acknowledged, but "that fact alone does not entitle Kennedy to experiment on housing conditions in low-income neighborhoods of Baltimore without assuming a duty to minimize the risks to the subjects."[38]

The university's arguments "simply miss the point," she went on. The State's obligation was to protect human subjects despite potential benefits to the population at large. "It is not legally, ethically, nor morally acceptable to spare the health of even a few innocent children for the advancements of science or the future benefit of others in society." She took on the university's rejection of the comparisons with Tuskegee and Nazi human experimentation as well. While KKI might take "offense" at these comparisons "it is important for this court to understand that the very reason medical ethics codes and federal regulations have evolved for the protection of subjects of research is directly in response to these types of past abuses of poor and vulnerable populations by medical researchers." Citing other notorious examples—such as the case of mentally retarded children at New York's Willowbrook School in the early 1970s who were used as subjects in hepatitis research, the Jewish chronic disease study where patients were injected with cancer cells, the human radiation experiments at Vanderbilt University in which primarily poor women suffering from cancer were injected with plutonium without their knowledge or consent, and the then-recent University of Pennsylvania gene therapy experiment in which a young research subject slipped into a coma and died after injection with a genetically altered cold virus—Shapiro warned that "the twentieth and twenty-first centuries have witnessed specific cases where the social benefits of research have come at the expense of desperate or unknowing participants drawn from the most vulnerable groups in society." Like the victims in these other cases, parents and their children in the KKI study—"children who are voiceless and who are unable to determine for themselves whether they wish to be part of this research"—were "not on an equal footing" with the researchers and their institutional backers. Shapiro specifically rejected any utilitarian argument that positioned the benefits to society over the rights of the individual. "No matter what Kennedy's end goal was in trying to better the greater good of society or advance science," she concluded, "this does not abrogate its duty that all citizens share, to ensure that it act reasonably [so] as not to bring harm to another."[39] The simple fact was, she said, some children entered a renovated home with low blood lead levels and in the course of the study their blood lead levels rose to dangerous heights.[40]

In oral arguments before the Maryland Court of Appeals, Shapiro argued that to have at least begun to fulfill its responsibility to fully inform study participants of potential dangers, Johns Hopkins would have had to use a consent form that explicitly stated the dangers of exposure to lead. Referring to the very first sentence of the Johns Hopkins's consent form, she noted its inadequacy as a warning to parents. It stated that "lead paint is a known problem in Baltimore City and other communities around the country," but the document "never defines what that problem is," Shapiro pointed out.[41]

Shapiro then zeroed in on the fatal flaws in the experiment. First, Johns Hopkins did not "protect the research subject from unreasonable harm," and second, the study was "not just examining the world as it already existed. Kennedy actually wanted to control the environments of these homes." In other words, this was not just an observational surveillance study of children and parents living in their preexisting home environments. Far from being passive observers, KKI recruited "landlords [asking them to] give [KKI] homes that have lead in them." Then the Kennedy Krieger researchers "decide[d] to randomly assign these homes to three different groups, and give different levels of minimal repair to each home."[42]

Further, the KKI researchers already knew the answers to the questions the study was meant to address, Shapiro charged. "Kennedy is not trying to find the safest way to prevent children from getting lead poisoning. Kennedy already knows that the safest way ... is to fully and completely abate homes or put children in homes that were built after 1980 that don't have any lead paint in them." The real "purpose of the study," Shapiro argued, "was to see if there was anything cheaper that could be done [because] landlords say it is too expensive to fully abate these homes."[43] There was a line between "ethical" and "unethical" experimentation, and KKI had crossed it. KKI researchers, Shapiro pointed out, "could have done a different experiment" that would have been observational in nature, based on information gleaned from the records of the Baltimore Health Department: "They could have gone to the homes where those children were poisoned and ... measured the dust in those homes." If they had done that, Johns Hopkins would have had a legitimate argument that "they were just passively observing the collected data."[44]

Shapiro avowed that far from protecting the children, KKI had actually put children in harm's way.[45] The court asked Shapiro, was there "an agreement between the landlord and Kennedy that the landlord must rent the premise to a family that had young children?" She pointed to the deposition of landlord Polakoff, where he had said "he was supposed to rent the house to a [family] with healthy children," a point confirmed by the study's principal investigators. The court asked whether "Kennedy was recruiting children, healthy children to live in these homes," to which Shapiro answered, "Exactly." Furthermore, the lead research community in general and Kennedy Krieger researchers in particular understood that "even if paint was intact to the naked eye ... it could still be shedding dust particles into the air and ... this dust could harm children." As a result of this knowledge, Shapiro argued, it was "one hundred percent foreseeable to Kennedy that there was a risk . . . an unreasonable risk . . . that these children were going to get poisoned, were likely to get poisoned."[46]

Shapiro insisted that it was precisely for situations like this that federal regulations aimed at protecting human research subjects existed. History had taught, she pointed out, that "the researcher's interest in advancing science conflicts sometimes with the duty to protect the research subject." In this specific case, the mothers were never told directly by KKI that "we believe inherent in the study a child living in that home may be poisoned. And that means permanent, irreversible brain damage to your child."[47] The parents and children were "volunteers" and they were "benefiting Kennedy," Shapiro said, yet they were "not getting any benefit from this at all."[48]

The attorney for KKI, Michael Joseph of Godard, West & Adelman, objected. He thought it was "disingenuous" to argue that "to be able to live in a home that had these repairs done to it" did not count as a benefit. The court responded, "You're talking about a child that had no lead paint, is normal for lead paint *[sic]*, . . . and end[s] up with elevated lead paint levels *[sic]*, and you say that's a benefit?" Playing on the fact that the children's baseline blood lead levels were taken shortly after the study began, Joseph answered that "we don't know what this child's lead levels were before moving into this home, nor do we know where this child was poisoned." The court asked, "I thought your study required healthy children to be included in the study," and Joseph answered, "Because that was the only way to measure if the children did get poisoned."[49] Whatever lead hazard existed in the house amounted to an improvement over what had existed before, Joseph asserted. "These homes were in disrepair. Kennedy went in there and improved the homes," reducing the dust to "permissible lead levels. And in this case, the home was repaired so that it was below" Maryland's legal standard. Far from being hazardous, "there was no lead hazard in the home. This home was made safe. And Kennedy instructed the landlords, put children in these homes that we've made safe." The court was skeptical. "If they're safe, then why test children's blood," the court asked. To which Joseph responded, "Because . . . they were testing to see which levels worked best. . . . I think they suspected that all [levels of partial abatement] were going to be effective. . . . Each level made some improvement to the home."[50] All of these improvements, Joseph argued "were for the benefit of society at large and these children," to which the court added, "and the landlords."[51]

By improving the property so that the levels of lead were below the legal maximum allowed at the time, KKI maintained that the researchers were absolved from any legal liability. But Shapiro countered that new research had uncovered the devastating effects of low-level lead exposure on children. KKI's researchers knew better than to argue that the legal standards were adequate to protect children from lead's harm, she pointed out. Because they had this specialized knowledge, they had an obligation to warn the parents of the potential danger that their children faced as part of the experiment.[52]

In the end, Shapiro acknowledged that the KKI study might have been socially valuable in showing how the level of lead to which children were exposed could be reduced in a way that would minimize landlord abandonment of Baltimore's housing stock. "It might even be noble and beneficial," she said. But none of this overrode the rights of research subjects. "Our society has made a value judgment," she argued. "And that value judgment is that the rights of the individual research subject to autonomy, to dignity, to protection overrides the right of our society to advance science." The reason for this societal decision was rooted in the sixty-year-old debate in the history of science: "The reason we've made that judgment is based on lessons we've learned from history . . . that scientific research can cause harm, unreasonable harm to research subjects." Shapiro reminded the court of the Nuremberg Code, the Declaration of Helsinki, and the more recent Belmont Report, *Ethical Principles and Guidelines for the Protection of Human Subjects of Research*, that had been issued in 1978 by the U.S. Department of Health, Education and Welfare (now Health and Human Services). Together, these defined "the duty that we owe to research subjects" and that duty "overrides the advancement of science. We don't sacrifice [an] individual's health to advance science. That's a judgment that we've made and that creates the duty."[53]

THE COURT DECISION

It was a hot August day when the Maryland Court of Appeals, the state's highest court, filed its opinion in the now-joined cases of Enid G. and Michael H. versus the Kennedy Krieger Institute.[54] In a detailed, very lengthy decision written by Dale R. Cathell, considered one of the more conservative judges on the bench,[55] the court began by reviewing the KKI study that was the subject of the civil suit. The study was important to look at closely, because "nontherapeutic research using minors" was an issue that has "been virtually unanalyzed by courts and legislatures" since 1977, when the National Commission for the Protection of Human Subjects of Biomedical and Behavioral Research had issued its report on research involving children. The court noted that Kennedy Krieger, "a prestigious research institute," had "encouraged" and even "required" landlords to rent houses with lead paint to families with young children "in order for his or her blood to be periodically analyzed." The moral question that was at the heart of the study, according to the court, was whether it was appropriate to use children of "lower economic strata" to determine if specific abatement methods were effective.[56]

The court observed that researchers Mark Farfel and Julian Chisolm understood the dangers of exposing young children to lead in their homes, citing their 1990 study in the *American Journal of Public Health* in which they had reported that "lead-bearing dust is particularly hazardous for children." The court continued that "after publishing this report, the researchers began the present research project in which children were encouraged to reside in households where the possibility of lead dust was known to the researchers to be likely." Thus, the court asserted, "apparently, it was anticipated that the children . . . would, or at least might, accumulate lead in their blood."[57]

Much of the decision was a scathing critique of Johns Hopkins that paralleled the arguments Suzanne Shapiro had made.[58] Judge Cathell questioned the judgment of both the researchers and the university's institutional review board. Either they "apparently saw nothing wrong with the [re]search protocols that anticipated the possible accumulation of lead in the blood of otherwise healthy children as a result of the experiment, or they believed that the consents of the parents of the children made the research appropriate." Judge Cathell was particularly critical of the IRB at Hopkins, which had the responsibility to guarantee the safety of the human subjects of any experiment, especially children and other vulnerable subjects. The IRB's function, he pointed out, "is *not* to help researchers seek funding for research projects."[59]

The court decision explored the intricacies of the ethical, moral, and legal issues raised by the case, but its angry tone reflected six of the seven judges' views that "the very inappropriateness of the research itself cannot be overlooked." Whatever the specific defenses of the research methods, the protocols, the IRB's actions, or compliance with applicable safety requirements, the court rejected the argument that the personal rights of the children could be put at risk "for the greater good." In particular, the court discarded the idea that children's health could be "put at risk in order to develop low-cost abatement methods that would help all children, the landlords, and the general public as well."[60]

The court pulled out all of the rhetorical stops by comparing KKI's actions with those of several infamous cases mentioned by the plaintiffs' attorney:

"the Tuskegee Syphilis Study . . . the intentional exposure of soldiers to radiation . . . the tests involving the exposure of Navajo miners to radiation . . . and the secret administration of LSD to soldiers by the CIA and the Army." The court acknowledged that "in the present case, children, especially young children, living in lower economic circumstances," might not be "as vulnerable as the other examples," but they were "vulnerable as well."[61]

The court rejected the basis for the lower court's dismissal of the case, which had sided with Johns Hopkins's argument that its actions were benevolent and therefore the institution was not responsible for unforeseen and unintended consequences of its good works. In the end, the court of appeals held that universal principles were needed, rather than judgments based on the prestige or ostensibly good intentions of researchers, because "history is replete with claims of noble purpose for institutions and institutional volunteers."[62]

"The very nature of nontherapeutic scientific research on human subjects can, and normally will, create special relationships out of which duties arise," the appeals court maintained; indeed, the Nuremberg Code had been established to assert the principle that researchers had a duty to their research subjects.[63] Further, while the State of Maryland might not have specific requirements regarding the obligations of researchers in general, and specifically when that research involved children, the federal government did. And because KKI's research was funded by the EPA, that research was therefore subject to these federal regulations.[64]

The court also criticized Johns Hopkins for the inadequacy of what it conveyed to the study families: "there was no complete and clear explanation" to either the parents or the children that the whole purpose of the research was "to measure the success of the abatement procedures by measuring the extent to which the children's blood was being contaminated." In summary, the court opined, "it can be argued that the researchers intended that the children be the canaries in the mines but never clearly told the parents."[65] Legally, the court maintained, the consent form laid out a "reciprocal set of obligations" that constituted a contract between the parents and KKI. For participating in the research study, the parents and their children would receive "all the information necessary for the subject to freely choose whether to participate, and continue to participate, and receive promptly any information that might bear on their willingness to continue to participate in the study." In return for this information, the court noted, "KKI received a measuring tool—the children's blood."[66] In the court's view "a reasonable parent would expect to be clearly informed that it was at least contemplated that her child would ingest lead dust particles" and that the child's blood was the measure of the experiment's success or failure. If parents were given this information "it might be difficult to obtain human subjects for the research," but that did not change the fact that the researchers "needed to supply the information." Nor did it "alter the ethics of failing to provide such information."[67]

In the end, the court believed that the federal regulations "strike right at the heart of KKI's defense" because "*fully informed* consent is lacking in these cases. There clearly was more than a minimal risk involved. Under the regulations, children should not have been used for the purpose of measuring how much lead they would accumulate in their blood while living in partially abated houses to which they were recruited initially or encouraged to remain, because of the study."[68]

The court's condemnation of the research went beyond the issue of informed consent or narrow legalistic arguments, however. In its view, "otherwise healthy children should not be the subjects of nontherapeutic experimentation or research that has the potential to be harmful to the child." Not only was the consent inadequate, but its very premise was unacceptable because, the court held, children were an especially vulnerable special class and in nontherapeutic research their rights could not be signed away, even by their parents.[69] It did not matter, the court said, that "the general motives of all concerned in these contested cases, were, for the most part, proper, albeit in our view not well thought out."[70] Knowingly putting children in harm's way was not acceptable.

THE DECISION'S AFTERMATH

Many were shocked by the tone of the decision and the comparisons with such egregious past instances of research impropriety. Contributing to that tone may have been the timing of the court's deliberations, a tumultuous period of judicial and professional self-examination following two dramatic moments in the history of human experimentation. In September 1999, two years before the Maryland court wrote its opinion, the world learned of the death of Jesse Gelsinger, an eighteen-year-old volunteer at the University of Pennsylvania, who died during an experiment testing gene therapy to correct a metabolic problem.[71] The Food and Drug Administration found that the university's consent form had failed to provide the patient all relevant information, including the fact that monkeys that had received the same treatment had died.

And just weeks before the court of appeals heard oral arguments in the KKI case, the medical community at Johns Hopkins had been rocked by another emerging scandal. On June 2, 2001, Ellen Roche, a twenty-four-year-old medical school employee at Johns Hopkins's Asthma and Allergy Center, died after she had volunteered in a research study conducted there. Roche had inhaled 1 gram of hexamethonium as part of a study on the effect of this substance on bronchial nerve ganglia. Soon thereafter she developed a dry cough and then flu-like symptoms, fever, and shortness of breath. She entered Johns Hopkins Bayview Medical Center, but her symptoms worsened and she died three weeks later. When the federal Office for Human Research Protections investigated, it found the Hopkins human subject protection system deficient and discovered numerous transgressions of good research protocol by both the researchers and the university's institutional review board. The asthma researchers had not properly informed volunteers of the potential risks; they had referred to the experimental material as "a medication," leading research subjects to believe there was little danger; they failed to tell subjects that hexamethonium had been identified as a dangerous material in the 1970s and had "never been approved by the FDA for administration via inhalation"; and they had not reported that the material had previously been noted in the medical literature as causing "cough, shortness of breath, and decreased lung function." The Office for Human Research Protections also found that the Hopkins IRB had failed to do a good literature review that would have identified many of these problems, had not held "properly constituted meetings," and had not included laypersons or experts from fields other than the medical sciences.[72] As a result of these findings, the federal agency shut down hundreds of clinical trials at Johns Hopkins for five days.[73]

Cognizance of these cases may have contributed to the tone of the Maryland court's decision in the KKI case, but probably not to its substance. The Kennedy Krieger decision received national attention in the *Washington Post*, the *New York Times*, the Associated Press, National Public Radio, and other media outlets. While the court "could have limited its remarks to a narrow legal question," the *Post* noted, it chose instead to issue "a scathing ... opinion that broadly admonished research methods in the state" and the actions of the Johns Hopkins IRB. In its defense, Kennedy Krieger told the *Post* that it had more than two decades of research experience in lead poisoning that had "resulted in proven ways to help reduce the problem of childhood lead poisoning and have benefitted children and families by reducing their exposure to lead."[74] The co-principal investigator, Mark Farfel, took particular offense at the comparison with Tuskegee, since the broader community was doing very little to protect poor children from the scourge of lead paint. He told a reporter for the *Baltimore Sun* that "society was already doing a Tuskegee experiment. Very little if anything was happening to remove lead while children were being poisoned."[75]

In a subsequent interview with the Associated Press, Gary Goldstein, chief executive of KKI, maintained that understanding the context within which the research was conducted was all-important. The children were at high risk of lead poisoning in any case: "If you come into East Baltimore," Goldstein said, "it's not like one child in 100 is exposed. It's everyone, and we're trying to fix it." He argued that "if a child is lead-poisoned in one of those houses, is that our fault and are we doing something wrong by studying those children?"[76] Goldstein denounced the court for suggesting that KKI and its doctors would purposely put children in harm's way: "We were not trying to put children in houses and get them get lead-poisoned. We did not expect anyone to get lead-poisoned." Rather, the intentions were noble and benevolent, he said. Baltimore's poor were stuck in neighborhoods "where 95 percent of the houses contain lead" and where "35 percent of the kids have lead poisoning." The research was aimed at finding a way to provide housing that residents could move into "and not get lead-poisoned." In fact, that is exactly what happened: "for the majority of kids in the study, lead levels did go down."[77]

Contrary to the court's statements, KKI was providing a relatively safe environment for children who were otherwise fated to live in peril in homes polluted with lead paint, Goldstein told the *Washington Post*. "It's not that we intercepted people who were on their way to some treasure trove of lead-safe houses in Baltimore and directed them to houses with lead paint," he pointed out.[78] Farfel said, "The kids in the study [were] so much better off than the average kid in the city. . . . They benefited and society benefited as well." Farfel, who along with Julian Chisolm had dedicated his life to addressing the lead-poisoning plague in Baltimore, argued that the research design was not indifferent to the well-being of the children. "We made the environment better in every one of those houses," Farfel told the *Baltimore City Paper*.[79]

A week after the court's ruling, the Office for Human Research Protections of the Department of Health and Human Services announced that it had opened an investigation into KKI's Repair and Maintenance study.[80] The decision, particularly the court's allusions to Nazi science and Tuskegee, "rocked" pediatric and public health researchers around the country, according to two prominent lead researchers, Kim Dietrich and David Bellinger.[81] All wondered whether they faced a similar predicament in their own studies. What a number of them had in common with the KKI researchers was observing children in less than fully abated homes and recognition that these children were at some risk. Unlike Farfel and Chisolm's research, however, other studies had not actively intervened in the creation of the children's environments. Lead researchers were also faced with reconciling the traditional public health commitments to protection and prevention against disease with the desire to make at least some positive difference, given that governing institutions seemed unwilling to spend the money to protect primarily poor African American and Hispanic children.

Others in the public health and medical fields worried about the legal implications of the court's decision.[82] Michael Weitzman, director of the American Academy of Pediatrics' Center for Child Health Research, called the KKI lawsuit "a profoundly important, ironic and sad case." He worried that the court's decision could make it more difficult to conduct similar types of research in the future. Here was the dilemma: "You never, ever want to hurt a child or put a child in harm's way. But for very large numbers of America's children, the only way that we can protect them from lead, at this particular point in history, is to do this type of research."[83]

Ellen Silbergeld, who had done pioneering toxicological work on lead and other toxic substances, gave a troubled commentary on the issues raised by the KKI study. In a *Washington Post* op-ed titled "A Necessary Paradox," she noted the special resonance the case held in light of Ellen Roche's recent death in the Johns Hopkins asthma study and Jesse Gelsinger's death in 1999 in the University of Pennsylvania's gene therapy experiment. All such cases raised difficult issues of a university's obligation to protect human subjects, and, Silbergeld argued, the KKI lead study illustrated the problem most clearly as one of "putting an individual at risk so that society can benefit." There were "tensions inherent in almost all such investigations." All public health efforts entailed some risk to the individual, Silbergeld argued, "but these risks paled in comparison to the benefits to the overall society." Vaccination campaigns, for example, asked individuals who might never come down with the disease to assume the small danger of having a bad reaction to the vaccine itself. "Yet, by participating in the societal commitment to vaccination, you protect the public at large," she wrote. The history of public health confirmed the value of this trade-off, and Silbergeld pointed "to the successful eradication of smallpox through a world-wide vaccination program."[84]

Such trade-offs between the potential for harm to the individual and the potential benefits to society were particularly important in lead poisoning in Baltimore, since so many "generations of children" had suffered needlessly from this terrible condition. "Throughout the 25 years I've worked in this field," wrote Silbergeld, "I've been continually angered by the complacency with which politicians, as well as many members of the medical profession, and public health community, accept the reality that as many as 5 percent of all American children continue to be poisoned by lead-based paint in their homes resulting in lowered IQs and brain damage." Silbergeld praised efforts "by investigators to devise new methods of prevention." She noted, however, that individuals in research settings had "the right to expect honorable and honest conditions of research" and that it was "the responsibility of institutional review boards to insure that this process works." But however stringent and responsible the IRBs and the researchers were, the paradox of public health was that the safeguards could "never resolve the tension inherent" in such research. Said Silbergeld, "These tensions are best settled by greater openness by researchers and subjects, between the medical community and the public."[85]

Other researchers agreed that there was an important rationale and need for studies like the Johns Hopkins one. "It's very important if these minor tune-ups of houses have any protective effect," Herbert Needleman commented to *U.S. News and World Report*. But, he said, "I happen to think most of them are useless."[86] Bruce Lanphear, an avid advocate for protecting children from lead who had recently published an important article suggesting that there may not be any level of lead exposure safe for children, captured the unhappiness of much of the research community with the court's denunciation of the KKI study. Lanphear argued that good, rigorous science demanded well-controlled studies such as Farfel and Chisolm's was intended to be. There was simply no other means of scientifically evaluating the effectiveness of specific lead-control efforts in stemming the epidemic other than "testing blood lead levels in children."[87]

The *Washington Post*, in a September 29, 2001, editorial, presented the most pointed defense of the KKI study and became the strongest critic of the court of appeals decision. "The Kennedy Krieger Institute in Baltimore took a brutal and unjustified walloping last month from Maryland's highest court," declared the *Post*. While the court characterized the "[KKI] study as an amoral experiment that put children at risk and offered them no benefit," the editorial maintained that KKI had done "nothing unethical." There may have been some mistakes, the paper suggested, but "none of this brings the study within a country mile of serious ethical lapses let alone the horrendous abuses at Tuskegee or Buchenwald." The *Post* contended that "far more offensive [than the study] is the social indifference that has let generations of children suffer the insidious menace of lead poisoning."[88]

But not everyone thought that the ostensible ends (for most of the children) justified the means (which ended up hurting a few). A reporter for the *Baltimore City Paper* criticized Farfel and Goldstein, pointing out that "what's better for the average child or better for the city—isn't necessarily good for the individual." The reporter argued that "the children were [used as] simply measuring devices like the vacuum cleaners that picked up dust samples, to test how much lead was left in the building."[89]

For the mother of one of the children in the study, the rationale for the research and the way it was carried out embodied some of the worst paternalistic aspects of black-white relations. The *Washington Post* reported that Joan M.'s worries about the "increasing lead levels in the blood of her 2-year-old daughter," Annabel M., were casually handled by "Miss Ruth," a member of the research team, who would simply give her "another supply of cleanser." Ms. M. was told to "mix it with water and the lead dust will go away. . . . Clean the windowsills. Clean the floors. Everything will be OK. But it wasn't. Annabel's lead levels got worse. . . . 'I felt betrayed [said Ms. M.] . . . I felt like my kids were used like guinea pigs.'"[90] According to the *Post*, one child's blood lead levels went from 6 to 21 micrograms per deciliter; another's went from 9 to 32 µg/dl; and a third's went from 10.7 to 24 µg/dl. For the families whose children's blood lead levels went up, the rationale that children were generally being poisoned anyhow gave little solace. They argued that their children should have been protected, not just observed, because the consequences were so severe. The *Post* reported that Enid G.'s mother wondered "whether the lead is responsible for her daughter's learning disabilities, attention problems and troubles at George Washington Elementary School," where her daughter repeated second grade. Enid's mother said that she wondered "most on the days when Enid comes home crying and asks: 'Mommy, I'm stupid?' I'm like, 'no, baby, you're not stupid. We just have to work harder.'"[91]

Enid's mother herself had been an honors student at Baltimore's Dunbar High School, had steady employment as a warehouse worker, and had grown up in a solid working-class family. Her mother worked in the Social Security Administration and her father was a construction worker. She had felt fortunate to live in the renovated, previously abated apartment on North Monroe. She had been living in a drug-infested, high-crime public housing project when she saw an ad for a $450-per-month row house in West Baltimore. "It's really getting bad. Every day somebody is getting killed. It's time for you to go," Enid's grandmother had said. "[Enid's mother] was thrilled to have fled that dangerous environment," a *Baltimore Sun* reporter wrote. "Her landlord assured her the home was lead free when she moved there in 1990. She later felt an extra layer of protection . . . from the presence of Kennedy Krieger researchers, who frequently visited to take samples for lead dust." Enid's mother told the *Sun*, "I thought, 'lead poisoning? How could this be when the scientists from Kennedy Krieger were coming in here to test it all the time?'"[92]

THE QUANDARY OF PUBLIC HEALTH RESEARCH

In September 2001, the Kennedy Krieger Institute, Johns Hopkins University, and the University of Maryland Medical System, along with others, asked the Maryland Court of Appeals to "reconsider or modify aspects of its August 16th ruling." They specifically asked the court to clarify its "ruling on the issue of parental and guardian consent for research on children," because if the ruling "were allowed to stand" it would "cripple pursuit of critical medical and public health research." The brief did not ask for the court to reverse its decision; the defendants argued, despite evidence to the contrary, that when the case was returned to the lower court, it would be made clear that the Repair and Maintenance study "brought benefits to all participating children and their families."[93]

This position had a great deal of support within the broader research and medical ethics community. Ruth Faden, a prominent Johns Hopkins ethicist, reflected on the history and implications of a narrow interpretation of the court's decision. She noted that the 1977 report of the National Commission for the Protection of Human Subjects of Biomedical and Behavioral Research had argued against a complete ban on experiments on children because of such experiments' potential importance for children's health. "There has been a big push in recent years to increase the amount of drug testing on children because we need to know how to treat sick kids," Faden told the *Baltimore Sun*, although the court had made a distinction between therapeutic and nontherapeutic research experiments.[94] The president of Johns Hopkins, Dr. William R. Brody, said he was worried that the court's decision "could have enormously broad implications, because almost all studies involve risk. The polio vaccine could never have been developed with this court decision." But he also had practical concerns. Brody worried that the court's decision "could drive tens of millions of dollars in research grants out of the state." According to the *Sun*, "Hopkins officials worry that 40 percent of their pediatrics research . . . could be disrupted."[95]

On October 11, 2001, the court of appeals reaffirmed its August ruling but clarified one of the most contentious issues raised by its decision. The court had said that children could not be subjected to "any" risk in nontherapeutic research, even with their parents' approval. This language had led many researchers to fear that "hundreds of on-going and planned studies involving children" could be shut down. In the course of reaffirming the decision, the court defined "any risk" as "any articulable risk beyond the minimal kind of risk that is inherent in any endeavor." This assuaged much of the fear but still caused worry for some.[96] Coming as it did at a moment when the generally accepted limit of safe exposure to lead was declining, and many researchers were arguing that no level of lead exposure was safe, even this clarification was likely to be a source of controversy among lead researchers.

The court's clarification also caused concern for those outside the world of lead research. Other forms of observational research, in the view of some, put certain people at risk: for example, epidemiological studies of obesity and diabetes, where surveillance of dietary habits and lifestyles of high-risk populations raised ethical questions about research designs that required subjects to be followed without intervention in order to reach statistically valid conclusions. This question became even more complicated around the time of the Kennedy Krieger study because many constituencies *wanted* to be included in medical research. Many believed that research protocols that left out women, children, the elderly, and ethnic and racial minorities were profoundly flawed. Ironically, much of the modern public health ethics that had been spelled out in the Belmont Report of the late 1970s were built around the rights of research subjects to be protected from "conscription" into studies that might prove harmful. But the AIDS crisis in particular had fundamentally altered the discourse, such that specific groups now insisted that it was their right to be included in research.[97]

This can be seen as a culmination of fifty years of defining biomedical and public health ethics in the wake of World War II, the revelations of Nazi medical experiments, and the subsequent development of the Nuremberg Code, whose first principle was the importance of the informed consent of voluntary participants.[98] More recently, public health advocates have extended this principle to broader concerns over the disproportionate pollution of poorer communities, developing the concepts of environmental justice and environmental racism. They have also focused on the role of researchers in exploiting vulnerable populations at home and abroad.[99]

The growing importance of environmental pollutants as a subject of research has raised new and troubling issues for academic researchers. For example, the 2004 decision of the Environmental Protection Agency, partially funded by the American Chemistry Council, to study the effects of pesticides on infants and toddlers by exposing them to the chemicals in their homes raised widespread outrage among environmental and consumer groups who argued that such activities violate central tenets of the

Nuremberg Code.[100] Revelations about the project led to its condemnation in Congress and then to its abandonment in 2005.[101] And the recent revelation of the purposeful infection of Guatemalan prisoners with syphilis in the 1940s is a shocking example of research malfeasance and the abuse of vulnerable (and in this case, foreign) populations by American researchers and public health authorities.[102]

While there are obviously vast differences between the problematic above-mentioned studies and what happened in Baltimore, it is significant that many in the lay public and some scholars have seen all these issues through the lens of human rights abuses. The questions for these instances of practice-based research (and other studies that are far less controversial) are, What is the boundary between ethical and unethical research? And How does one separate scientific questions from the societal pressures of a moment?[103]

LEAD SPECIALISTS AND THE KKI STUDY RULING

In the months following the Maryland Court of Appeals decision, scholars in the lead and medical research communities tried to unravel its meaning and its implications for research. The journal *Neurotoxicology and Teratology* devoted a special section to these questions in the summer of 2002. David Bellinger, one of the deans of lead toxicology, and Kim Dietrich, an important investigator of the effects of low-level lead exposure on children, convened an array of commentators to examine the "ethical issues in the conduct of pediatric environmental health, using the Kennedy-Krieger study ruling as a starting point." They brought together bioethicists, environmental health researchers, clinicians, and representatives from an environmental justice organization to examine the "ineluctable tension [that] exists at the intersection of bioethics and public health."

The tension that Bellinger and Dietrich identified reflected differences between public health and medical ethics: "Bioethical systems largely worked out in the context of clinical medicine, generally focus on the individual and his or her rights." But, Dietrich and Bellinger argued, "public health focuses on populations and more universalist conceptions of the 'common good.'" Public health was in a quandary and "it remains to be determined how, or whether, the canons of human subject protection will need to be amended in light of this tension."[104] Was the "greater good" that public health research promised in fact so important that harming a few individuals in the process was acceptable? Public health from the time of Edwin Chadwick, the nineteenth-century English official often credited with transforming the field by reforming urban sanitation in Great Britain, had been rooted in utilitarian principles that had to be reconsidered in light of the questions raised by suspect studies of vulnerable populations.

Paul Mushak, the toxicologist whose own work had been central to the discovery of airborne lead dust as a serious threat, argued that the logic and conclusions of the KKI decision were sounder than its hyperbolic rhetoric: "The matter of some intemperate judicial hyperbole aside, the Court's concerns reasonably align with accepted (albeit often somnolent) guidelines in the health science communities." The issues that arose at Kennedy Krieger emerged from a set of common "realities" that framed all research on any "pervasive toxic contaminant such as environmental lead." The "realities," Mushak posited, were that such toxins were ubiquitous throughout the environment and will cause "toxic harm . . . in the absence of effective remedial interventions becoming fundamental public health and regulatory policies." "Primary prevention of toxic exposures" is the "ideal societal and health science option," but it is not always politically possible. The "design and implementation of interim, i.e., not total or permanent, remedial interventions in the case of childhood lead exposures result in" real contradictions because "partial interventions require that children be studied in the absence of any empirical certitude as to total subject safety." In such research, Mushak believed, the safety of the children "requires an added set of safeguarding methodologies that avert development of toxic risk to children" as a "toxicological artifact of the research from the research itself."[105]

The most critical statement of the KKI research came from Howard Mielke, a researcher at Xavier University in New Orleans who had focused on how leaded gasoline exhaust affected children. He believed it was "unconscionable to use children as bioindicators of environmental lead" because children who were lead poisoned "are left with various degrees of intellectual and social disabilities." This was an "unethical and senseless practice," Mielke maintained. Primary prevention was the only ethically and scientifically acceptable approach to this environmental danger, in his view.[106]

Of those who contributed to the journal's special section, Don Ryan of the Alliance to End Childhood Lead Poisoning and Nick Farr of the National Center for Healthy Housing were the most sympathetic to the dilemmas that Kennedy Krieger researchers confronted. Ryan and Farr asked the research community to understand the real-life problems housing advocates faced: "Environmental health hazards are rampant in older low-income housing," but "for the most part, housing related health hazards go unexamined and unattended until disease occurs."[107] As a practical reality, they said, it was essential that research not lose sight of the economic costs of any measure that was promoted. Science would not provide "benefit to communities at risk unless [the recommendations and conclusions] are accessible, easy-to-use, and relatively low cost." Ryan and Farr argued that "lofty demands by scientists that substandard housing be upgraded to conform to risk models' ideals of safety are more likely to spawn cynicism and paralysis than spark actual public health gains." They pointed to Chisolm's and Farfel's work on the dangers of power sanding and open flame burning in lead paint removal as examples of practical research that led to meaningful change in federal regulations and actual practice. "Without such real world research of health hazards pervasive in substandard housing," they wrote, "unproven and even dangerous interventions can gain acceptance in practice or regulation."[108]

Lynn Pinder, the founder and executive director of Youth Warriors, a nonprofit community environmental justice organization working in Baltimore with young African Americans, provided counterpoint to the Ryan and Farr position.[109] Because of Johns Hopkins's and KKI's decades of effort in lead-poisoning prevention and treatment, she acknowledged, "poor children in urban cities, like Baltimore, are no longer dying from excessive amounts of lead poisoning." Yet, "Baltimore children live in the same neglected, lead-contaminated row houses that claimed lives decades ago. Despite the efforts of the university researchers, children in the poorest quarters of the city are being poisoned over and over at the same addresses."[110] She described how community organizations, including her own Youth Warriors, had examined the KKI study and had specific concerns about its very conception as well as about how it was implemented: "Families were recruited to participate in the R&M Study without a clear understanding that the risks of the R&M Study far outweighed the benefits." She reminded readers of the parents' expressed assumptions that because Johns Hopkins and Kennedy Krieger were involved, their children were at least going to be protected from harm and would possibly benefit from the study. Furthest from their minds was the possibility that the Hopkins researchers would put their children at risk.[111]

Pinder voiced more fundamental objections to the study as well. She believed that it sent the wrong signal to researchers and the public alike: "The R&M Study sent an erroneous message worldwide that 'alternative abatement methods' and/or 'interim controls' are long-term strategies for ending childhood lead poisoning." In fact, she argued, such approaches "are short-term strategies that only put off for a few years the inevitable—another lead-poisoned child." Quoting Herbert Needleman, she asserted that there was only one way to make sure that future generations were not harmed by lead: "the permanent removal of lead paint from dwellings . . . using safe work protocols."[112]

In his own contribution to the journal's special section, Needleman asked how good people ended up asking questions that were compromised from the beginning: "Why did it become necessary or desirable to conduct studies looking for the least expensive means of removing lead from houses?" Needleman traced the ways that human subjects research had evolved in the past few decades as statistical and epidemiological methodologies created abstractions of their clients and "subjects." He acknowledged the problems of early medical methods where physicians regularly "practiced" on patients, applying nostrums and experimental procedures "of uncertain efficacy and unknown risk." As practitioners and researchers had become more aware of patients' rights, and their own professional obligations to inform patients of the risks and benefits of medical procedures, some positive changes had occurred.[113]

Institutional review boards were certainly a part of this reform. But, Needleman pointed out, such efforts to oversee the activities of well-meaning practitioners and researchers were resented both by the medical and the public health communities, which considered the oversight an intrusion into the relationship "between us and the subjects of our inquiry, or of digressions between us and the answers we seek." But Needleman persisted. Despite the good intentions and noble ambitions of investigators, he said, such institutional oversight was necessary, "not because investigators are callous or evil, but because clinical studies by their nature do not grant subjects full status as persons." He cast his gaze specifically at epidemiological studies, which he said search "for normative content in *samples*, and deal with the differences in *people* by the use of summary variables such as standard deviations or confidence limits." Distancing was inherent in such epidemiological studies: "There is simply no room in spread sheets for the 'I-Thou' relationship that Martin Buber described. It is in the spreadsheets, not in the people, that the principle investigator finds the information he seeks, and in them, the 'Thou' of an individual is replaced by 'It.'"[114] Every aspect of a research project reinforces this disembodiment of the individuals in the study: "As a study is designed, the proposal written, the administrative structure to conduct it shaped and recruiting done, the patient as individual becomes more distant. As deadlines approach, problems appear and are dealt with, and subjects' singular identities fade." "It requires a strenuous effort to keep their personhood in mind and a vigilant external force to assure it," Needleman reminded his readers. This was not just the problem of researchers at Hopkins but, rather, "this distancing happens to everyone who has undertaken a clinical study."[115]

Needleman criticized the Maryland Court of Appeals for comparing what happened at Kennedy Krieger with Tuskegee and Nazi science. Whatever happened at KKI, the conduct of the research did not rise to the level of a crime such as took place at Tuskegee. The problem at Kennedy Krieger was nevertheless profound and went to the heart of American medical and public health science. For a brief moment in the early 1990s, at the very moment that the KKI study was being formulated and implemented, Needleman argued, the federal government had been on the verge of making a commitment "for the elimination of childhood lead poisoning," when government officials had told him that deleading the nation was a goal. But then strong opposition "from a number of quarters" undermined this possibility. As Needleman lamented, "It was not long before the vision of the early 1990s, true primary prevention, eradication of the disease in 15 years, was replaced by an enfeebled pseudopragmatism."[116]

It was "in this climate" Needleman continued, that research limited its vision and constricted its goals: "The question became, 'how little can we spend and still reduce blood lead levels in the short term?'"[117] Needleman's frustration at the time can perhaps be traced to his recognition that by the 1990s the vast majority of public health officials and researchers already knew that lead had to be removed from the child's environment to prevent injury from low-level exposure. If the KKI researchers had been looking for ways to completely and safely abate the lead hazard, the rationale for the study may have been acceptable to Needleman, and later, to the court and the public at large. But there was not the political will to confront either the culture's racial and class prejudices or the power of real estate interests by insisting that the children of poor, often minority populations be freed of the scourge of lead poisoning. Society as a whole had retreated from its responsibility to protect the most vulnerable. Public health practitioners and researchers alike, in this circumstance, could only get funding to work at the margins and by and large would not confront the deeper social inequalities that were destroying children's lives.

8   Lead Poisoning and the Courts

> The trial as a public gathering—a public airing—in and of itself, win,
> lose, or draw, had tremendous positive benefit.
>
> JOHN MCCONNELL 2011

The Baltimore Kennedy Krieger case and the controversy surrounding it
brought into high relief the contradictory strands of public health thought
at the turn of the twenty-first century. Traditionally, public health had been
a discipline that took prevention of disease as its primary, in fact vaunted,
mission. That academic public health researchers at perhaps the leading
research institution in the country could knowingly—without much internal questioning or debate—accept "amelioration" rather than prevention as
a legitimate goal, and could use "vulnerable" children as study subjects,
indicated how far the field had moved from its historical roots.

While numerous members of the public health community were ceding
the principle of prevention when it came to lead poisoning, a group of lawyers and politicians in Rhode Island in the late 1990s were taking it up. In
what would become a landmark case, initially filed in 1999 as *State of
Rhode Island v. Lead Industries Association*, the attorney general of Rhode
Island, working with one of the nation's premier plaintiffs' law firms, Ness
Motley (now Motley Rice), decided to take on not a landlord, not a university, but the lead industry itself. Public health efforts and government regulations had been able to remove lead from new paint and gasoline but thus
far had been unable to address the legacy of a century's use of lead products,
a legacy that was slowly and silently harming children. As long as the
poison remained, children of present and future generations would be at
risk. It was this problem that Sheldon Whitehouse, then Rhode Island's
attorney general, and attorneys from Ness Motley decided to take on.

Taking up the public health mantle of prevention was a prime motivation for the suit, as Fidelma Fitzpatrick, one of the two lead attorneys for
the State, recalls. Prevention "would eliminate the need for children to ever
sue for damages." It "was a much greater gift that you could give to future

generations than just compensating and giving money for . . . the injuries that they had." And for the young attorneys taking on this case, developing precedents that would embody public health principles was paramount.[1] In testimony before Congress, Sheldon Whitehouse (whose own children had been identified with elevated blood lead levels during the renovation of their house) summarized the thinking that went into filing: "If Rhode Island is considered to be the lead paint capital of the United States, then let it as well be considered the capital of lead paint solutions—solutions to a silent public health menace to our children and to children throughout the United States."[2] In the lawsuit, the State asked for enough money from the lead pigment manufacturers—primarily Sherwin-Williams, National Lead, Glidden, and Anaconda—to develop permanent means to abate the lead hazard in Rhode Island homes. This would once and for all time end virtually all childhood lead poisoning in the state.

The modern dance between public health workers and lawyers on the theme of lead dated back to the 1960s. While researchers in the 1970s and early 1980s were documenting the subtle long-term damages from lead, those filing suit around the country sought to hold landlords accountable for the damage done to children by the lead paint on the walls of substandard housing. Newspaper photographs brought to broad public awareness the dilapidated conditions found in many buildings, symbolized by peeling paint in the slums of the nation's large cities. In the 1960s and 1970s, as the Young Lords and other civil rights groups focused on lead poisoning as a symptom of inequality, racism, and poverty, municipalities passed ordinances aimed at improving living conditions for the urban poor. Baltimore, for example, passed a housing code in 1966 stipulating that landlords maintain their properties in a condition suitable for human habitation, and the presence of peeling and flaking paint indicated a failure to meet this requirement.[3] This mandate became the basis for lawsuits brought by families of lead-poisoned children that began in the late 1970s and 1980s in Baltimore and cities that had passed similar ordinances.

Saul Kerpelman, the attorney whose law firm filed the lawsuits against the Kennedy Krieger Institute, recalls that in 1981, when he was a young attorney starting out in a law firm, he was given what was considered a hopeless case: that of a child who had been poisoned from ingesting lead paint in his home. At the time, "the word on the street among plaintiffs' lawyers . . . was that lead cases were unprovable and not worth anything," Kerpelman said. "You had to show that the landlord had actual knowledge of the hazard" to prove liability. "Common law was very harsh . . . and gave all the advantages to the landlord," while landlord-tenant relations were based on "literally a medieval idea. . . . The gist of it was that someone was nice enough to give you a place to live, and you should just be thankful that you have a place to live in." Kerpelman recognized, however, that the times and the law were changing and that the civil rights and housing movements of the previous decades had left room for a new kind of lawsuit based on Baltimore's 1966 housing code.[4]

Kerpelman's case involved a toddler named Jeremy who lived in one of Baltimore's impoverished neighborhoods.[5] Referred by the Kennedy Institute (as it was then called), Jeremy had been admitted to Metropolitan Washington Pediatric Hospital for weeks of chelation and other lead-poisoning treatment, costing at the time well over thirty thousand dollars. Kerpelman was personally eager to take the case, for he had grown up in a primarily African American Baltimore neighborhood and had visited his friends in their homes, which were typically neglected by their landlords: "just typical slumlords who don't even care about the property. They only care about the source of cash flow."[6]

Jeremy was severely mentally retarded, with terrible learning disabilities and an enormous hospital bill. Legally, there were two pieces of the puzzle that had to be fitted together for a successful lead-poisoning lawsuit against a landlord. The first was to show that the housing in question was not "fit for human habitation" because of chipping and peeling paint. And the second was to show that the landlord's responsibility to *maintain* the home in good condition was not being met. Kerpelman argued that by failing to maintain the house, the landlord had allowed the child to be exposed to lead paint and was therefore responsible for the child's injuries. At the time, many cases were coming up in which it was held that "the breach of an ordinance or statute is evidence of negligence on the part of the landlord," Kerpelman recalls. The landlord's insurance company had thus realized it had a big problem: slumlords could no longer hide behind older notions of tenant responsibility but were themselves now being held liable for poorly maintained properties. The insurance company's lawyers decided to settle the case out of court for the value of the insurance policy that the landlord held.[7]

But Kerpelman's sense of victory was short-lived. Landlord lawyers soon realized that there were hundreds, perhaps thousands of potential lead-poisoning victims who might sue and that settling each case would cost their clients millions. The defense attorneys thus began seeking summary judgments to dismiss the cases on the grounds that there was no evidence of landlord negligence because the landlord accused did not understand that the peeling paint in his property contained lead. Over an eighteen-month period, Kerpelman estimates, he brought forty to fifty cases before one circuit court judge and lost most of them on summary judgment. He and his new associate, Suzanne Shapiro, began to appeal these verdicts to the appellate court, which consistently upheld the lower-court decisions on the grounds that the landlords needed to have "notice" that there was lead paint in the house, even though the housing ordinance did not excuse landlords on the basis of ignorance.[8] For the next decade Kerpelman was nevertheless deluged with lead lawsuits from the many families whose children were poisoned, and in the process he was able to settle scores of cases against Baltimore landlords, even though he lost many others in court.[9]

A critical element in Kerpelman's landlord-tenant cases was attaining a diagnosis of lead poisoning from perhaps the world's top lead-poisoning expert, J. Julian Chisolm. Kerpelman estimates that Chisolm testified, was deposed, or gave evidence in hundreds of his cases and saw it as part of his ethical responsibility to help obtain justice for these poisoned children.[10] Throughout the mid- to late 1980s and early 1990s, "Chisolm was the treating doctor in virtually every lead-poisoning case in Baltimore," Kerpelman maintains, and "the Kennedy Institute was the main referral center" for all these cases. In 1993, however, even Kerpelman's modest ability to win compensation for individual children was undermined by a Maryland Court of Appeals decision, the same court that would rule in the KKI case eight years later. In *Richwind Joint Venture 4 v. Brunson* the court ruled that, not only was it necessary for plaintiffs to show that landlords had not kept their properties in livable condition, but—in line with the lower courts' decisions— they had to show that landlords knew that the peeling paint contained lead and that lead paint was likely to damage children.[11]

The landlord-tenant cases brought by Saul Kerpelman and others like him in other cities and states, though occasionally successful in attaining justice for a limited number of clients, could not address the national epidemic of lead-poisoned children, which had been the focus of local citizen advocacy campaigns such as Baltimore's Coalition to End Childhood Lead Poisoning, headed by Ruth Ann Norton. The number of children hurt was huge, in the 1980s through the mid-1990s estimated at more than a million. More importantly, the liability system these cases depended on could only aid children already damaged. How, then, could the law be used to protect children from harm in the first place? Another approach was needed. In that search, a young history major turned litigator would play an important role.

REFOCUSING ON THE LEAD INDUSTRY

Neil Leifer graduated from Clark University in 1976, where he majored in American history, with a special focus on the plight of American Indians. It was not surprising, then, that after graduating from Northeastern Law School in 1981 he took a job with the Native American Rights Fund, a legal practice representing the Penobscot Nation and the Passamaquoddy Indian Tribe who were seeking to reclaim tribal lands in northeastern Maine. Among the issues he took on was community pollution in the Portland area, including asbestos cases of workers in a nearby paper mill. After two years he moved to Boston to join the law firm of Thornton and Early (now Thornton and Naumes), where he specialized in toxic tort litigation representing workers, neighborhoods, and children who had been exposed to environmental and occupational toxins. He focused on asbestos, which had emerged as a major issue following publication of Paul Brodeur's riveting *New Yorker* articles and book on the Johns Manville company and its cover-up of the link between asbestos exposure and cancer, specifically mesothelioma.[12]

For decades asbestosis and mesothelioma had been mostly the concern of physicians. The conditions had escaped scrutiny by the courts because workers' compensation legislation prevented those affected from bringing actions against their employers. In the late 1970s, however, innovative plaintiffs' lawyers found a way around this obstacle. While workers' comp laws prevented workers from suing their employers for on-the-job injuries, they did not rule out lawsuits against manufacturers of a workplace material—in this instance, asbestos—who failed to warn about its dangers. Johns Manville, Raybestos, and other manufacturers of asbestos and asbestos products were soon deluged with lawsuits brought by workers in construction, shipbuilding, steam fitting, and dozens of other trades that used asbestos products for insulation, siding, or other purposes.

In 1985, as a lawyer with experience in asbestos litigation, Neil Leifer was invited to a meeting of the Massachusetts Child Advocacy Center to speak about product liability lawsuits. Lawyers for the center were looking for a way to address what they saw as a major problem in Boston's poor neighborhoods: childhood lead poisoning. "Candidly, at the time I did not think that lead poisoning even existed . . . and thought it was pretty much limited to pencils," Leifer recalls. But he went to the meeting anyway. There he learned that despite a 1971 statute that required landlords to maintain their properties as lead-safe, thousands of Boston children were still exposed to lead paint in their homes. Up to this point, suing landlords had "had mixed success" because lawyers and public health officials "were really fighting house to house"; and where they had been successful, they were only able to help children who had been permanently damaged by this toxic material. "Because of the asbestos litigation and . . . other environmental litigation," Leifer recalls, "people started thinking about whether there was a toxic tort case" that could be brought against the industry for having manufactured a dangerous product without a warning.[13]

Shortly after this meeting, a new chapter in lead litigation began to take shape. Leifer was sent a 1950s decision on a Federal Trade Commission (FTC) suit against six white-lead manufacturers for price-fixing. At this point Leifer's historical sensibility came into play: "I kid you not. Thinking about this was like the closing scene of *Raiders of the Lost Ark* .... I imagined this crate of documents [in Washington] because, having done Indian law, I knew how the Justice Department did litigation. . . . Once they took your papers they never destroyed them." Sure enough, a huge store of historical materials drawn from the FTC case had been preserved in the National Archives. Leifer went to Washington and the archivist "rolled out pretty much what Indiana Jones would have expected. We pried open these old musty folders" that included the minutes of the Lead Industry Association and other invaluable documents. "These were voices from the past who were telling us how they thought about the problem," he commented. It was clear that for decades the lead industry had looked on childhood lead poisoning as a public relations problem, not a public health crisis.[14]

Childhood lead poisoning had "all the elements of a serious products liability case," Leifer realized; and the right case could mark a transitional moment in the legal history of the issue. Soon thereafter, Leifer met Monica Santiago, a teenage girl who had been severely lead poisoned in the early 1970s, and he and her parents decided to try, for the first time, to hold the lead industry itself rather than the landlord responsible for her poisoning. "We thought long and hard about it because it had never been done before," Leifer remembers. "It was going to be expensive. Our clients are poor, and were not able to underwrite any of it." Along with Trial Lawyers for Public Justice, a group of progressive lawyers led by Arthur Bryant, Leifer filed what became known as the *Santiago* case in November 1987 in Boston's federal court. The problem the plaintiffs faced was that liability cases depended on being able to show that a specific product, made by a specific company, was responsible for the harm suffered. But in this and other lead-poisoning cases the technology did not exist to discriminate whose lead pigment was responsible. Most lead-poisoning cases involved slum dwellings that had multiple layers of lead paint, sometimes many decades old.

The Santiago legal team decided to draw on a precedent set in a series of cases of young women who had developed cervical cancer years after their exposure in the womb to diethylstilbestrol (DES), a synthetic form of estrogen that doctors prescribed in the 1940s–60s to help women with certain complications of pregnancy. During the 1970s and early 1980s, as the young women developed cancer, a slew of lawsuits were filed in which manufacturers were successfully held accountable for individual injuries in proportion to the market share of each company manufacturing DES at the time of the injury. "A number of courts had reasoned that through no fault of their own, neither the mother nor the daughter knew who made the DES that the particular mother took . . . yet all those companies shared the knowledge of the risk," Leifer noted. With lead, Leifer said, "we have six companies here. DES had scores of companies." All the lead companies were members of the same trade association, the Lead Industries Association, and their products were indistinguishable. As in the DES cases, the members of the LIA knew about the dangers that lead held for children, but none of them had warned the public about these dangers.[15]

At the time, the late 1980s, Trial Lawyers for Public Justice had been involved in the Woburn environmental pollution case that later became the subject of *A Civil Action*,[16] the book and film that traced a cluster of families in a small Massachusetts community whose children had developed leukemia and who had sued the multinational corporation W. R. Grace for polluting area wells with carcinogens. The legal effort was unsuccessful and led to the financial ruin of the plaintiffs' head attorney, Jan Schlictmann, and his law firm. Schlictmann did not have the staff and financial resources to survive the lengthy legal process and compete with Grace's huge corporate law firms that hired experts, filed motions, challenged every brief and delayed proceedings literally for years.

In light of the Woburn experience, Leifer recalls, the lawyers at his firm, Thornton and Early, "were all really worried that we would descend into a [financial] black hole and never come out." But with support from Ellen Silbergeld, Philip Landrigan, Herbert Needleman, and John Graef, the head of the Lead Toxicology Program at Boston's Children's Hospital, the firm went ahead and filed suit on behalf of Monica Santiago against Sherwin-Williams in 1987. From the beginning, the industry lawyers understood the potential significance of this case, which for the first time sought to hold the lead industry responsible for the damage it had done to children over the decades. During depositions, the defense counsel for Sherwin-Williams "spent most of the time obstructing my examination," recalls Leifer.[17]

By 1991, after years of legal wrangling, Leifer and his team felt they had finally put together a compelling liability and damages case on childhood lead poisoning. The next year, the defense—the lead pigment manufacturers—asked the judge to dismiss the case before it reached trial. In a motion for summary judgment, the companies argued that market-share liability should not apply in this case. The courts were at the time becoming wary of environmental and occupational lawsuits, Leifer recalls, because of the potential for huge settlements and awards and the damage such costs would potentially cause to American industry. There had already been a flood of asbestos litigation as well as large settlements in cases concerning industrial pollution in Love Canal, New York, and Times Beach, Missouri, in which industries and state governments had been held liable for the costs of cleanup.

In the background of the summary judgment hearing, then, was the collective understanding that far more was at stake than the damage inflicted upon one child. Rather, there were thousands upon thousands of kids who could bring lawsuits against major companies such as Sherwin-Williams, NL Industries (formerly the National Lead Company), and other manufacturers of lead pigment. Industry lawyers communicated this fear "in a very effective way," Leifer recalls. They implored the judge not to "open the door here. You open the door [and] let Monica Santiago through, [and] you have 10,000 kids behind her." But the judge granted the summary judgment for a different reason: there was a critical difference between the lead-poisoning and DES cases, and thus market-share liability did not apply. Unlike DES, where the damage was unequivocally caused by one specific product, in lead-poisoning cases there were non-lead-paint sources, such as leaded gasoline and lead plumbing, that could be associated with the damage to the child.[18]

The failure of the *Santiago* case strategy, and that of market-share liability more generally, was another disappointing conclusion to the efforts at using the court system as a lever to prevent childhood lead poisoning. For much of the 1990s, lawyers advocating for lead-poisoned kids and the removal of lead from the nation's homes hunted for an approach that would avoid the pitfalls of earlier litigation strategies.

FROM PRIVATE SUITS TO PUBLIC HEALTH

It was in 1998 that lawyers in Providence, Rhode Island, fresh from recent victories against the asbestos and tobacco industries, decided to take on big lead. That year, Jack McConnell, Fidelma Fitzpatrick, and the law firm of Ness Motley began to talk to Rhode Island's attorney general, Jeffrey Pine, about initiating an innovative legal strategy to finally end the lead-poisoning epidemic in his state. Pine, a Republican, was passionate about using his office to force landlords to clean up the lead paint in their properties, so he was receptive when McConnell approached him. McConnell came armed with historical documents from lead-industry files that showed the industry's deep involvement in promoting the use of what now constituted a major health hazard. Intrigued by the parallels with tobacco and asbestos, Pine asked McConnell to prepare, along with Fitzpatrick, an "initial legal memo and binder with the documents in it with just the facts." The major problem the attorney general's office faced was overcoming the legal stumbling block that had been identified in the *Santiago* case: "If you can't identify whose paint is on what wall, then how do you sue?"[19] Because his term was ending, Pine left the development of the case to his successor, the Democrat Sheldon Whitehouse, who took office in 1999.

Whitehouse became engrossed in the various legal theories that might be used to hold the lead pigment manufacturers accountable. He slowly settled on using public nuisance law as the basis for action. Holding individual landlords accountable had proven virtually useless in affecting public health policy. There were too many children harmed and too many landlords to sue for that approach to be effective on a large scale. The *Santiago* decision had shot down the use of market-share liability when it came to lead paint. Nuisance law was a body of common law that addressed public or private actions that affect the peace, safety, or health of others. Using it seemed possible because it provided not only a means of holding the lead industry accountable but also of financing a true lead-poisoning prevention program that would once and for all end the blight. Unlike liability laws, which only provided a financial remedy for damages already incurred, nuisance law could be used to remove the danger before damage was done to future generations of children.[20] Historically, nuisance law had been used to prevent factories, for example, from dumping waste into waterways or even near their property line, because such acts, even on private property, created a threat to the health of those living nearby or downstream.[21]

Taking on the lead industry was a formidable task and presented numerous problems for Whitehouse and the State of Rhode Island. Where, for starters, would the resources come from, both human and financial, to mount the legal challenge? Research aides, paralegals, secretaries, and lawyers would have to devote years to this one case alone. Office space and equipment would be required to sort and analyze the hundreds of thousands of pages of documents that would inevitably be produced through the legal process of discovery. Medical, public health, technical, and historical experts would have to be found to help the lawyers understand the many-sided issues that would inevitably come up. Doctors and specialists in lead would be needed to explain the latest research in low-level lead exposures to a lay jury. All of this was beyond the capabilities of the relatively small cadre of lawyers and staff that composed the Attorney General's Office. Too many other issues occupied the AG's workforce. As in the tobacco lawsuits brought on behalf of the nation's attorneys general just a few years earlier, an alliance with plaintiffs' attorneys would be necessary for such a major effort to have any chance of success.

It was here that Ness Motley, flush from its victories in tobacco and asbestos lawsuits, could provide the needed support. Until the 1980s, law firms that represented consumers were generally small, often with at most a handful of attorneys working on behalf of individual clients. Taking on major industries was typically a difficult, if not quixotic enterprise that at best recovered small monetary settlements. But a sea change occurred in the late 1970s and early 1980s when lawyers found the way to successfully sue asbestos manufacturers for producing a product they knew to be dangerous. With these victories, the largest plaintiffs' law firms used a portion of the settlements to fund a new challenge against the tobacco industry, which by the 1990s had become the focus of consumer and government agencies concerned with the health dangers of tobacco use.[22] By 1999, Ness Motley and a handful of other such plaintiffs' law firms were as large and well financed as the defendants' firms.

Jack McConnell was hired by Ness Motley following his graduation from Case Western Reserve Law School in 1983, and by the end of the decade he was handling mainly asbestos cases for the firm. In the early 1990s, McConnell relates, he and Ron Motley "tried the largest civil case ever in U.S. jurist history in Baltimore," which involved fifty-two hundred plaintiffs suffering from asbestos-related diseases "against fifteen defendants in a single courtroom, in a case that lasted eight months." They won a huge victory. Shortly thereafter, Motley and McConnell began working with Dickie Scruggs, a Mississippi plaintiffs' lawyer who wanted help developing new ways to bring the tobacco industry to court. Up to that point, individual smokers had sued tobacco companies, but these cases "were burdened by 'free choice,'" that is, the tobacco industry lawyers successfully argued that smokers had chosen to smoke and therefore were responsible for their own illnesses.[23] As the *New York Times* summarized the argument of Steven C. Parrish, vice president and chief counsel for Phillip Morris, "through years of litigation the tobacco industry has never paid anything in a judgment or settlement, chiefly because companies have always been able to show that smoking is a matter of choice."[24]

What Scruggs and Motley sought to do was to change the frame, from a question of individual free choice to one of the economic burden levied on states by tobacco-related diseases such as certain cancers, emphysema, and heart disease.[25] This legal strategy would lead to four class action lawsuits filed by private attorneys against the tobacco industry; and in May 1994 the attorney general of Mississippi, Michael Moore, would bring suit, "seeking reimbursement for the cost of medical program[s], including Medicaid, that support victims of smoking-related illnesses."[26] As the *New York Times* pointed out, it was "the first [suit] initiated by a government on behalf of taxpayers to hold tobacco companies directly accountable for the health consequences of their products."[27] This would ultimately result in a $365 billion settlement in 1998 between twenty-six states and the tobacco industry, including a huge windfall for the plaintiffs' law firms, a portion of which some of these firms later used to fund lead lawsuits.[28]

Today, it seems obvious that the tobacco industry would have been "an easy target" for plaintiffs' lawyers. But in the early 1990s, not only had the industry never lost a lawsuit, but various plaintiffs' law firms had been forced into bankruptcy because of the great cost of litigation. Defense firms for Phillip Morris, R. J. Reynolds Tobacco Company, Brown and Williamson Tobacco Corporation, and Lorillard Tobacco Company were too large, too powerful, and too well connected for individual plaintiffs and states to mount a successful challenge. And in fact, had it not been for the victories in asbestos cases, attorney Fidelma Fitzpatrick pointed out, "Ron Motley would not have had the ability to commit the firms' funds to what turned out to be a multi-million dollar battle. . . . It was more than just a set of brains and good lawyering. It was also the fact that we had the money to do it."[29]

In the same way that asbestos set the table for tobacco, the enormous victory against big tobacco by the states' attorneys general set the table for the lead case in Rhode Island.[30] And in many ways the initial Rhode Island lead case was modeled on the victory over tobacco. But there were major differences. In the tobacco litigation, the states primarily sought reimbursement for the cost of caring for millions of Americans damaged by tobacco products. They also sought money to organize smoking prevention and cessation programs. In the evolving lead case, the situation was different. "In lead," McConnell points out, "the primary damage isn't very great to the State Medicaid coffers" unless a patient has to be chelated. But by the 1990s chelation was not the major burden, as relatively few children by that time experienced extremely high lead exposure. Unlike tobacco, where the primary motivation was recovery of damages, not the promotion of public health, in the Rhode Island lead case the focus was less on recovery of damages and more on achieving, as Fitzpatrick characterized it, "a better public health solution"—that is, prevention of future damages through abatement funded by companies shown to have knowingly put children and others in harm's way.[31] The goal of this strategy was nothing less than the complete removal of all lead paint from both public and private housing in Rhode Island.

Another major difference between the tobacco and lead cases was that in the tobacco suits states attorneys general banded together, whereas in lead Rhode Island decided to go it alone. Michael Moore, the attorney general for Mississippi who was the driving force behind the tobacco cases, believed he would need many allies to counter the enormous political and economic power of one of the nation's (perhaps the world's) largest industries, which meant actively recruiting other AGs to join in the lawsuit. With lead, a strong moral focus led Rhode Island AG Sheldon Whitehouse to try the case in one state. As McConnell notes, Whitehouse was focused on the larger public health issue, not the recovery of money at issue in the tobacco case. He "showed incredible statesmanship," said McConnell of Whitehouse, "because his focus was really on a bigger picture than oftentimes you see [among lawyers] or among public servants." Fitzpatrick observes that "obviously, dollars weren't driving him [Whitehouse]. . . . This was a tough political issue" because the "business community was up in arms about it."[32] And Fitzpatrick said there were risks in this strategy: "all of the eggs were in one basket with one court and the way one court would or wouldn't go was going to dictate how things were going to happen."[33] As the lawsuit went forward in the coming years, Rhode Island became a battleground in a war between the nation's business community and 122 attorneys of record representing the lead industry versus a small band of lawyers from the Rhode Island AG's office and seven lawyers, four paralegals, and staff from the newly renamed Motley Rice in downtown Providence.[34]

The suit centered on the historical responsibility the lead industry had incurred by knowingly creating a statewide crisis that had put tens of thousands of Rhode Island's children at risk for lead poisoning. Since the early twentieth century, documents presented at the trial revealed, companies had reported in their internal memos and newsletters that lead paint was a "deadly cumulative poison" that as early as 1914 had resulted in convulsions, comas, and deaths as well as loss of appetite, irritability, unsteadiness afoot, abdominal pain, and vomiting among children. Despite extensive discussion of childhood lead poisoning in the late 1920s and 1930s in the meetings of their trade association, the companies continued to market their leaden products and even sought to undermine the growing medical literature that documented cases of lead poisoning throughout the nation. In advertisements in mass-market publications like the *National Geographic* and the *Saturday Evening Post*, the National Lead Company, for example, claimed that "Lead Helps to Guard Your Health" and "Lead

Takes Part in Many Games." The Lead Industries Association organized massive "white lead promotion" campaigns in the 1930s and 1940s (and even into the 1950s) to promote the deadly product. When the publicity about childhood lead poisoning increased in the 1940s, and when Maryland in particular passed legislation to stop the use of lead paint on toys, cribs, and children's furniture, the industry successfully lobbied that state's legislature to overturn the law. When political opposition to the use of lead paint grew in the 1950s, the LIA leadership argued that lead poisoning was the fault of "ignorant" "Negro and Puerto Rican families" rather than of the companies that had sold, marketed, and profited from the decades-long pollution campaign.[35]

The first Rhode Island trial took place in 2002 and ended in a hung jury. But a second trial, which began in late 2005, would become the longest civil trial in the state's history. *Rhode Island v. Sherwin-Williams, NL Industries, Millennium Holdings, and Atlantic Richfield* in the Superior Court for the State of Rhode Island emerged as a landmark case when a jury held the first three companies liable for cleaning up and detoxifying hundreds of thousands of homes in Rhode Island. In a verdict handed down on February 22, 2006, that might "cost the companies billions of dollars," in the words of the *Providence Journal*, lead pigment manufacturers were for the first time held responsible, not only for the harm they had already inflicted on tens of thousands of children, but also for preventing damage to the many more children living in 240,000 lead-infested homes.[36]

In the wake of the verdict, the trial judge, Michael Silverstein, began a search for public health experts capable of developing a master plan for the identification of housing and methods for abating the lead hazard. For close to two years, plans proceeded to implement what some saw as an enormous public health victory and others viewed as a dastardly misuse of nuisance law. Community groups such as ACORN, the Childhood Lead Action Project, and the Alliance to End Childhood Lead Poisoning hailed the Rhode Island decision as pointing the way to finally resolving the century-long public health crisis created by lead pollution. But large-circulation newspapers throughout the country bemoaned the potentially enormous cost to the industry that this suit foretold, as California and Ohio had already initiated their own suits and other states' attorneys general were sure to follow.

The *Wall Street Journal* had followed the trial and had editorialized that the suit was nothing more than an attempt by Motley Rice to extort money from the lead industry. "Even as its asbestos and silicosis scams are unraveling," the *Journal* lamented, "the trial bar is looking for its next industry to loot. It may have found it last week in a state court in Providence, Rhode

Island, where a jury found three paint companies liable for creating a 'public nuisance' by selling lead paint many decades ago."[37] Virtually all the big newspapers around the country saw the Rhode Island decision solely through the lens of the lead industry and the financial impact it could have. Few understood or cared about the public health crisis that had spurred the state to sue in the first place and few gave credit to the state for trying to protect the health of children. The *Chattanooga Times Free Press* argued, for example, that "it would have been better to compensate those who were actually harmed, rather than place a huge financial burden on companies that sold a legal product" decades ago. The *Toledo (Ohio) Blade* complained that "frivolous law suits have become a national disgrace," citing the effort by the City of Toledo to join other Ohio cities "to recover money to help pay for past and future remediation of lead paint in older buildings."[38] The *New York Times* Sunday business section summarized the dread that plagued the business community, featuring a quarter-page image of a paint can covered by dollar signs and the headline "The Nuisance That May Cost Billions."[39]

The nationwide attention was not a chance event. Rather, the lead industry hired lobbyists and media people to promote its view of the case. Among the most important lobbyists was Bonnie Campbell, who, in the years preceding and following the trial, was the liberal face of the industry. A Democrat, she had been Iowa's attorney general between 1990 and 1994 and then had run (unsuccessfully) for governor. In 1995 President Clinton appointed her director of the newly created Office on Violence against Women in the U.S. Department of Justice; in early 2000 he nominated her for a judgeship, but Senate Republicans on the Judiciary Committee blocked the vote on her nomination. By 2003 Campbell had abandoned her political ambitions, turning her focus instead to public relations and lobbying for the lead industry. The focus of attention in lawsuits, she told *Newsweek* in early 2003, should not be the industry's past malfeasance but landlords' current violations of existing housing codes. Of the then-upcoming Rhode Island trial, Campbell said, "This kind of litigation sends the wrong message to an industry that has been very responsible and it won't help one child."[40] In a refrain that would be repeated over and over again in the coming barrage of blog posts, editorials, and articles, the industry portrayed itself as the victim of specious attacks by greedy lawyers and misinformed advocates.

The victory in Rhode Island severely shook the confidence of industry lawyers and representatives, especially as Judge Silverstein carefully addressed and rejected all of the industry's post-trial appeals that sought to overturn the jury verdict. But the battle was not over. The paint companies appealed the decision to the Supreme Court of Rhode Island, and in July

2008, more than two years after the jury verdict, the higher court's stunning reversal undercut ten years of litigation. The supreme court rejected the legal basis of the plantiffs' suit. Nuisance law, the court maintained, did not apply. "However grave the problem of lead poisoning is in Rhode Island, public nuisance law," the court said, "simply does not provide a remedy for this harm."[41] The State had worked hard to find a means of preventing future generations of children from developing lead poisoning through the use of nuisance law, but the court ruled that only *past* harm rose to the level of a civil suit. The proper basis for this suit, the court claimed, should have been liability laws, which provide a possible remedy for harm already done but do not address future injuries. Ignoring the fact that the industry had been aware of the harmfulness of its products when it sold lead paint to homeowners, landlords, and renters, the court said that the responsibility for prevention rested on individual landlords and that individual landlords should be the focus of any lawsuits.

Responses to the ruling fell along more or less predictable lines. "Today's ruling is a landmark victory for common sense," one of the lawyers for Sherwin-Williams told the *New York Times*. "The responsibility of making sure children aren't exposed to lead paint remains squarely on property owners." Jack McConnell, Motley Rice's lead attorney for the State, by contrast told the *Times* of the dire public health consequences of the supreme court's decision: "Children in Rhode Island will continue to be poisoned by lead in paint and the companies that put the poisonous paint in Rhode Island [will be considered by the court to] have no responsibility for cleaning up the mess that they created in the first place."[42] The court was aware of the harm lead had done. In its conclusion to its lengthy decision, the court noted that it did not "mean to minimize the severity of the harm that thousands of children in Rhode Island have suffered as a result of lead poisoning." Nor were the justices unfeeling: "Our hearts go out to those children whose lives forever have been changed by the poisonous presence of lead."[43] But these were crocodile tears, some would say. Never did the justices acknowledge the future generations whose lives they could have protected.

The Rhode Island Supreme Court ruling disappointed public health advocates, the plantiffs' lawyers, and the State, but in a peculiar way the initial trial itself proved to be an enormous public health victory. As Jack McConnell put it, "The trial as a public gathering—a public airing—in and of itself, win, lose or draw, had tremendous positive benefit." Through the numerous news articles and television and radio reports—along with the national attention from health professionals and activists throughout the nation—the public as well as the public health community seemed reenergized to combat lead's devastating effects on children. Even the constant drumbeat of negative articles in the mainstream press that lambasted the State's lawyers, Motley Rice in particular, as little more than ambulance-chasing, money-hungry opportunists alerted thousands of people in Rhode Island and millions of parents around the country to the issue of lead poisoning.[44]

While the Rhode Island case was the marquee event in the lead wars of the first decade of the new century, and spurred other states to explore similar suits, the Rhode Island Supreme Court's decision discouraged most other states from proceeding. This does not mean that the legal battles are over. In fact, as of the winter of 2012–13, a new and potentially much bigger lawsuit was moving ahead in several cities and counties in California, including San Francisco, Oakland, Los Angeles, and San Diego.[45] As in Rhode Island, the suit argues that lead paint is a public nuisance threatening future generations of California's children and asks that the lead industry clean up the mess it made. But this time some of the key issues that allowed the Rhode Island Supreme Court to reverse the jury decision have already been decided. Because of an initial favorable ruling about the use of nuisance law by the California Supreme Court, it is likely that this suit will go forward.

The lead wars from the 1960s through the 1980s involved street-level organizing by community organizations, the regulatory fights over the definitions of what constituted dangerous lead exposure, and legislative battles to ban certain uses of lead. The movement into the courts during the past two decades presumes a legislative and regulatory failure, not just in Rhode Island. Other state legislatures and the U.S. Congress generally have not been able to resolve the complex politics of lead abatement.

But lead poisoning is an issue that will not just die. While there may be little movement in the public health community, legislatures, and regulatory bodies of late, the issue is still moving forward through various courts. A July 2011 jury verdict in St. Louis highlights how lead pollution continues to haunt Americans. In that case, brought by attorney Gerson Smoger and his colleagues at the law firm of Newman, Bronson and Wallis, residents of the town of Herculaneum, Missouri, the site of the last (and historically the largest) primary lead smelter in the country, sued its owners, the Fluor Corporation, for having polluted the town and having poisoned their children, giving them among the highest blood lead levels in the state. In one of the longest civil cases in Missouri's history, the jury heard historical and contemporary evidence about the company's knowledge of lead dangers faced by residents and the company's efforts to manipulate state and federal officials in order to avoid regulatory actions. The jury, in the words of the *St. Louis Post-Dispatch*, sent "a clear message" when it awarded the town's residents $38 million for compensatory damages and $320 million for punitive damages.[46]

In September 2011, ten years after the Maryland Court of Appeals issued its rebuke of Johns Hopkins, lawyers in Baltimore filed a class action lawsuit against the Kennedy Krieger Institute for, in the words of the *New York Times,* "knowingly exposing black children as young as a year old to lead poisoning in the 1990s as part of a study exploring the hazards of lead paint." This reprise of the legal battle that stirred such controversy a decade ago is a reminder that the legacy of lead and of an industry that polluted the nation remains with us still, at tremendous human cost.

9 A Plague on All Our Houses

> We are allowing industry to profit by using our children as
> uninformed research subjects of a vast experiment.
>
> BRUCE LANPHEAR, 2009

In 1992, just as the Kennedy Krieger Institute research was getting under way, prominent lead researcher Herbert Needleman and Richard Jackson, soon to be head of the CDC's Center for Environmental Health division, bemoaned the ineffectual attempts to end the century-old affliction of lead poisoning. They were concerned that the size of the lead-poisoning problem, and the money and work required to solve it, had led to a "wave of pessimism. Self-styled realists, when confronted with [the high cost] to de-lead and improve the [millions of] dangerous houses in which children live . . . shrug and turn away." They felt that public health practitioners had a moral calling, however. "It should not be necessary to place a price tag on the eradication of a serious childhood illness; the presence of the disease and owning the means to eliminate it should be enough."[1]

In the two decades since Needleman and Jackson made this statement, hundreds of thousands of children in the United States have been diagnosed, and many others undoubtedly have gone undetected, with elevated blood lead levels that have transformed their life chances.[2] These children's ability to succeed in school has been undercut by reduced IQ, increased behavioral problems, attention deficit disorders, and neurological problems such as dyslexia and hyperactivity. If these problems had been linked to meningitis or another viral disease, the mere dimension of the damages—and threat of contagion—would likely have resulted in a national mobilization to protect this vulnerable population. The sheer number of children adversely affected by lead over the past twenty years, not to mention the past century, dwarfs the number of U.S. residents affected by SARS, West Nile virus, Legionnaires' disease, anthrax, smallpox, and other diseases that have led to broad national efforts to eliminate them as threats.[3]

Yet little such effort at the national scale—beyond the work of some dedicated scientists, public health workers, public interest lawyers, politicians, and community groups—is evident in the case of lead. From today's perspective, the ten billion dollars that Needleman and Jackson identified in 1992 as necessary for removing lead from the walls of the nation and ending the threat of lead, "this blunter of children's cognition and silent thief of their futures," seems a small price to pay. Yet that investment did not happen then, and it looks unlikely to happen anytime soon. Lacking such a commitment, lead will remain an ever-present threat to children for years to come, and one day we will look back with wonder at our crass willingness to sacrifice so many children, particularly those who just happen to be born into poor and minority families.[4]

The issues that Needleman and Jackson identified in 1992 lay at the heart of the controversy that consumed Johns Hopkins and the Maryland Court of Appeals in the early years of the twenty-first century. As the lead industry self-servingly proclaimed in the 1950s, as long as there are slums and as long as children could get to the paint, lead poisoning would continue to "plague us." The industry took no responsibility then and still refuses to acknowledge its culpability today. In the end, the industry counted on society's willingness to accept that damage would be done, decade after decade, to children. And so far, lead companies have not been disappointed.

The Kennedy Krieger experiment emerged from the frustration of scientists and activists who had for decades searched for a solution that would not disrupt the status quo relationships among landlords, industry, government, and public health scientists. By the mid-1990s, the work of Mark Farfel and J. Julian Chisolm, among others, such as David Jacobs at the U.S. Department of Housing and Urban Development, had contributed to the development of techniques to remove lead safely from children's home environment. Further, by this time technological advances had led to routine tests capable of inexpensively identifying much lower levels of lead in children's blood. The impediment to finally eliminating childhood lead poisoning was not technological: it was cost and commitment. Who would bear the costs of complete lead removal—landlords, industry, government, or some combination of the three? Who would bear the financial risks if this was not done—city, state, and federal governments, in the form of special-education classes, Medicaid, and welfare, and the families themselves? Who would bear the costs in silently stolen futures, lower IQs, lost productivity, narrowed life chances and well-being, in emotional distress, and physical damage—poor white, Hispanic, and black children?

What is it about lead poisoning that makes it different from epidemics of SARS, influenza, and the like? One difference is that, unlike these other deadly threats, lead poisoning is not an infectious disease; we need not fear contact with strangers or friends. Moreover, lead poisoning today is not, except in relatively rare acute cases, a condition whose symptoms are obvious and immediate. We know that lead interferes at least with blood production, which may be the beginning of greater biochemical and neurological effects. But we primarily know of its subtler impact because of the abstract epidemiologic studies that tell us that lead-poisoned children, as a group, do worse than those who are not poisoned. We can rarely "prove," in a common-sense meaning of proof, who has and who has not been affected.

Finally, lead poisoning as it has been commonly portrayed does not affect all of us in society evenly but rather is particularly damaging to those who live in the older, rundown, more dilapidated neighborhoods of our fading urban centers, where lead paint is most likely to be exposed. As such, those who make the decisions about what our priorities are as a society and what risks we are willing to take with our children's lives often feel immune from the consequences of lead, especially now that lead has been removed from gasoline. We can take some solace in the observable fact that the number of children diagnosed with blood lead levels above 10 micrograms per deciliter has continually declined since systematic surveillance began in the 1990s. We can applaud the victories of public health workers and housing advocates and those legislators and officials whose actions have brought lead to the nation's consciousness and who have themselves helped to dramatically reduce the number of children affected. We can believe that lead poisoning—along with other environmental childhood threats such as asthma linked to mold and cockroaches, for example—will at some future date be all but eradicated as the rebuilding of our urban infrastructure, the gentrification of older neighborhoods, and the movement of peoples out of dilapidated structures eliminates the primary source of lead poisoning: the nation's leaded housing stock.

But self-satisfied complacency born of the successes of the past thirty years must be tempered by the growing body of research that shows lead to be a multiheaded hydra whose dangers are constantly being revealed in new forms. Each time we believe we have one lead danger under control, we are forced to confront another set of problems that challenge our science, our epidemiology, our morality, and our sense of social justice. Today's science shows that lead poisoning can be understood as a contributing cause of juvenile delinquency and crime. Recent studies even suggest a possible link between the decline in lead poisoning and a decline in serious crime over the last thirty years.[5]

In light of recent epidemiological evidence of lead's broad social impacts and its biological effects—from learning disabilities and crime to psychiatric disturbance, heart disease, and even schizophrenia[6]—the science behind our definitions of lead poisoning has changed dramatically. From the 1960s through the early 1990s, blood lead levels considered dangerous to children declined from 60 to 10 µg/dl. And more recent research indicates that even the lower blood lead level considered safe in the 1990s offers children inadequate protection. In fact, the CDC in mid-2012 lowered its level of concern—the level at which children should be considered at risk—to 5 µg/dl, thereby increasing the estimated number of endangered children from 250,000 to 450,000. Even this may not be a safe level. The CDC's Advisory Committee on Childhood Lead Poisoning Prevention itself acknowledged that there may not be any "safe" level of lead exposure for children.[7]

Our common-sense assumptions, long held by toxicologists as well as the general public, that the higher the level of a poison, the more damage it causes, may not always be true. New research shows that the most serious damage from lead occurs at some of the lowest levels of exposure, often in utero or in the first years of life, when the neurological structures of the brain are forming.[8] For example, compared to children with virtually no evidence of lead in their blood, the greatest effect of lead on IQ occurs in children with blood lead levels below 5 µg/dl. As blood lead levels climb above 5 µg/dl, IQ continues to decline but at a much slower rate.[9] Similarly, endocrine disruptors such as bisphenol A have their greatest impact on physiological structures at the lowest levels of bioaccumulation, if exposure occurs at critical moments in fetal development. This raises troubling issues for toxicology and for society, because these data imply that other toxins may also defy the traditional dogma that the "dose makes the poison" and that lowering exposures lowers the risk.[10] Unlike toxins whose acute effects disappear with the elimination of the poison, lead's effect on the child's brain is immediate and often permanent.

DOSE AND DISEASE

The ongoing controversy over what constitutes low-level lead poisoning is paradigmatic of the broader social debate that has been brewing for the past thirty years over a host of other industrial toxins that have been introduced into our world. At least since the publication of Rachel Carson's *Silent Spring* a half a century ago, we have been weighing the costs to our health and well-being of various products and processes of our industrial economy.

Should saccharine be used as a sweetener, DDT as an insecticide; should bisphenol A and vinyl chloride be the mainstays of plastics, glues, and other consumer products; should mercury, cadmium, and other heavy metals be eliminated from light bulbs, batteries, and from the effluent of smelters and coal-using power plants. In all of these cases we face the same overall question as that raised in the century-old debate over lead: are diseases with clinical symptoms the only problems we should be concerned about or do we need to expand the concept of disease to include behavioral changes like attention deficit/hyperactivity disorder (ADHD), altered social behavior, and lowered IQ?

We readily accept clinical disease in individual patients and psychological problems as legitimate medical issues. But what happens to our consensus when we measure changes in behavior, IQ, or school success on a population level? How do we ascribe responsibility for harm and how do we remedy permanent damage? How do we define what is a poison? Are poisons only those things that produce acute damage or death in one person, or can we talk meaningfully about environmental poisons that produce physiological or subtle behavioral changes invisible to the clinician or even the victims or entire populations themselves? How do we ascribe responsibility in an industrial society when the harms produced appear many years after the exposure to the toxin? And whose lives and futures should or should not be put at risk in the name of profit and industrial progress?

The developing science of lead's effects on the human body may be a harbinger of things to come in other arenas, of the challenge that awaits us as we confront new materials and exposures whose effects are unlike those we have experienced before. Endocrine disruptors such as bisphenol A (BPA) have already been identified as part of this brave new world as we learn of their impact on human physiology and biological processes.[11] Like low-level lead, BPA challenges our traditional understanding of disease: it has measurable biological impacts, but the symptoms are usually not obvious and not commonly understood as pathological. Endocrine disruptors affect animals' hormonal systems, leading to a variety of biological changes. Some of these are widely seen as pathological, such as cancer, birth defects, and physiological abnormalities; others are subtler and can easily be ascribed to social or other factors, such as learning disabilities, attention deficit disorders, and subtle developmental anomalies. Still other physiological changes are linked to exposures to endocrine disruptors, but their import is less well understood. Does it matter that "feminine" characteristics are more prevalent in frogs and mice as a result to exposures to endocrine disruptors, and does this have implications for humans? Would it matter if more girls than boys were born every year? Are the cancer rates changing because we have been exposed to increased amounts of chlorinated hydrocarbons?

Even people whose professional lives have been shaped by the lead-poisoning controversy described in this book are startled by the continuing revelations of lead's dangers. Ellen Silbergeld, whose early studies in the 1970s provided the toxicological basis for the behavioral changes that Herbert Needleman and others were observing in children, recalls her reaction when a younger colleague said to her, "What your problem is, Ellen, is that you don't understand how toxic lead is." She replied, "Me? I don't understand? Those are fighting words." Silbergeld's research had shown that adults whose blood lead levels were in the 10 to 30 μg/dl range had a higher risk of dying of stroke and mild heart attacks, but this young researcher said that Silbergeld had dramatically underestimated lead's impact. He told her that when blood lead levels go from 0.5 μg/dl—one-tenth of the existing 5 μg/dl standard for children, established in 2012—to 2 μg/dl, two-fifths of that standard, "the odds of getting a stroke go up four times." Silbergeld is now convinced that lead is a major cause of arteriosclerosis and heart disease. What is shocking for her is that the new data indicate the presence of clinical disease, not subtle behavioral change or statistical associations: "I'm talking about stroke; I'm talking about clinically diagnosed hypertension after arteriosclerosis."[12]

Beginning in the mid-1990s, understanding of the true dimensions of the lead crisis expanded dramatically. The generation of children who had been identified with what Jane Lin-Fu had described in the early 1970s as "undue lead absorption" (which became "elevated blood lead levels" by the early 1980s) had reached maturity. Through studies of the social histories of these children, longer-term effects of low-level exposures could begin to be traced. It became apparent that the first cognitive symptoms that had been associated with low-level lead exposure—hyperactivity, attention deficit, lowered IQ, problems with verbal competency, growing rates of reading disabilities, and academic failure—were the proverbial tip of the neuropathological iceberg. Herbert Needleman once again led the way in expanding the scope of the research community. In 1996 he and his colleagues looked at children they had been following for decades and found that those with lead exposures early in life showed antisocial and even delinquent behavior. In a study of 850 first-grade boys in Pittsburgh public schools, Needleman and his colleagues controlled for a variety of socioeconomic, racial, and family factors and found that parents' and teachers' reports on children's behavior correlated closely to teeth and blood lead levels.[13] This suggestive study spurred new epidemiological and observational research that explored the multiple social impacts of lead and questioned the idea that any level of lead exposure in a developing child was safe.

Researchers had suspected since the 1990s that even the then newly lowered 10 µg/dl threshold was inadequate to protect children. In the first decade of the new century considerable research confirmed this. In 2005 Bruce Lanphear and colleagues pooled data from seven international studies to evaluate the effects of blood lead levels below 10 µg/dl on intellectual functioning. They found that "environmental lead exposure in children who have maximal blood-lead levels <7.5 µg/dL is associated with intellectual deficits," specifically lower IQ.[14] "Existing data indicate that there is no evidence of a threshold for the adverse consequences of lead exposure," they concluded.[15] The following year Joe Braun and his colleagues showed that even extremely low levels of lead were associated with hyperactivity and attention deficits in children. Indeed, children with blood lead levels of 5 µg/dl had an increased risk for ADHD when compared with children whose blood lead levels were below 0.8 µg/dl.[16]

In 2001 Kim Dietrich produced the first study that measured lead exposure during pregnancy through a child's sixth birthday, the results of which confirmed earlier clinical and other retrospective studies that indicated that early exposure was correlated with delinquent and antisocial behavior in later childhood and adolescence.[17] And, in 2005, economist Rick Nevin followed up with a study of the relationship between lead exposure in the preschool years and later crime records. Using data from the United States and eight other countries, Nevin, controlling for class and other socioeconomic variables, found "a very strong association between preschool blood lead and subsequent crime rate trends over several decades." He made the unsettling suggestion that "murder rates across USA cities suggest that murder could be especially associated with more severe cases of childhood lead poisoning."[18] Stunning on its surface, Nevin's work was bolstered by a prospective study that criminologist John Paul Wright and his colleagues published in *PLoS Medicine* in 2008 that showed that "prenatal and postnatal blood lead concentrations are associated with higher rates of total arrests and/or arrests for offenses involving violence."[19] Even more shocking correlations began to emerge at the end of the last decade as Maryse Bouchard and colleagues, as well as Tomás Guilarte and Ezra Susser, began to document the correlation of tiny lead exposures—levels above 2.1 µg/dl, with a median of 3 µg/dl—with later development of major depressive disorder and panic disorder in young adults in the United States.[20] Other studies correlated "prenatal lead exposure" with "a significant deficit in cognitive

TABLE 1. Health effects of low-level lead (Pb) exposure

Health Area	Population or Exposure Window	NTP Conclusion	Principal Health Effects	Blood Pb Evidence	Bone Pb Evidence
Neurological	Children	Sufficient*	Decreased academic achievement, IQ and specific cognitive measures, increased incidence of attention-related behaviors and problem behaviors	Yes, <5µg/dl	Tibia and dentin Pb are associated with attention-related behaviors, problem behaviors, and cognition
	Children	Sufficient	Decreased IQ, decreased hearing	Yes, <10µg/dl	No data
Immunological	Children	Sufficient	Increased hypersensitivity/allergy by skin prick test to allergens and increased IgE† (effect, not a health outcome)	Yes, <10µg/dl	No data
Cardiovascular	Adults	Sufficient	Increased blood pressure, increased risk of hypertension, and increased incidence of essential tremor	Yes, <10µg/dl	Association between bone Pb and cardiovascular effects more consistent than for blood
Renal	Adults	Sufficient	Decreased glomerular filtration rate	Yes, <5µg/dl	Yes, in one study
Reproductive and Developmental	Children	Sufficient	Delayed puberty, reduced postnatal growth	Yes, <10µg/dl	No data

Source: Adapted from National Toxicology Program (NTP), *NTP Monograph on Health Effects of Low-Level Lead*, prepublication copy (U.S. Department of Health and Human Services, June 13, 2012), xix, available at http://ntp.niehs.nih.gov/?objectid=4F04B8EA-B187-9EF2-9F9413C68E76458E (accessed September 28, 2012).

* Sufficient = adequate data support NTP conclusion

† IgE = immunoglobulin E; increased serum IgE is associated with hypersensitivity

function" that was apparent by the time the child entered the third year of life.[21]

The cascade of research findings from a variety of disciplines has dramatically shifted the scientific politics of lead. From celebrating public health's "success" in lowering blood lead levels, scientists have moved to warning about the uncertain future of the magnitude of this problem. In October 2011, the National Toxicology Program of the U.S. Department of Health and Human Services issued a draft report that evaluated the accumulating data. There was "sufficient evidence," the report concluded, to believe that lead caused an "increased diagnosis of attention deficit disorder, greater incidence of problem behaviors, and decreased cognitive performance" as measured by "lower academic achievement and specific cognitive measures." In the measured, removed tone of a medical treatise, the report noted that blood lead levels even below 10 µg/dl were associated with "delayed puberty, reduced postnatal growth, and decreased cognitive performance as indicated by lower IQ." Not only children were affected but also adults. Data showed that adult blood lead levels below 5 µg/dl are associated with kidney disease and below 10 µg/dl with increased blood pressure, hypertension, and high rates of heart disease.[22] At a peer review meeting sponsored by the National Institute of Environmental Health Sciences in December 2011, one of the panel members, Eliseo Guallar from Johns Hopkins, predicted that still other deleterious effects of even lower lead levels would be found: "The lower we go, we still find effects of lead, and I think we still haven't seen the end of it."[23]

THE CONSERVATIVE ATTACK ON SCIENCE

The lead controversy has reached the highest levels of the political and health hierarchies and has led to dramatic conflicts over the very institutions that define our understanding of danger, including the Centers for Disease Control. Since the 1970s, the CDC, the nation's primary agency for the protection of the public's health, has depended on scientific panels made up of independent scientists, policy consultants, and experts in a wide range of fields to gather information and provide advice regarding policy for a variety of toxic materials.

One of the most important safeguards of the scientific integrity of governmental policy and research has been the independence of the 258 scientific advisory committees to the various branches of the CDC that presently help policy makers decide on the appropriate means of addressing serious health issues. These advisory committees, while not possessing the actual power to reshape policy, are a font of influential expert opinion available to various CDC chiefs. Soon after the year 2000, the CDC's Advisory Committee on Childhood Lead Poisoning Prevention became the focus of an intense political battle that reflected the growing importance of low-level environmental exposures to national public health policy. As the CDC's committee began to consider the new research that questioned the safety of the 10 µg/dl blood lead standard for children, the George W. Bush administration sought to short-circuit the traditional manner in which appointments to the CDC committees had been made, substituting instead a partisan selection process conducive to the administration's well-known antiregulatory and antienvironmental agenda.

The federal government established the U.S. Department of Health, Education and Welfare (the predecessor of today's Department of Health and Human Services) in 1954, while the Environmental Protection Agency, the Occupational Safety and Health Administration, and the National Institute of Occupational Safety and Health were formed in 1970, only four decades ago. As money and research opportunities that were independent of industry control began to expand, independent researchers asked new questions and provided new and troubling data that marked a transformation in our understanding of the potential dangers of lead and other toxic substances. One of the most important changes in research and policy formation to occur was the establishment of government agencies freed from industry control, and the creation of those 258 CDC scientific advisory panels during the past forty years has been integral to this process.

The law establishing the advisory structure was passed in 1972. It "require[s] the membership of the advisory committee to be fairly balanced in terms of the points of view represented and the functions to be performed by the advisory committee" and to "assure that the advice and recommendations of the advisory committee will not be inappropriately influenced by the appointing authority or by any special interest, but will instead be the result of the advisory committee's independent judgment."[24] For the first decades of its existence, members of the CDC's lead advisory committee had been the scientific community's leaders in the field. They had pioneered new methodologies for lead measurement, epidemiology, and for lead's effects on children as well as applying that research knowledge to CDC recommendations.

In 2002 the Bush administration announced that it was rejecting the recommendations of CDC staff and existing panel members regarding new appointments to the lead advisory committee. "The last time anything like this happened was under Reagan," noted Ellen Silbergeld.[25] Health and

Human Services secretary Tommy Thompson rejected the recommended reappointment of Michael Weitzman, a member of the Department of Pediatrics at the University of Rochester, pediatrician in chief of the Rochester General Hospital (now at New York University), a member of the lead advisory committee since 1997, and author of numerous publications on lead poisoning in peer-reviewed journals. Thompson also rejected new nominations of Bruce Lanphear and Susan Klitzman, professor of urban public health at the City University of New York School of Public Health and author of numerous peer-reviewed publications on lead poisoning.[26] In their stead, the Bush administration nominated individuals whose ideological commitments, pronouncements, or connections to the lead industry virtually guaranteed that they would not be amenable to lowering the standard of acceptable lead exposure despite the mounting evidence of the adverse effects of very low levels.

Perhaps the most blatantly ideological nomination was that of William Banner, at the time an attending physician at Tulsa's St. Francis Hospital and clinical professor of pediatrics at the University of Oklahoma College of Medicine. Not only were his research credentials in lead thin, but he served as an expert witness on behalf of the lead industry in the landmark lead-poisoning lawsuit brought by Rhode Island's attorney general against lead pigment manufacturers. Banner's deposition in that case—and in another, in Milwaukee, Wisconsin—were revealing of his belief that the effects of lead poisoning in children had been grossly overemphasized. Despite the fact that the CDC had progressively lowered acceptable blood lead levels from 60 to 10 µg/dl, for example, Banner, when he was deposed in the Rhode Island case, argued that there were no "central nervous system deficits or injuries" at levels below "70 and closer to 100, probably."[27] Banner rejected the conclusions reached by investigator after investigator that there was a relationship between low levels of "lead ingestion and adverse cognitive, behavioral or emotional status."[28] More recently, at a 2011 trial about the poisoning of children in the town of Herculaneum, Missouri, by the Fluor Corporation's lead smelter, Banner rejected the significance of the relationship between low-level lead and behavioral and psychological measures, arguing that these measures did not constitute lead poisoning because only "demonstrable clinical effects on a human system is lead poisoning [and] that occurs as you start to interfere with hemoglobin, metabolism, at about forty [µg/dl]." Whatever "associations" existed between low-level lead exposure and behavioral, psychological, and educational deficits were "tiny," he claimed, when compared to the effects of social factors such as "the home environment and parenting interactions."[29]

The lead industry's close ties to the nation's presidential administrations has a long history. In the 1950s, President Eisenhower appointed the former head of the Lead Industries Association as assistant secretary of the interior for mineral resources, the office that controlled lead procurements and policy for the federal government. During the George W. Bush administration, Gale Norton, who, until her nomination was a lobbyist for the lead industry, served as the secretary of the interior. When questioned at her confirmation hearing in January 2001 about the role of her company, NL Industries (formerly the National Lead Company), she maintained that the lead industry, unlike the tobacco industry, had "a record of responsible corporate behavior."[30]

The Bush administration's attempts to undermine the purpose and safeguards established under the Federal Advisory Committee Act did not go unnoticed by the scientific and technical community. David Michaels, former assistant secretary of the Department of Energy in the Clinton administration and under the Obama administration the assistant secretary of labor for OSHA; Eula Bingham, former administrator of OSHA under President Carter; Sheldon Krimsky, professor of environmental sciences and long-time writer on environmental policy; Celeste Montforton, former assistant to the administrator of the Mine Safety and Health Administration; David Ozonoff, professor of public health at Boston University; and Anthony Robbins, one of the first chiefs of NIOSH, among others, wrote an editorial for *Science* magazine that laid out their concerns. The Bush administration's appointments were undermining the "vital role" that the CDC advisory committees played in developing and guiding the federal government's science policy: "Instead of grappling with scientific ambiguity and shaping public policy using the best available evidence (the fundamental principle underlying public health and environmental regulation), we can now expect these committees to emphasize the uncertainties of health and environmental risks, supporting the administration's anti-regulatory views and in those areas where there are deeply held conflicts and values, we can expect only silence. Regulatory paralysis appears to be the goal here, rather than the application of honest, balanced science."[31]

The Bush administration's strategy, often shared by the lead industry, was to prey upon natural uncertainty and a misunderstanding of science. The inherent uncertainty of epidemiology, which often leads to multiple statistical associations between different factors linked to disease outcomes, and careful application of the scientific method, which encourages skepticism and constant refinement and rethinking, become—in the hands of those opposed to regulation and complete lead abatement—a tool for maintaining the status quo and, as a consequence, for allowing children to be poisoned. The historical attempt by those who have leveraged scientific uncertainty to undermine the importance of evidence helps to explain why lead researchers like Julian Chisolm and Mark Farfel felt compelled to use a controlled experiment to "prove" what could otherwise seem self-evident: that the less lead dust present in the child's environment, the better for the children.[32]

Since the 1970s, conservative analysts have often been successful in using epidemiological studies to raise doubts about the dangers of industrial pollution in their communities. The inability to pinpoint the specific pollutant or source of exposure that leads to cancer clusters in chemically polluted communities in Massachusetts, Louisiana, and elsewhere, for example, has been used to deny the culpability of the chemical industry.[33] In part, this reflects a difference in the understanding of what constitutes epidemiological and scientific proof and a difference in perspective as to how much evidence is enough to justify imposing protective regulations.[34] It is the accumulation of evidence and the direction of that evidence, however, that shows causality. Even tobacco's relationship to lung cancer was not "proven" by a single study, epidemiological or otherwise. Rather, it was the accretion of epidemiological and clinical evidence that leaves few, if anyone, in doubt of the reality of this causal link.

David Michaels in *Doubt Is Their Product*, Thomas McGarity and Wendy Wagner in *Bending Science*, and Naomi Oreskes and Erik Conway in *Merchants of Doubt* have broadly analyzed the ways that numerous industries have used the inherent processes of science (in which new questions arise in light of new evidence) to create scientific uncertainty about even the most obvious relationships between toxic products and outcomes. They show how the tobacco, chemical, and oil and gas industries, among others, manipulate science and scientists to undermine awareness of the connection between their industry's activities and issues ranging from cancer to global warming.[35] Although the Obama administration appointed department heads, administrators, and advisory committee members who were respected for scientific integrity and who understood the stakes involved in the battles over science, many of the same antiregulatory tactics used in previous decades continued to haunt important issues such as the root causes of global warming and air pollution. In fact, in 2012 funding for the CDC's lead program was virtually eliminated. Also important in stifling reform has been the paralyzing inability of regulatory agencies such as the EPA to even evaluate the environmental dangers of thousands of chemicals. According to the EPA, in 1998 only 43 percent of twenty-eight hundred chemicals produced in volumes of 1 million pounds a year or more had basic toxicity data, and only 7 percent had a complete set of basic screening-level toxicity data.[36] (According to the EPA website in 2011, such data have not been updated and are no longer being collected—itself indicative of the problem.)[37]

Unfortunately for the public's health, when it comes to potential toxins the absence of evidence is not evidence of absence of risk. Bruce Lanphear points out the implications of policy that allows us to be exposed to these untested chemicals: "We are finding that exceedingly low levels of exposure to the most widely studied chemicals," including lead, mercury, tobacco, plastics, DDT, and pesticides, "are associated with learning problems and behavior problems such as reading deficits and ADHD and pre-term birth." By allowing new and untested chemicals to be introduced into our environment, "we are allowing industry to profit by using our children as uninformed research subjects of a vast experiment."[38]

BATTLES OVER SCIENCE AND EPIDEMIOLOGY

Until the late 1990s, most environmental critiques focused on local or national disputes. But in the first years of the twenty-first century, the arguments have taken on international dimensions, especially concerning the role of human activity in climate change. These international discussions have significantly raised the stakes in what was once a relatively limited debate about how to respond to particular crises like Love Canal in New York, Bhopal in India, or specific threats like lead. The World Health Organization in 2010 said that "acute and chronic lead poisoning remain problems of enormous importance for child health and development worldwide," for "16% of all children worldwide [are] estimated to have [blood lead] levels above 10 µg/dl."[39] Issues that were once of concern to particular companies and local communities are now of concern to multinational corporations and the world. In recent years, lobbying groups ranging from the American Petroleum Institute and its corporate sponsors in the oil and gas industry to the American Enterprise Institute, along with some major funders of the Republican Party, including billionaire brothers David and Charles Koch, have argued that the climate question is still unresolved and that much more research is needed before this "theory" can be addressed through changes in U.S. energy policy.[40]

The scientific community itself has no doubt about lead's terrible effects or the reality of global warming caused by human actions, despite efforts to cloud these issues. But even for less certain science—nanotechnologies, for example—we still need to develop policies that protect the public's health while we accumulate and evaluate the evidence for and against potential harm. Some argue that "progress" demands that industries remain free from regulatory constraints until dangers are proven, a process that can take decades. Does this mean that policy making should remain paralyzed as we seek more and more information? Perhaps we need a different approach, one that takes science's uncertainty not as a sign that there is no danger but as a sign that serious danger might well exist. If we took this approach, we would have a policy model that emphasizes restraint and caution rather than unchecked technological advancement. Such an approach (called by some the "precautionary principle") might become ever-more important as we contemplate the newer health issues that industry presents us. Perhaps we should consider the admonition of the National Research Council in 1991: "Until better evidence is developed prudent public policy demands that a margin of safety be provided regarding potential health risks. . . . We do no less in designing bridges and buildings. We do no less in establishing criteria for scientific credibility. We must surely do no less when the health and quality of life of Americans are at stake."[41]

But it is difficult to envision adopting a precautionary approach when confronted with legislative paralysis and a broad antiregulatory ideology that equates government action with individual repression. The logic of the public health model depends on the belief that good empirical evidence leads to good policy. But if good empirical evidence demands a level of certainty that the methodologies of science in general, and the sciences of epidemiology and statistics in particular, are not capable of providing, then, ironically, politicians can use public health science to delay, deny, and obscure scientific consensus. Science can thus be turned against itself. More than thirty-five studies were done during the 1980s and 1990s about various lead-abatement strategies. Yet, despite the evidence compiled, by the turn of the twenty-first century policy makers were unwilling to commit the needed resources to finally remove lead from children's homes, and the courts were unwilling to hold accountable the companies responsible for this ecological and human tragedy.

This was, perhaps, most poignantly expressed by Julian Chisolm himself in an article published in the midst of the Maryland Court of Appeals consideration of the Kennedy Krieger Institute case and three months before his death of congestive heart failure. His piece had a special irony, for it captured the sad hundred-year history of this completely preventable national tragedy, and perhaps Chisolm's own role in it. Chisolm identified the bitter political obstacles that were placed on this road. Observing that "the total removal of lead in the United States has long been rejected by the authorities as too expensive," he lamented that children were still being used as the "biological indicators of substandard housing" and that "this must stop!" But while the "ultimate goal" might be primary prevention, Chisolm accepted the political limitations that were imposed on public health and argued for "introducing interim measures" that could "protect thousands of children until we can eliminate this preventable disease altogether."[42]

The inability of public health by itself to marshal the forces needed to get rid of lead and truly protect children moved the actions of the 1990s through the present day out of the professional and political arenas and into the courts, in the hope that the courts could impose on politicians what the public health field could not.[43] One message from this story is that those who create the risks should have a responsibility in eliminating them, even in the face of uncertainty about the breadth and seriousness of those risks.

Presently, the public health profession faces a conundrum: as the threats from industrial and environmental pollutants multiply, will the profession of public health remain true to its traditional mission of working to prevent disease or will it accommodate itself time and again to the politics of "economic feasibility"? And what will we as a society insist upon? As public health researchers, environmental activists, and those concerned with environmental justice have documented for more than fifty years, those without power—poor whites, African Americans, and Latinos, among others—bear the disproportionate burden of risks that shorten their life spans, destroy the life chances of their children, and burden them with heart disease, hypertension, stroke, diabetes, and multiple other consequences of social inequalities.

But, even if the powerless bear a disproportionate burden, we are all at risk: the pollution of our homes, land, air, streets, and waterways and the injection of chemicals into our everyday lives through food itself are now deeply engrained in our national economy and even culture. Public health workers, researchers, and advocates, faced with the depressing realities of an antigovernment and antiregulatory ideology, and the ongoing suffering of people, will in future years continue to confront the dilemma that the researchers at Kennedy Krieger did. Will people working in public health re-create the earlier alliances with the poor, the disenfranchised, and political activists, which transformed the nation's health through a radical restructuring of the nation's housing, food distribution, and industrial and urban infrastructure? Or will they retreat into their professional shell, defining the role of public health as doing more and more studies in the hope that others will be convinced to act? We all have a stake in rethinking the danger, risk, and responsibility that the story of lead reveals. If the threats from low levels of lead and other toxins continue to multiply in the environment, and if we continue to accept that scientific uncertainty about danger can trump precaution and prevention, we all remain research subjects in a grand experiment without purpose.

Many world and moral leaders, from Mahatma Gandhi to Hubert Humphrey, have noted that a society is measured by its treatment of its children. If this is true, we must ask whether we in the United States have passed this measure. For more than a hundred years, we have knowingly poisoned our children and destroyed the futures of millions of our citizens. Lead poisoning, we remind ourselves, is a completely preventable disease that we have had foisted on us by rapacious industries that have knowingly profited from our human suffering. We have avoided holding them accountable and by doing so have ensured that future generations of children will be sacrificed as well. We have created a false and morally bankrupt equation that has judged the ill health of our citizens to be less costly than removal from our environment of this dangerous neurotoxin. The lessons learned from our sad history of lead poisoning should not be forgotten, for in future years we will again and again face the Faustian bargain in which today's technological "progress" will be paid for with the health and well-being of future generations.

Notes

PREFACE

1. State of Rhode Island v. Lead Industries Association Inc., Case No. PC 99-5226, 2007 R.I. Super LEXIS 32 (2007), *rev'd*, 951 A.2d 428 (R.I. 2008).

2. *Rhode Island v. Lead Industries Assoc.*, 951 A.2d at 455–59 (this revised ruling held that the defendants' actions were not cognizable as a public nuisance).

3. See the video *Harmless to Humans* (1946), available at www.youtube.com/watch?v=nP3ZLNSJu5g (accessed March 20, 2012).

4. John Ruddock, "Lead Poisoning in Children with Special Reference to Pica," *Journal of the American Medical Association* (hereafter *JAMA*) 82 (May 24, 1924): 1684.

CHAPTER 1

1. Ericka Grimes v. Kennedy Krieger Institute Inc., No. 128, and Myron Higgins et al. v. Kennedy Krieger Institute Inc., No. 129, 366 Md. 29, 782 A.2d 807, 2001 Md. LEXIS 496 at *16 (2001).

2. Ibid. at *114.

3. Sarah Vogel, *Is It Safe?: Bisphenol A and the Struggle to Define the Risks of Chemicals* (Berkeley: University of California Press, 2013).

4. Hibbert Hill, *The New Public Health* (New York: Macmillan, 1916), 8 (emphasis in original).

5. This section is based on Amy Fairchild, David Rosner, James Colgrove, Ronald Bayer, and Linda Fried, "The Exodus of Public Health," *American Journal of Public Health* 100 (January 2010): 54–63.

6. This tension between environmental/social reform and laboratory science continued even within these universities for decades. For example, at Yale, C-E.A. Winslow continued until the 1930s to fight for the more radical vision of public health, while Johns Hopkins biologist Raymond Pearl

and others provided intellectual support for the new, politically more conservative public health vision—eugenics in particular—until the late 1920s.

7. Fairchild et al., "Exodus of Public Health."

8. Centers for Disease Control, "Blood Lead Levels Keep Dropping; New Guidelines Proposed for Those Most Vulnerable" (1997), available at www.cdc.gov/nchs/pressroom/97news/bldlead.htm (accessed September 28, 2011); U.S. Environmental Protection Agency, "Chapter 1: Executive Summary" in *Air Quality: EPA's Integrated Science Assessments* (draft report), available at http://oaspub.epa.gov/eims/eimscomm.getfile?p_download_id=505107 (accessed March 12, 2012).

9. Bruce Lanphear, "Editorial: The Conquest of Lead Poisoning; A Pyrrhic Victory," *Environmental Health Perspectives* 115 (October 2007): A484–85.

10. John Ruddock, "Lead Poisoning in Children with Special Reference to Pica," *JAMA* 82 (May 24, 1924): 1684.

11. National Lead Company, *The Dutch Boy Conquers Old Man Gloom* (National Lead Company, 1929) (pamphlet).

12. Gerald Markowitz and David Rosner, *Deceit and Denial: The Deadly Politics of Industrial Pollution* (Berkeley: University of California Press; New York: Milbank Memorial Fund, 2013), chapters 2 and 3.

13. This estimate is based on a review of the history of lead poisoning Julian Chisolm wrote near the end of his life. He noted that Baltimore, the only city that had attempted any systematic surveillance of lead poisoning prior to the 1960s, reported forty-nine deaths during the 1930s for a population of children that represented 0.65 percent of the "total child population of the United States." J. Julian Chisolm, "Evolution of the Management and Prevention of Childhood Lead Poisoning: Dependence of Advances in Public Health on Technological Advances in the Determination of Lead and Related Biochemical Indicators of Its Toxicity," *Environmental Research*, Section A, vol. 86 (2001): 113.

14. In 1937, Johns Hopkins University founded the Children's Rehabilitation Institute primarily to treat children with cerebral palsy. In 1968, its name was changed to the Kennedy Institute, and in 1992 it was renamed the Kennedy Krieger Institute.

15. See Markowitz and Rosner, *Deceit and Denial*.

16. *Grimes v. Kennedy Krieger Institute* and *Higgins v. Kennedy Krieger Institute*, 366 Md. 29, 782 A.2d 807, 2001 Md. LEXIS 496 at *6.

17. Ibid. at *114.

18. "John T." is a pseudonym. We use pseudonyms in the chapter text for individual plaintiffs; source citations retain true names.

19. Unless otherwise noted, quotations and medical information about John T. are from the medical record of J.T., Johns Hopkins Hospital, Harriet Lane Home for Invalid Children, May 21, 1940, through July 20, 1943, Rec. No. A-14795, Medical Records Department, Johns Hopkins Hospital, Baltimore.

20. In January 2012 the CDC's lead advisory committee recommended that the level of concern for lead poisoning in children be reduced from 10 to 5 micrograms per deciliter of blood.

21. Baltimore Health Department, radio broadcast [October 15, 1935], transcript, Baltimore Health Department Archives, LIA Papers.

22. Since the 1970s the issue of the relative responsibilities of the individual, the government, and society for controlling chronic disease has been the source of a critical debate among policy makers, ethicists, and public health practitioners, stimulated in part by the appearance of Marc Lalonde's 1974 report, *A New Perspective on the Health of Canadians* (Ottawa: Department of National Health and Welfare, 1974).

23. See Vogel, *Is It Safe?: Bisphenol A and the Struggle to Define the Risks of Chemicals.*

24. Public health also faced internal crises that did not help its cause. The swine flu vaccination program, organized during the administration of Gerald Ford as a national effort to protect against a perceived potential epidemic, was broadly considered a fiasco when the disease failed to appear. Many see this moment as a "cause" of the decline in public health authority, but it must be seen within a larger historical perspective. See Richard Neustadt and Harvey Fineberg, *The Epidemic That Never Was: Policy-Making and the Swine Flu Scare* (New York: Vintage, 1983).

25. Herbert Needleman, "The Future Challenge of Lead Toxicity," *Environmental Health Perspectives* 89 (1990): 87–88.

26. "Sam T." is a pseudonym.

27. Jury trial transcript, October 5, 2007, vol. 5, 1138–39, in Steven Thomas v. Clinton L. Mallett et al., Case No. 99CV006411, State of Wisconsin Circuit Court, Milwaukee Branch.

28. Ibid., 1139–40.

29. Ibid., 1141.

30. Ibid., 1141–42.

31. Ibid., 1144–45.

32. Ibid., 1143–44.

33. Ibid., 1146.

34. Ibid., 1148.

35. On top of these physiological and neurological problems, it could not have helped that when he was eight years old Steven witnessed the murder of his two sisters, gunned down in front of his house, and when he was sixteen his mother died from lung cancer.

36. See Vogel, *Is it Safe?: Bisphenol A and the Struggle to Define the Risks of Chemicals.*

37. See Joe Thorton, *Pandora's Poison: Chlorine, Health and a New Environmental Strategy* (Cambridge, MA: MIT Press, 2000); and Theo Colburn, Diane Dumanoski, and John Peterson Myers, *Our Stolen Future: Are We Threatening Our Fertility, Intelligence and Survival? A Scientific Detective Story* (New York: Plume, 1997).

38. David Rosner and Gerald Markowitz, "The Politics of Lead Toxicology and the Devastating Consequences for Children," *American Journal of Industrial Medicine* 50 (October 2007): 740–56; Gerald Markowitz and David

Rosner, "Standing Up to the Lead Industry: An Interview with Herbert Needleman," *Public Health Reports* 120 (May–June 2005): 300–337. See also Lydia Denworth, *Toxic Truth: A Scientist, a Doctor and the Battle over Lead* (Boston: Beacon Press, 2008).

39. J. S. Lin-Fu, "Modern History of Lead Poisoning: A Century of Discovery and Rediscovery," in *Human Lead Exposure*, ed. H. L. Needleman (Boca Raton, FL: CRC Press, 1992), 23–43.

40. Jane S. Lin-Fu to leadnet@mail-list.com, "Re: Holier than thou—what we did not know until the 1970s and later," July 3, 2007.

41. Gerald Markowitz and David Rosner, "Politicizing Science: The Case of the Bush Administration's Influence on the Lead Advisory Panel at the Centers for Disease Control," *Journal of Public Health Policy* 24 (Summer 2003): 101–24.

42. Mike Stobbe, "Panel Urges Lower Cutoff for Child Lead Poisoning," Associated Press, available at www.google.com/hostednews/ap/article/ALeqM5iAwIoBG7rtcz5eJ6CLjWuhcCc86Q (accessed January 5, 2012).

43. U.S. Department of Health and Human Services, Public Health Service, Centers for Disease Control (CDC), *Strategic Plan for the Elimination of Childhood Lead Poisoning* (Atlanta: U.S. Department of Health and Human Services, Public Health Service, Centers for Disease Control, 1991).

44. Herbert L. Needleman, "What Is Not Found in the Spreadsheets," *Neurotoxicology and Teratology* 24 (2002): 460.

45. CDC, *Strategic Plan for the Elimination of Childhood Lead Poisoning*.

46. Needleman, "What Is Not Found in the Spreadsheets," 461.

47. *Grimes v. Kennedy Krieger Institute* and *Higgins v. Kennedy Krieger Institute*, 366 Md. 29, 782 A.2d 807, 2001 Md. LEXIS 496.

48. Battelle, *Quality Assurance Project Plan for the Kennedy Krieger Institute Lead-Based Paint Abatement and Repair and Maintenance Study* (draft report to Office of Pollution Prevention and Toxics, U.S. Environmental Protection Agency, June 22, 1992).

49. Mark Farfel, "Third-Year Renewal: RPN No. 91-05-02-01, Lead-Paint Abatement and Repair and Maintenance Study in Baltimore," received by Joint Committee on Clinical Investigation, Johns Hopkins University, April 21, 1995.

50. Robert M. Nelson, "Nontherapeutic Research, Minimal Risk: The Kennedy Krieger Lead Abatement Study," *IRB: Ethics and Human Research* 23 (November–December 2001): 7–11, reprinted as "Appropriate Risk Exposure in Environmental Health Research: The Kennedy Krieger Lead Abatement Study," *Journal of Law, Medicine and Ethics* 30 (Spring 2002): 445–49.

51. An out-of-court settlement occurred before a trial took place, eliminating any chance for a public hearing of the issue, although the Maryland Court of Appeals records are, of course, publicly available. In 2011 a new class action lawsuit was filed against Johns Hopkins on behalf of all the children in the study.

52. National Commission for the Protection of Human Subjects of Biomedical and Behavioral Research, *The Belmont Report: Ethical Principles*

and Guidelines for the Protection of Human Subjects of Research, DHEW Publication No. (OS) 78-0012 (Washington, D.C.: GPO, 1978), available at http://videocast.nih.gov/pdf/ohrp_belmont_report.pdf (accessed March 16, 2012).

53. David R. Buchanan and Franklin G. Miller, "Justice and Fairness in the Kennedy Krieger Institute Lead Paint Study: The Ethics of Public Health Research on Less Expensive, Less Effective Interventions," *American Journal of Public Health* 96 (May 2006): 784.

54. Lainie Friedman Ross, "In Defense of The Hopkins Lead Abatement Studies," *Journal of Law, Medicine and Ethics* 30 (Spring 2002): 53–54.

55. Nelson, "Appropriate Risk Exposure in Environmental Health Research: The Kennedy Krieger Lead Abatement Study."

56. Nelson, "Appropriate Risk Exposure in Environmental Health Research," 448.

57. Ibid., 449.

58. Loretta M. Kopelman, "Pediatric Research Regulations Under Legal Scrutiny: *Grimes* Narrows Their Interpretation," *Journal of Law, Medicine and Ethics* 30 (2002): 42.

59. Merle Spriggs, "Canaries in the Mines: Children, Risk, Non-Therapeutic Research, and Justice," *Journal of Medical Ethics* 30 (2004): 179. Such debates prompted the National Academy of Sciences to issue a report arguing that with strong protections such research could proceed if benefits to other vulnerable children were anticipated. Committee on Ethical Issues in Housing-Related Health Hazard Research Involving Children, Youth, and Families, *Ethical Considerations for Research on Housing-Related Health Hazards Involving Children,* ed. Bernard Lo and Mary Ellen O'Connell (Washington, D.C.: National Academies Press, 2005), available at www.nap.edu/openbook.php?record_id=11450&page=R1 (accessed December 15, 2011).

CHAPTER 2

Epigraph: Austin Bradford Hill, "The Environment and Disease: Association or Causation?," *Proceedings of the Royal Society of Medicine* 58 (1965): 300.

1. Randolph K. Byers and Elizabeth E. Lord, "Late Effects of Lead Poisoning on Mental Development," *American Journal of Diseases of Children* 66 (November 1943): 477.

2. See Gerald Markowitz and David Rosner, *Deceit and Denial: The Deadly Politics of Industrial Pollution* (Berkeley: University of California Press; New York: Milbank Memorial Fund, 2013), 95–107.

3. Elizabeth Fee, "Public Health in Practice: An Early Confrontation with the 'Silent Epidemic' of Childhood Lead Paint Poisoning," *Journal of the History of Medicine and Allied Sciences* 45 (October 1990): 570. This section on the Baltimore experience is drawn largely from Fee's pioneering work.

4. LIA, directors' meeting, minutes, September 28, 1932, papers of the Lead Industries Association and Associated Companies, New York City Law

Department, Affirmative Litigation Division, in authors' possession (hereafter LIA Papers).

5. Fee, "Public Health in Practice," 579.

6. "Death Brings Warning on Lead Poisoning," *Baltimore American*, October 13, 1932, Huntington Williams Collection, Chesney Archives, Baltimore.

7. Fee, "Public Health in Practice," 581.

8. Billianman A. Alli, "Lead Poisoning in Children," *Journal of the National Medical Association* 69 (1977): 797.

9. Baltimore Health Department, radio broadcast, [October 15, 1935], transcript, Baltimore Health Department Archives, LIA Papers.

10. In the decades before World War II, the "estimation of lead in [one] 24-hr urine specimen occupied a technician for two full days." Randolph K. Byers, introduction to *Low Level Lead Exposure: The Clinical Implications of Current Research*, ed. Herbert L. Needleman, (New York: Raven Press, 1980), 1.

11. J. Julian Chisolm, "Evolution of the Management and Prevention of Childhood Lead Poisoning: Dependence of Advances in Public Health on Technological Advances in the Determination of Lead and Related Biochemical Indicators of Its Toxicity," *Environmental Research*, Section A, vol. 86 (2001): 116.

12. Fee, "Public Health in Practice," 584.

13. Ibid., 585. See also Mark R. Farfel, "Reducing Lead Exposure in Children," *Annual Reviews of Public Health* 6 (1985): 339, which notes that Baltimore's "Ordinance on the Hygiene of Housing provided a legal base for lead paint removal from housing as a health hazard" and that "public health nurses began investigating cases and educating parents in the late 1940s."

14. J.M. McDonald and E. Kaplan, "Incidence of Lead Poisoning in the City of Baltimore," *JAMA* 119 (July 11, 1942): 870.

15. M.Q. McDonald, "Maryland—Toxic Finishes," July 14, 1949, LIA Papers.

16. LIA, "Lead Hygiene and Safety Bulletin #79," December 1, 1950, LIA Papers.

17. LIA, "Report of the Secretary," annual meeting, April 13–14, 1950, LIA Papers.

18. Bowditch to Aub, December 21, 1949, LIA Papers.

19. LIA, "Lead Hygiene and Safety Bulletin #79," December 1, 1950, LIA Papers.

20. A. Jefferis Turner, "Lead Poisoning in Childhood," *Australasian Medical Congress* (1908): 2–9.

21. Mark R. Farfel, "Reducing Lead Exposure in Children," *Annual Reviews of Public Health* 6 (1985): 334. See also J. Edmund Bradley et. al., "The Incidence of Abnormal Blood Levels of Lead in a Metropolitan Pediatric Clinic," *Journal of Pediatrics* 49 (July 1956): 1–6.

22. Regulation quoted in Fee, "Public Health in Practice," 588.

23. Huntington Williams, Emanuel Kaplan, Charles Couchman, and R.R. Sayers, "Lead Poisoning in Young Children," *Public Health Reports* 67 (March 1952): 230.

24. LIA, "Report of the Secretary," annual meeting, April 13–14, 1950, LIA Papers.

25. LIA, "Lead Hygiene," annual meeting, April 9–10, 1953, LIA Papers.

26. J. Julian Chisolm Jr. and Harold Harrison, "The Exposure of Children to Lead," *Pediatrics* 18 (1956): 955.

27. "Dietary Habits of Baltimore Babies," editorial, *American Journal of Public Health* 41 (December 1951): 1528.

28. Interview with Robert Mellins, New York City, January 10, 2012.

29. Bowditch to Ziegfield, December 16, 1952, courtesy of Christian Warren.

30. *New York Times*, November 9, 1954, 26. Wheatley later worked with Metropolitan Life as a consultant and principal designer of major medical coverage for chronic diseases.

31. Bowditch to Ziegfield, December 16, 1952.

32. Ibid.

33. Kehoe to Herbert Hillman, September 4, 1953, courtesy of Christian Warren.

34. Manfred Bowditch to Reginald Atwater, December 19, 1951, LIA Papers.

35. Bowditch to Wormser, July 11, 1956, LIA Papers.

36. Manfred Bowditch, Director, LIA, "Report of Health and Safety Division," 29th Annual Meeting, April 24–25, 1957, LIA Papers.

37. Bowditch to Kehoe, December 26, 1957, courtesy of Christian Warren.

38. Jane S. Lin-Fu, untitled article in *Children Today*, January–February 1979, 11.

39. Ibid.

40. Ibid.

41. BAL was first used in 1946 to treat children, CaEDTA in 1950.

42. J. Julian Chisolm, "Synopsis of Medical Aspects of Childhood Lead Poisoning," paper presented at the Conference on Lead Poisoning in Children, Rockefeller University, May 26, 1969, LIA Papers.

43. Melvin W. First, "Possibilities of Removal of Sources of Lead Contamination in the Environment," in *Symposium on Environmental Lead Contamination*, by U.S. Public Health Service (Washington, D.C.: GPO, March 1966), 91.

44. Roy O. McCaldin, "Estimation of Sources of Atmospheric Lead and Measured Atmospheric Lead Levels," in *Symposium on Environmental Lead Contamination*, by U.S. Public Health Service (Washington, D.C.: GPO, March 1966), 8.

45. First, "Possibilities of Removal of Sources of Lead Contamination in the Environment," 92.

46. Robert A. Kehoe, "Under What Circumstances Is Ingestion of Lead Dangerous?," in *Symposium on Environmental Lead Contamination*, by U.S. Public Health Service (Washington, D.C.: GPO, March 1966), 54.

47. Harry Heimann in "Discussion of Harry Heimann," transcript of discussion following Heimann's presentation of "Risk of Exposure and Absorption of Lead," in *Symposium on Environmental Lead Contamination*, by U.S. Public Health Service (Washington, D.C.: GPO, March 1966), 147–48. See also William Graebner, "Hegemony through Science: Information Engineering and Lead Toxicology, 1925–1965," in *Dying for Work: Workers' Safety and Health in Twentieth-Century America*, ed. David Rosner and Gerald Markowitz (Bloomington: Indiana University Press, 1987), 140–59.

48. Dr. Radford in "Discussion of Harry Heimann," following Heimann's "Risk of Exposure and Absorption of Lead," in *Symposium on Environmental Lead Contamination*, 151.

49. Ibid.

50. LIA, "Minutes of Special Committee on Health and Safety," January 14, 1966, Wormser MSS, American Heritage Center, University of Wyoming, Cheyenne (hereafter Wormser MSS). Included on the committee were S. D. Strauss, chairman, American Smelting and Refining Company; A. H. Drewes, National Lead Company; John Englehorn, St. Joseph Lead Company; and Burt Goss and Carl Thompson, Hill & Knowlton.

51. LIA, "No Public Hazard from Lead Seen, Muskie Sub-Committee on Pollution Told," press release, June 9, [1966], Wormser MSS.

52. *Air Pollution—1966: Hearings Before a Senate Subcommittee on Air and Water Pollution of the Committee on Public Works*, 89th Congress (1966) (statement of Robert Kehoe), 205.

53. Ibid., 205–7.

54. LIA, "Opinion Research Corp. Caravan Survey on Lead: Summary Report," in J. L. Kimberly to Board of Directors, March 7, 1967, papers of the Manufacturing Chemists Association (later, the Chemical Manufacturers Association) and several individual chemical companies obtained in discovery proceedings by the law firm of Baggett, McCall, Burgess, and Watson, Lake Charles, Louisiana. The summary report was prepared by Hill & Knowlton, the LIA's public relations counsel.

55. David M. Borcina, Secretary, Treasurer, LIA, to members of the LIA, January 18, 1968, LIA Papers.

56. LIA, *Facts about Lead and the Atmosphere* [1968], LIA Papers. The early ads included such headlines as "Lead Helps to Guard Your Health," "Lead Takes Part in Many Games," "Why Paint Saves Lives," "Color—Yes . . . for Every Part of the Hospital," and other booklets and promotional materials aimed at linking lead with modernity and healthfulness. See Markowitz and Rosner, *Deceit and Denial*, chapter 3, "Cater to the Children: The Promotion of White Lead."

57. LIA, *Facts about Lead and the Atmosphere*.

58. Clair C. Patterson, "Contaminated and Natural Lead Environments of Man," *Archives of Environmental Health* 11 (September 1965): 350. This section on Patterson and Hardy is based on our book *Deceit and Denial*, chapter 4.

59. Patterson, "Contaminated and Natural Lead Environments of Man," 350.

60. Christian Warren, *Brush with Death: A Social History of Lead Poisoning* (Baltimore: Johns Hopkins University Press, 2000), 210–11; Patterson, "Contaminated and Natural Lead Environments of Man," 344.

61. Patterson, "Contaminated and Natural Lead Environments of Man"; Warren, *Brush with Death*, 307n4.

62. Patterson, "Contaminated and Natural Lead Environments of Man," 344.

63. Warren, *Brush with Death*, 214.

64. Patterson, "Contaminated and Natural Lead Environments of Man," 344, quoted in Warren, *Brush with Death*, 212.

65. Patterson, "Contaminated and Natural Lead Environments of Man," 344–60. See also Warren, *Brush with Death*, 216–17. Indeed, as Warren has noted, news of and interest in Patterson's challenge to prevailing ideas about environmental lead extended beyond the scientific and technical communities by the late 1960s. Saul Bellow modeled Albert Corde, the central character of his novel *The Dean's December* (New York: Harper and Row, 1982), on Clair Patterson.

66. LIA, "News from Lead Industries Association," press release, September 10, [1965], LIA Papers.

67. LIA, "Annual Review—1974," [1975], LIA Papers.

68. Harriet Hardy, "Lead," in *Symposium on Environmental Lead Contamination*, by U.S. Public Health Service (Washington, D.C.: GPO, March 1966), 74–82,

69. See Markowitz and Rosner, *Deceit and Denial*, 36–63.

70. Hardy, "Lead," 74–82, cited in Warren, *Brush with Death*, 217.

71. Warren, *Brush with Death*, 216–17.

72. Hardy, "Lead," 149. See also Hardy, "What Is the Status of Knowledge of the Toxic Effect of Lead on Identifiable Groups in the Population," 713–22. Hardy was quoting Hill's famous lecture before the Royal Society of Medicine that became a basic statement of the evolving field of environmental epidemiology. See Austin Bradford Hill, "The Environment and Disease: Association or Causation?," *Proceedings of the Royal Society of Medicine* 58 (1965): 295–300.

73. Warren, *Brush with Death*, 262.

74. Lin-Fu, untitled article in *Children Today*, 11–12; Nicholas Freudenberg and Maxine Golub, "Health Education, Public Policy and Disease Prevention: A Case History of the New York City Coalition to End Lead Poisoning," *Health Education Quarterly* 14 (Winter 1987): 389–90; Frank P. L. Somerville, "Harlem Park Group Rapped," *Baltimore Sun*, December 6, 1964, 28; "Panthers Set Sickle Cell Tests," *Baltimore Sun*, October 26, 1971, A7.

75. Freudenberg and Golub, "Health Education, Public Policy and Disease Prevention," 390. See also Judy Klemesrud, "Young Women Find a Place in High Command of Young Lords," *New York Times*, November 11, 1970, 78.

76. Jack Newfield, "Silent Epidemic in the Slums," *Village Voice*, September 18, 1969, 3. See also Freudenberg and Golub, "Health Education, Public Policy and Disease Prevention," 390.

77. Mark R. Farfel, "Reducing Lead Exposure in Children," *Annual Reviews of Public Health* 6 (1985): 340.

78. We are indebted to Merlin Chowkwanyun, a doctoral candidate at the University of Pennsylvania, whose pioneering work on the history of the health Left details the untold contributions of numerous groups around the country to reform health care in its various aspects.

79. Lin-Fu, untitled article in *Children Today*, 11–12.

80. Billianman A. Alli, "Lead Poisoning in Children," *Journal of the National Medical Association* 69 (1977): 797.

81. Ibid., 797–98.

82. Chisolm, "Evolution of the Management and Prevention of Childhood Lead Poisoning," 114. Interestingly, Chisolm began his lead research career with a grant from the Lead Industries Association. The LIA believed that the Baltimore Health Department was vastly overestimating the number of children who were lead poisoned and hoped that Chisolm's research would confirm this. It did the opposite.

83. J. Julian Chisolm, *A Manual of Military Surgery for the Use of Surgeons in the Confederate States Army* (Richmond, VA: West & Johnson, 1862).

84. Robert B. Welch, "Julian John Chisolm, M.D. Confederate Surgeon, Ophthalmologist and Hospital Founder," *Documenta Ophthalmologica* 99 (1999): 273–84. We are indebted also to Faye Haun for her research on the Chisolm family; see http://tres.ancestry.com/tree/22492056/person/1247209184/family/pedigree (accessed February 6, 2011). See also William Garnett Chisolm, *Chisolm Genealogy* (Knickerbocker Press, 1914).

85. *Johns Hopkins University Circular*, January 1917; "Dr. Chisolm Rites Today," *Baltimore Sun*, February 27, 1969, A15.

86. Interview with Ellen Silbergeld, March 25, 2010, Baltimore.

87. Interview with Connie Nathanson, December 1, 2009, New York City. See also Stephanie E. Farquhar, "Making a University City: Cycles of Disinvestment, Urban Renewal and Displacement in East Baltimore" (PhD diss., Johns Hopkins University, 2012), for a detailed look at the history of Johns Hopkins's relationship with East Baltimore: "Across the 20th century East Baltimore was subject to a complex web of disinvestment and profiteering, all aided by the actions or inactions of Baltimore City and Johns Hopkins. Hopkins wanted its faculty, students and staff to replace the blighted conditions and poor black people that the university felt made its East Baltimore institutions less attractive to the 'world class' faculty, students and staff that maintained Hopkins' reputation and its ability to attract funding. Baltimore City wanted to ensure Hopkins' fiscal wellbeing and wanted residents who paid more tax dollars" (13).

88. Farquhar, "Making a University City," 35.

89. Nathanson, interview.

90. Chisolm, "Synopsis of Medical Aspects of Childhood Lead Poisoning."

91. Ibid.

92. J. Julian Chisolm Jr., "Is Lead Poisoning Still a Problem?" *Clinical Chemistry* 23 (1977): 255.

CHAPTER 3

Epigraph: Herbert L. Needleman, "Exposure to Lead: Sources and Effects," *New England Journal of Medicine* 297 (October 27, 1977): 945.

1. The details of Jane Lin-Fu's early and professional life are from an interview with her, April 16, 2009, Potomac, MD, amended by interviewee August 24, 2009.

2. Both of Lin-Fu's parents emigrated to the United States in 1972. Her father's brother, Lin Yutang, was a prominent author in the 1940s–1960s, whose books, written in English and translated into many languages, introduced Chinese culture and philosophy to the West.

3. Lin-Fu, interview.

4. Ibid. See also Jane Lin-Fu, *Lead Poisoning in Children* (Washington, D.C.: Department of Health Education and Welfare, 1967).

5. Lin-Fu, interview.

6. Christian Warren, *Brush with Death: A Social History of Lead Poisoning* (Baltimore: Johns Hopkins University Press, 2000), 199. See also Lin-Fu, *Lead Poisoning in Children.*

7. Alondra Nelson, *Body and Soul: The Black Panther Party and the Fight against Medical Discrimination* (St. Paul: University of Minnesota Press, 2011).

8. Lin-Fu, interview.

9. Ibid.

10. Ibid.

11. Ibid.

12. CDC, "Lead," available at www.cdc.gov/nceh/lead/default.htm (accessed July 27, 2010).

13. "U.S. Campaign Urged on Lead Poisoning," *New York Times*, November 8, 1970, 95. For the surgeon general's statement, see Jesse L. Steinfeld, "Medical Aspects of Childhood Lead Poisoning," *Pediatrics* 48 (September 1971): 464–68.

14. Lin-Fu, interview.

15. Ibid.

16. See J. Julian Chisolm Jr., "Chronic Lead Intoxication in Children," *Developmental Medicine and Child Neurology* 7 (1965): 531: "Beyond infancy there is general agreement that the median value in unexposed subjects is approximately 27µg. Pb per 100 g. of whole blood and that the upper limit is 40 µg. Pb per 100 g. of whole blood. In the past, 50 to 60 µg. has been cited as the upper limit of 'normal.' . . . Indeed, it has been suggested that intoxication may occur in the presence of normal blood lead values!"

17. Lin-Fu, interview.

18. Ibid.

19. Warren, *Brush with Death*, 198.

20. See U.S. General Accounting Office, *Report by the Comptroller General of the United States: HUD Not Fulfilling Responsibility to Eliminate Lead-Based Paint Hazard in Federal Housing*, CED-81-31 (Washington, D.C.: U.S. GAO, December 16, 1980), 8.

21. Jack Newfield, "Let Them Eat Lead," *New York Times*, June 16, 1971, 45. See also Nancy Hicks, "Officials Differ on Best Way to Halt Lead Poisoning," *New York Times*, August 14, 1971, 21; and Jane S. Lin-Fu, untitled article in *Children Today*, January–February 1979, 9.

22. Hicks, "Officials Differ on Best Way to Halt Lead Poisoning," 21.

23. Ibid.

24. Jane S. Lin-Fu, "Undue Absorption of Lead Among Children: A New Look at an Old Problem," *New England Journal of Medicine* 286 (March 30, 1972): 705.

25. Ibid., 706.

26. Lin-Fu, interview.

27. Herbert L. Needleman, Orhan C. Tuncay, and Irving M. Shapiro, "Lead Levels in Deciduous Teeth of Urban and Suburban American Children," *Nature* 235 (January 14, 1972): 111.

28. Herbert Needleman and Irving Shapiro, "Lead in Deciduous Teeth: A Marker of Exposure in Heretofore Asymptomatic Children," in *Proceedings: International Symposium; Environmental Health Aspects of Lead, Amsterdam, October 2–6, 1972* (Luxemburg: Commission of the European Communities, May 1973), 775.

29. Walter Sullivan, "Babies Surveyed for Strontium 90," *New York Times*, November 25, 1961, 2. See also Les Leopold, *The Man Who Hated Work and Loved Labor* (White River Junction, VT: Chelsea Green, 2007).

30. Needleman, Tuncay, and Shapiro, "Lead Levels in Deciduous Teeth of Urban and Suburban American Children," 111.

31. "List of Participants," in *Proceedings: International Symposium; Environmental Health Aspects of Lead, Amsterdam, October 2–6, 1972* (Luxemburg: Commission of the European Communities, May 1973), 1139–55.

32. Denworth, *Toxic Truth*, 81.

33. Needleman and Shapiro, "Lead in Deciduous Teeth," 775.

34. Ibid.

35. Ibid. See also Herbert Needleman, I. Davidson, E. M. Sewell, and Irving Shapiro, "Subclinical Lead Exposure in Philadelphia School Children," *New England Journal of Medicine* 290 (January 31, 1974): 244–48.

36. See Robert Proctor, *The Golden Holocaust* (Berkeley: University of California Press, 2011); and Allan Brandt, *The Cigarette Century* (New York: Basic Books, 2008).

37. "Discussion" of Needleman and Shapiro, "Lead in Deciduous Teeth," in *Proceedings: International Symposium; Environmental Health Aspects of Lead, Amsterdam, October 2–6, 1972* (Luxemburg: Commission of the European Communities, May 1973), 780.

38. David Rosner and Gerald Markowitz, "Standing Up to the Lead Industry: An Interview with Herbert Needleman," *Public Health Reports* 120 (May–June 2005): 331.

39. Denworth, *Toxic Truth*, 31.

40. Ibid., 32.

41. Rosner and Markowitz, "Standing Up to the Lead Industry," 331. See also Denworth, *Toxic Truth*, 77.

42. Rosner and Markowitz, "Standing Up to the Lead Industry," 331.

43. Ibid. Needleman noted that "there actually had been one paper in the 1960s on high tooth lead levels in kids who had been poisoned": L. F. Altshuller, D. B. Halak, B. H. Landing, and R. A. Kehoe, "Deciduous Teeth as an Index of Body Burden of Lead," *Journal of Pediatrics* 60 (1962): 224–29.

44. Oliver David, Julian Clark, and Kytja Voeller, "Lead and Hyperactivity," *Lancet* 2 (October 28, 1972): 900.

45. Ibid.

46. For example, see ibid., 902–3.

47. Among the participants were industry spokespeople such as Gary Ter Haar; academics; pediatricians; scientists such as Herbert Needleman, Julian Chisolm, Oliver David, John Rosen, Henrietta Sachs, and Ellen Silbergeld; and government lead experts such as Kathryn Mahaffey and Robert Goyer.

48. Henrietta K. Sachs, "Effect of a Screening Program on Changing Patterns of Lead Poisoning," *Environmental Health Perspectives* 7 (May 1974): 44.

49. Gary Ter Haar and Regina Aronow, "New Information on Lead in Dirt and Dust, as Related to the Childhood Lead Problem," *Environmental Health Perspectives* 7 (May 1974): 83.

50. E. K. Silbergeld, J. T. Fales, and A. M. Goldberg, "Evidence for a Junctional Effect of Lead on Neuromuscular Function," *Nature* 247, no. 5435 (1974): 49–50.

51. Interview with Ellen K. Silbergeld, March 25, 2010, Baltimore.

52. E. K. Silbergeld and A. M. Goldberg, "Hyperactivity: A Lead-Induced Behavior Disorder," *Environmental Health Perspectives* 7 (May 1974): 227.

53. For examples, see Markowitz and Rosner, *Deceit and Denial*, chapters 6–7; and David Rosner and Gerald Markowitz, "Persistent Pollutants: A Brief History of the Discovery of the Widespread Toxicity of Chlorinated Hydrocarbons," *Environmental Research* (September 21, 2012), available at http://dx.doi.org/10.1016/j.envres.2012.08.011.

54. Silbergeld, interview.

55. *Ellen K. Silbergeld, Papers, 1968–1994: A Finding Aid* at the Arthur and Elizabeth Schlesinger Library on the History of Women in America, Cambridge, MA, available at http://oasis.lib.harvard.edu/oasis/deliver/deepLink?_collect ion=oasis&uniqueId=sch00906 (accessed April 1, 2010). Silbergeld was even arrested following a federal employees' peace rally in Lafayette Square in 1971.

56. Denworth, *Toxic Truth*, 91.

57. Ibid., 91–92. Silbergeld subsequently published many other studies confirming and expanding on this early work. See, for example, Ellen K. Silbergeld, John T. Fales, and Alan M. Goldberg, "Evidence for a Junctional Effect of Lead on Neuromuscular Function," *Nature* 247 (January 4, 1974): 49–50; Ellen K. Silbergeld, John T. Fales, and Alan M. Goldberg, "The Effects of Inorganic Lead on Neuromuscular Junction," *Neuropharmacology* 13 (1974):

795–801; Ellen K. Silbergeld and Alan M. Goldberg, "Lead-Induced Behavioral Dysfunction: An Animal Model of Hyperactivity," *Experimental Neurology* 42 (1974): 146–57; and Ellen K. Silbergeld and A.M. Goldberg, "Pharmacological and Neurochemical Investigations of Lead-Induced Hyperactivity," *Neuropharmacology* 14 (1975): 431–44.

58. Lin-Fu, untitled article in *Children Today*, 36.

59. Sergio Piomelli, Bernard Davidow, Vincent F. Guinee [New York City health commissioner], et al., "The FEP (Free Erythrocyte Porphyrins) Test: A Screening Micromethod for Lead Poisoning," *Pediatrics* 51 (February 1973): 254–59. Don Ryan, then on a Senate committee staff, until he left to form the Alliance to End Childhood Lead Poisoning, recalls the impact of this new technology: "The prevailing response to childhood lead poisoning in the 1940s and '50s came in the emergency room, when kids showed up in extremis, with brain encephalopathy—tertiary prevention. Then in the 1960s, the system gradually moved upstream to secondary prevention by using blood lead screening—sticking the fingers of kids who were not symptomatic to identify those with elevated lead levels. When a child with a significantly elevated blood lead level was identified through blood lead screening, his or her home was investigated for lead hazards. Beginning in 1974 or '75, CDC began making grants to local, and some state, health departments to support blood lead screening programs. By 1980, about one hundred cities had blood lead screening and case-management programs funded primarily by CDC grants. As these screening programs identified thousands of EBL children [above the then thresholds of 30 or 25 µg/dl], recognition of the problem was growing." The free erythrocyte porphyrins (FEPs) test used small amounts of blood to indirectly measure blood lead levels. FEPs increased "exponentially" with increased blood lead levels. Interview with Don Ryan, Washington, D.C., February 5, 2010, amended by interviewee August 10, 2010.

60. Lin-Fu, untitled article in *Children Today*, 13. In 1973, Julian Chisolm hailed the development of the EP test in *Pediatrics*, citing Sergio Piomelli and his coauthors and his own experience as leaving "no doubt" that these new tests were "the simplest, least expensive and most practical method for primary screening of children for the prevention of lead poisoning." J. Julian Chisolm, "Screening for Lead Poisoning in Children," *Pediatrics* 51 (February 1973): 280. See also S. Granick et al., "Assays for Porphyrins, δ-Aminolevulinic-Acid Dehydratase, and Porphyrinogen Synthesase in Microliter Samples of Whole Blood: applications to Metabolic Defects Involving the Heme Pathway," *Proceedings of the National Academy of Sciences*, 69 (September 1972): 2381–83; and Larry P. Kammholz et al., "Rapid Protoporphyrin Quanitation for Detection of Lead Poisoning," *Pediatrics* 50 (October 1972): 625–31.

61. Joseph Perino and Claire Ernhart, "The Relation of Sub-Clinical Lead Level to Cognitive and Sensory Motor Impairment in Black Pre-Schoolers," *Journal of Learning Disabilities* 7 (December 1974): 616.

62. Brigitte de la Burdé and McLin S. Choate, "Does Asymptomatic Lead Exposure in Children Have Latent Sequelae?," *Journal of Pediatrics* 81 (December 1972): 1088–91.

63. Brigitte de la Burdé and Irving M. Shapiro, "Dental Lead, Blood Lead and Pica in Urban Children," *Archives of Environmental Health* 30 (1975): 281. Burdé and Shapiro's results confirmed their suspicion that low-level lead exposure had long-term effects, despite variations in blood lead levels at any specific point in time.

64. Brigitte de la Burdé and McLin S. Choate, "Early Asymptomatic Lead Exposure and Development at School Age," *Journal of Pediatrics* 87 (October 1975): 641.

65. R.G. Lansdown, J. Shepard, B.E. Clayton, H.T. Delves, P.J. Graham, and W.C. Turner, "Blood-Lead Levels, Behaviour, and Intelligence: A Population Study," *Lancet* 303 (March 30, 1974): 538.

66. Oliver J. David, letter re. "Blood-Lead Levels, Behaviour and Intelligence," *Lancet* 303 (May 4, 1974): 866.

67. D. Bryce-Smith and H.A. Waldron, letter re. "Blood-Lead Levels, Behaviour and Intelligence," *Lancet* 303 (June 8, 1974): 1166. In the same issue of the *Lancet*, Philip Landrigan, then at the CDC in the U.S. Public Health Service, along with two colleagues, criticized Lansdown's methodology for using "unquantified social factors [that] could have obscured any subtle ill-effects produced by chronic lead absorption." Philip J. Landrigan, Randolph H. Whitworth, and Robert W. Baloh, letter re. "Blood-Lead Levels, Behaviour and Intelligence," *Lancet* 303 (June 8, 1974): 1167.

68. R.G. Lansdown, B.E. Clayton, P.J. Graham, and H.T. Delves, letter re. "Blood-Lead Levels, Behaviour and Intelligence," *Lancet* 303 (June 8, 1974): 1168.

69. D. Bryce-Smith and H.A. Waldron, letter re. "Blood-Lead Levels, Behaviour and Intelligence," *Lancet* 303 (July 6, 1974): 44. The report about El Paso that the authors cite is R.H. Whitworth, B.F. Rosenblum, M.S. Dickerson, and R.W. Balch, "Epidemiologic Notes and Reports: Follow-Up on Human Lead Absorption—Texas," *Morbidity and Mortality Weekly Report*, no. 23 (1974): 157–59.

70. Edward B. McCabe, letter re. "Blood-Lead Levels, Behaviour and Intelligence," *Lancet* 304 (October 12, 1974): 896.

71. Herbert Needleman, Samuel Epstein, Bertram Carnow, John Scanlon, David Parkinson, Sheldon Samuels, Anthony Mazzocchi, and Oliver David, letter re. "Blood-Lead Levels, Behaviour and Intelligence," *Lancet* 305 (March 29, 1975): 751.

72. D.H. Beilstein, St. Joseph Lead Company, Smelting Division, to J.A. Wright, "ILZRO Budget Meetings—1980," September 22, 1980, p. 1, DR 2203652, Doe Run Papers, in authors' possession (hereafter Doe Run Papers).

73. At the time, the CDC was known as the Communicable Disease Center. It changed its name to the Center for Disease Control in 1970 and then to the Centers for Disease Control in 1980.

74. Philip Landrigan, Stephen Gehlbach, Bernard Rosenblum, Jimmie Shoults, Robert Candelaria, William Barthel, John Liddle, Ann Smrek, Norman Staehling, and JoDean Sanders, "Epidemic Lead Absorption Near an Ore

Smelter: The Role of Particulate Lead," *New England Journal of Medicine* 292 (January 16, 1975): 123.

75. Interview with Phil Landrigan, May 18, 2009, New York City.

76. Ibid.

77. Landrigan et al., "Epidemic Lead Absorption Near an Ore Smelter," 123. See Monica Perales, *Smeltertown: Making and Remembering a Southwest Border Community* (Chapel Hill: University of North Carolina Press, 2010), for a social history of this community.

78. Landrigan, interview.

79. Landrigan et al., "Epidemic Lead Absorption Near an Ore Smelter," 123. See also Whitworth et al., "Epidemiologic Notes and Reports: Follow-Up on Human Lead Absorption—Texas," the *Morbidity and Mortality Weekly Report* review of the El Paso data.

80. D. H. Beilstein, St. Joseph Minerals Corporation, Lead Smelting Division, to Gardner L. Brown, St. Joseph Minerals Corporation, September 27, 1972, DR 600193, Doe Run Papers.

81. Quoted in Marianne Sullivan, *Tainted Earth* (New Brunswick, NJ: Rutgers University Press, forthcoming). We are grateful to Dr. Sullivan for sharing her work.

82. Landrigan, interview.

83. Ibid.

84. Landrigan et al., "Epidemic Lead Absorption Near an Ore Smelter," 123–29; Philip Landrigan, Randolph Whitworth, Robert Baloh, William Barthel, Norman Staehling, and Bernard Rosenblum, "Neuropsychological Dysfunction in Children with Chronic Low-Level Lead Absorption," *Lancet* 1 (March 29, 1975): 708–12.

85. Landrigan et al., "Neuropsychological Dysfunction in Children with Chronic Low-Level Lead Absorption."

86. Ibid., 712. Joseph H. Graziano, et al., "Determinants of elevated blood lead during pregnancy in a population surrounding a lead smelter in Kosovo, Yugoslavia," *Environmental Health Perspectives* 89 (1990): 95-100. By 1972, Jane Lin-Fu had become the preeminent expert within the federal government on lead poisoning, fielding all lead-related issues for the government. Lead in gasoline was emerging as an important issue for both environmentalists and industry, as air pollution raised questions about lead's safety as well as its future as a gasoline additive. "The EPA called me and said that EPA was having a hearing and could I write up a statement about the issue of lead in dust," Lin-Fu recalls. Senator Phil Hart's (D-MI) office also wanted a statement for "a hearing on lead in dust and its relationship to lead poisoning in children." Lin-Fu remembers the complex political calculations that went into the public presentation of the science of lead toxicology to both the EPA and Hart's committee: "The statements needed to go through the DHEW secretary's office for clearance, and since both the EPA and Senate's hearings wanted the same information . . . [I] told both Senator Hart's office and EPA, 'I'll write one statement for both with different openings'." But Lin-Fu recalls that Secretary Elliot Richardson's office

wouldn't clear her statement because "it would be embarrassing" to have DHEW personnel impinge on the EPA's turf. She remembers that "Senator Hart's office was so upset [when they learned] that the secretary's office would not release [Lin-Fu's] letter that his staffers asked her, 'Couldn't you put a copy of the letter in the trash and we will pick it up from the trash?'" Lin-Fu refused to do that.

Whatever the bureaucratic machinations, the apparent attempt to keep Lin-Fu from presenting her testimony backfired when journalist Jack Anderson got wind of the story and wrote about it in his syndicated *Washington Post* column in late April 1972. He presented it as a scandalous attempt by the federal bureaucracy to cover up the danger that automobile exhaust posed to the public. "Health Education and Welfare officials temporarily blocked one of their most prominent pediatricians from warning the Senate that lead from car exhaust can poison ghetto children," Anderson began. Anderson claimed credit for having "broken the letter loose": "If the committee wants the letter, they'll have it." But the story was not over. Lin-Fu recalls that "the department wrote a [benign] statement . . . saying something like 'there was nothing really secret.' But it was not my statement and I refused to sign it." Hart's office was not pacified. Ultimately, Hart called another hearing at which Lin-Fu did testify, despite pressures placed on her at an unusual Sunday meeting with Health and Mental Health Administration officials "so they could find out what I was going to say," says Lin-Fu. "They told me, 'We have to be careful. We have to be discreet.' I told them, 'If I'm going to testify, I'm going to write my own statement.' Besides, much of what I would testify at the hearing had already been published in my paper in *NEJM*, and I had also shared the same info with EPA at EPA's request." In 1972 it was controversial for an official of the U.S. government to say that lead in gasoline was a threat to children's health. But the contest over Lin-Fu's testimony signaled the beginning of a long struggle over the importance of low-level lead exposures for white middle-class, as well as poor black, children. See Lin-Fu, interview; and Jack Anderson, "CIA Finds Bulgaria Involved in Drugs," *Washington Post*, April 28, 1972, D21.

87. LIA, "Minutes Meeting of Board of Directors," December 3, 1969, LIA Papers. In a 1972 letter to the editor of the *Washington Post*, the LIA maintained that "there was not a shred of evidence" to link "lead usage in gasoline with pediatric lead poisoning." In the process the trade group argued that all pediatric lead poisoning was due to lead paint "now chipping and flaking in substandard housing." J.F. Cole, Director, Environmental Health, LIA, to Editor, *Washington Post*, June 30, 1972, LIA Papers.

88. Warren, *Brush with Death*, 220.

89. Denworth, *Toxic Truth*, 95.

90. Warren, *Brush with Death*, 220–21. Even by 1986, nearly 40 percent of all gasoline sold in the United States still contained small amounts of lead. It would not be until late in the 1980s that lead would finally be removed from all gasoline.

91. Joseph C. Robert, *Ethyl: A History of the Corporation and the People Who Made It* (Charlottesville: University Press of Virginia, 1983), 295.

92. Telephone interview with Paul Mushak, March 16, 2009.

93. Ibid.

94. Gary Ter Haar, "Environmental Lead and Its Effect on Man: Sources and Pathways," paper presented at the Annual Meeting of the American Association for the Advancement of Science, January 26–31, 1975, abstract.

95. Ibid., 10.

96. Ethyl Corporation et al. v. Environmental Protection Agency, 541 F.2d 1 (D.C. Cir. 1976), available at www.openjurist.org/541/f2d/1 (accessed November 23, 2009).

97. Ibid.

98. Ibid.

99. Office of Research and Development, U.S. EPA, *Air Quality Criteria for Lead*, National Service Center for Environmental Publication, EPA 600/8-77-017 (Washington, D.C.: U.S. EPA, 1977), available at http://nepis.epa.gov (accessed October 3, 2011).

100. As reported in Edwin H. Seeger and Richard T. Witt, "Comments of Lead Industries Association, Inc., Before the Environmental Protection Agency," Proposed National Ambient Air Quality Standard for Lead, EPA Docket 0AQPS 77-1, March 17, 1978.

101. Denworth, *Toxic Truth*, 101.

102. Ibid., 102.

103. Ibid., 103.

104. International Lead Zinc Research Organization and Lead Industries Association Inc., "Comments on Air Quality Criteria for Atmospheric Lead—External Review Draft, November 1976, U.S.E.P.A." (January 20, 1977), 5, 6, Proposed National Ambient Air Quality Standard for Lead, EPA Docket 0AQPS 77-1, March 17, 1978.

105. Ibid., 7–8.

106. Mushak, interview.

107. Needleman, quoted in Denworth, *Toxic Truth*, 104.

108. Mushak, interview. Mushak points out that there was no formal relationship between the National Ambient Air Quality Standard and the amount of lead used in gasoline. E-mail to authors, October 1, 2011. The 1978 standard would remain in place for thirty years, until 2008, when it was lowered by a factor of ten to 0.15 µg/m^3.

109. "LIA Ambient Air Lead Standard Meeting of 1/16/78," minutes, January 17, 1978, DR 3802272–76, Doe Run Papers. In its official response to the EPA, the industry called for a standard "no lower than 5." See Seeger and Witt, "Comments of Lead Industries Association, Inc., Before the Environmental Protection Agency," 1.

110. "LIA Ambient Air Lead Standard Meeting of 1/16/78," minutes.

111. Ibid.

112. Jerome F. Cole to Official Members, Lead Industries Association Inc., Members, LIA Environmental Health Committee, "Subject: Public Hearing on EPA Proposed National Ambient Air Quality Standard for Lead," February 17, 1978, DR 3802189–90, Doe Run Papers.

113. See Julian Chisolm to Jerome Cole, March 2, 1978, appendix C of Seeger and Witt, "Comments of Lead Industries Association, Inc., Before the Environmental Protection Agency": "You asked me to keep a record of my time in relation to the hearings. I calculate that as a full day, if one takes into account travel, testimony and preparation time."

114. Seeger and Witt, "Comments of Lead Industries Association, Inc., Before the Environmental Protection Agency," 36.

115. "Increased Lead Absorption and Lead Poisoning in Young Children: A Statement by the Center for Disease Control, *Journal of Pediatrics* 87 (November 1975): 824.

116. Ibid., 825.

117. This level was selected because the commission, after opening up a series of paint cans, found that some were below 600 parts per million lead. Thus, they concluded, it was feasible to achieve this level of lead in paint. This exemplifies how most of the existing lead standards—for water and dust, in addition to paint—were established: based on what was thought to be feasible rather than on scientific evidence. We thank Bruce Lanphear for this insight.

118. Mushak, interview; CDC, *Preventing Lead Poisoning in Young Children: A Statement by the Center for Disease Control* (Washington, D.C.: CDC, April 1978).

119. CDC, *Preventing Lead Poisoning in Young Children*, 1.

120. Needleman, "Exposure to Lead: Sources and Effects," 943-45.

121. Chisolm, "Evolution of the Management and Prevention of Childhood Lead Poisoning," 118–20.

122. Herbert L. Needleman, Charles Gunnoe, Alan Leviton, Robert Reed, Henry Peresie, Cornelius Maher, and Peter Barrett, "Deficits in Psychologic and Classroom Performance of Children with Elevated Dentine Lead Levels," *New England Journal of Medicine* 300 (March 29, 1979): 689.

123. Ibid., 691.

124. Ibid., 694.

125. As examples of the new work that Needleman was building upon, see Burdé and Shapiro, "Dental Lead, Blood Lead, and Pica in Urban Children," 281–84; David, letter re. "Blood-Lead Levels, Behaviour and Intelligence"; Burdé and Choate, "Early Asymptomatic Lead Exposure and Development at School Age," 638–42; and J. Julian Chisolm Jr., "Is Lead Poisoning Still a Problem?" *Clinical Chemistry* 23 (1977): 253.

126. Jane S. Lin-Fu, "Lead Exposure among Children: A Reassessment (Editorial)," *New England Journal of Medicine* 300 (March 29, 1979): 732. See also Evan Charney, "Sub-Encephalopathic Lead Poisoning: Central Nervous System Effects in Children," in *Lead Absorption in Children: Management, Clinical, and Environmental Aspects*, ed. J. Julian Chisolm and David M. O'Hara (Baltimore: Urban and Schwarzenberg, 1982), 40; and Gail Bronson, "Modest Exposure to Lead Is Linked to School Troubles," *Wall Street Journal*, March 29, 1979, 20.

127. Jerome Cole, letter to the editor, Science Times, *New York Times*, June 3, 1980, C5.

CHAPTER 4

Epigraph: Jane S. Lin-Fu, "The Evolution of Childhood Lead Poisoning as a Public Health Problem," in *Lead Absorption in Children: Management, Clinical, and Environmental Aspects,* ed. J. Julian Chisolm and David M. O'Hara (Baltimore: Urban and Schwarzenberg, 1982), 9.

1. Jerome F. Cole, "Impact of Lead on Environmental Health: Conclusions Based on ILZRO Research," paper presented at the annual meeting of the American Association for the Advancement of Science, Toronto, January 5, 1981.

2. "Anne M. Gorsuch (Later Burford) (Served May 1981 to March 1983)," available at www.epa.gov/history/topics/epa/15e.htm#Gorsuch (accessed December 18, 2009).

3. D. V. Feliciano, "Gorsuch Cited for Contempt of Congress," *Journal (Water Pollution Control Federation)* 55 (February 1983): 119–22.

4. Samuel P. Hays, "The Role of Values in Science and Policy: The Case of Lead," in *Human Lead Exposure,* ed. Herbert L. Needleman (Boca Raton, FL: CRC Press, 1992), 269. In 1974 there were more than 2 grams of lead per gallon of gasoline. By 1985 this had been reduced to about 0.5 gram. See Richard G. Newell and Kristian Rogers, *The Market-Based Lead Phase Down,* Discussion Paper 03-37 (Washington, D.C.: Resources for the Future, November 2003), 22, available at http://ageconsearch.umn.edu/bitstream/10445/1/dp030037.pdf (accessed October 3, 2011).

5. William D. Ruckelshaus to vice president of the United States, "Inquiry Regarding EPA Policy on Industry-Supported Scientists as Members of Special Expert Review Panel," August 25, 1983, DR 0300941–42, Doe Run Papers.

6. EPA committee statement quoted in Jerome F. Cole, Chief Operating Officer, ILZRO, to Vice President George Bush, July 6, 1983, DR 0300937, Doe Run Papers.

7. Ibid.

8. Ruckelshaus to vice president of the United States, "Inquiry Regarding EPA Policy."

9. Jerome Cole to all members of the ILZRO Board of Directors, September 13, 1983, DR 0300936, Doe Run Papers.

10. Telephone interview with Paul Mushak, March 16, 2009.

11. Quoted in Lydia Denworth, *Toxic Truth: A Scientist, a Doctor, and the Battle over Lead* (Boston: Beacon Press, 2008), 104. See also J.F. Cole, "Subject: National Ambient Air Quality Standard for Lead," October 18, 1978, DR 11203332, Doe Run Papers; and Lead Industries Association Inc. v. Environmental Protection Agency, 647 F.2d 1130 (D.C. Cir. 1980).

12. Mushak, interview.

13. "Lead Balloon," *Wall Street Journal,* August 27, 1982, 16.

14. Jane S. Lin-Fu, untitled article in *Children Today,* January–February 1979, 12.

15. U.S. General Accounting Office, *Report by the Comptroller General of the United States: HUD Not Fulfilling Responsibility to Eliminate Lead-*

Based Paint Hazard in Federal Housing, CED-81-31 (Washington, D.C.: GAO, December 16, 1980), 9.

16. Nancy Nusser, "Affluent Kids Also Harmed by Toxic Lead," *Wall Street Journal*, July 24, 1981, 23.

17. K. R. Mahaffey, J. L. Annest, J. Roberts, and R. S. Murphy, "National Estimates of Blood Lead Levels: United States, 1976–1980; Association with Selected Demographic and Socioeconomic Factors," *New England Journal of Medicine* 307 (September 2, 1982): 573, 579; Mushak, interview. From 1973 through 1981, of the national sample of 3.9 million urban and rural children between six months and five years old who were screened nationally, 243,000, or 6.2 percent, were identified as lead poisoned by the standard of the time, with levels more than 30 µg/dl. *Morbidity and Mortality Weekly Report* 31 (March 12, 1982): 118–19.

18. Jane S. Lin-Fu, "Children and Lead: New Findings and Concerns," editorial, *New England Journal of Medicine* 307 (September 2, 1982): 615, 616. From 1978 to 1985 the CDC's level of concern was 30 µg/dl or above, which was considered poisoning; the older term, *undue lead absorption*, now referred to children whose blood lead levels were below 30 µg/dl. See also Kathryn R. Mahaffey and Joseph L. Annest, "Association of Erythrocyte Protoporphyrin with Blood Lead Level and Iron Status in the Second National Health and Nutrition Examination survey, 1976–1980," *Environmental Research* 41 (1986): 327–38.

19. Joseph L. Annest, James L. Pirkle, Diane Makuc, Jane W. Neese, David D. Bayse, and Mary Grace Kovar, "Chronological Trends in Blood Lead Levels between 1976 and 1980," *New England Journal of Medicine* 308 (June 9, 1983): 1373–77.

20. Paul Mushak and Annemarie F. Crocetti, "Methods for Reducing Lead Exposure in Young Children and Other Risk Groups: An Integrated Summary of a Report to the U.S. Congress on Childhood Lead Poisoning," *Environmental Health Perspectives* 89 (1990): 129. The NHANES II data led the EPA in 1982 to adopt "new rules that, among other things, reduced the lead content of gasoline to 1.1 [g] per liquid gallon" from the 1.5 grams per gallon that had been set in 1978. In 1984, the LIA objected to the EPA's proposal to reduce the lead content of gasoline to 0.1 gram per gallon. See Rosalind A. Volpe, Assistant Director, Environmental Health, LIA, to LIA Environmental Health and Regulatory Activities Committees, October 15, 1984, DR 4700903–47, Doe Run Papers. See also Christian Warren, *Brush with Death: A Social History of Lead Poisoning* (Baltimore: Johns Hopkins University Press, 2000), 222.

21. Sergio Piomelli, Carol Seaman, Dianne Zullow, Anita Curran, and Bernard Davidow, "Threshold for Lead Damage to Heme Synthesis in Urban Children," *Proceedings of the National Academy of Sciences* 79 (May 1982): 3335–39. In Piomelli's words, "The effect of Pb on EP [erythrocyte protoporphyrin concentration] reflects its interference with the last step in the heme biosynthetic pathway, at the level of the mitochondria in the erythrocyte precursors in the bone marrow. Thus, the elevation of EP has the same biological meaning as increased urinary AmLev, that is, damage to a biochemical step

beyond any hypothetical reserve capacity. The evidence of damage to a mito-chondrial function is obvious in the erythrocyte because blood is the easiest tissue to sample. However, the affinity of Pb is not limited to the mitochon-dria in the bone marrow but also to those in other tissues. Inhibition of heme synthesis affects all body tissues in which heme is the prosthetic group in the cytochrome system" (3339). This research also suggested a possible physio-logical basis for the observations of Herbert Needleman and others, who had found empirical correlations between blood lead levels and behavioral and neu-romotor disturbances. Piomelli and his colleagues noted as well that "subtle signs of neuropsychological disturbance have been recently demonstrated at [low] levels of exposure to Pb . . . in apparently normal suburban children by use of well-controlled experimental design" (3339). See also, John F. Rosen, Russell Chesney, Alan Hamstra, Hector F. DeLuca, and Kathryn R. Mahaffey, "Reduction in 1,25-Dihydroxyvitamin D in Children with Increased Lead Absorption," *New England Journal of Medicine* 302 (May 15, 1980): 1128–31.

In 1977, Julian Chisolm noted the following on heme synthesis: "Lead has adverse effects on the hematopoietic tissue, the kidney, and the nervous system. Currently available data indicate that erythroid tissue of the bone marrow is the critical organ for lead and that the critical effect is derangement in heme synthesis. Indicators of this effect are decreased activity of δ-aminolaevulinate dehydratase (porphobilinogen synthase, EC 4.2.1.24), increased accumulation and excretion in urine of δ-aminolaevulinate and coproporphyrin and increased concentration of protoporphyrin ix in erythrocytes)." J. Julian Chisolm Jr., "Is Lead Poisoning Still a Problem?" *Clinical Chemistry* 23 (1977): 254.

22. Lead was found to have, among other effects, "pervasive metabolic effects involving heme synthesis, red cell nucleotide metabolism, vitamin D and cortisol metabolism and renal function, and sub clinical neurobehavioral effects." Sergio Piomelli, John Rosen, J. Julian Chisolm Jr., and John Graef, "Management of Lead Poisoning," *Journal of Pediatrics* 105 (October 1984): 526.

23. Mushak, interview. See also Mahaffey et al., "National Estimates of Blood Lead Levels: United States, 1976–1980," 573, 579; and Lin-Fu, "Children and Lead: New Findings and Concerns," 616.

24. Evan Charney, "Sub-encephalopathic Lead Poisoning: Central Nervous System Effects in Children," in *Lead Absorption in Children: Management, Clinical, and Environmental Aspects*, ed. J. Julian Chisolm and David M. O'Hara (Baltimore: Urban and Schwarzenberg, 1982), 35–36.

25. U.S. EPA, Clean Air Scientific Advisory Committee, Science Advisory Board, "Open Meeting," Research Triangle Park, NC, April 26, 1984, p. 12, Paul Mushak Private Papers (hereafter Mushak Papers). Terry Yosie, a recent graduate of Carnegie Mellon's doctoral program in the humanities and social sciences, was appointed the SAB's director. Lester Grant, director of the EPA's Environmental Criteria and Assessment Office, and Morton Lippmann, chair of the SAB, explained that the purpose of the meeting was to "examine the data base and judge whether it serves as a scientific basis for later regulatory decisions."

26. U.S. EPA, Clean Air Scientific Advisory Committee, Science Advisory Board, "Open Meeting," April 26, 1984, p. 11.

27. Ibid., 12.

28. See Herbert L. Needleman, Charles Gunnoe, Alan Leviton, Robert Reed, Henry Peresie, Cornelius Maher, and Peter Barrett, "Deficits in Psychologic and Classroom Performance of Children with Elevated Dentine Lead Levels," *New England Journal of Medicine* 300 (March 29, 1979): 689–95.

29. Denworth, *Toxic Truth*, 141–42.

30. Claire B. Ernhart, Beth Landa, and Norman B. Schell, "Subclinical Levels of Lead in Developmental Deficit: a Multivariate Follow-up Reassessment," *Pediatrics* 67 (June 1981): 911. In a detailed letter of response to the editor of *Pediatrics*, Needleman and his coauthors criticized Ernhart's questioning of the "entire literature documenting the adverse effects of low levels of lead." In doing so, they said, Ernhart and her colleagues "contradict or ignore the findings of the earlier study by Perrino and Ernhart, misread a table from the one study they single out for criticism, and draw debatable conclusions from their own data." Herbert Needleman, David Bellinger, and Alan Leviton, "Does Lead at Low Dose Affect Intelligence in Children?" *Pediatrics* 68 (December 1981): 896. See also Ernhart's earlier study: Jay Perino and Claire Ernhart, "The Relation of Sub-clinical Lead Level to Cognitive and Sensory Motor Impairment in Black Pre-schoolers," *Journal of Learning Disabilities* 7 (December 1974): 616.

31. This is documented in ILZRO's summary of the grants it provided as well as its commentary on Ernhart's initial grant proposal, which was not funded but became the basis for ILZRO and Ernhart's future relationship. See ILZRO Project Summary, "LH-301A-Special Consultant," Claire B. Ernhart, July 1982, in ILZRO Lead Environmental Health Committee, "1983 ILZRO Catalog of Proposed Environmental Health Research," July 1982, Confidential, p. 24, DR 5302901, Doe Run Papers.

32. Ibid.

33. ILZRO Project Summary, "LH-227-Lead Level and Iron Deficiency in the Preschool Years," Claire Ernhart, PhD, June 1990, in ILZRO Lead Project Funding Committee, "1991 ILZRO Catalog of Proposed Research," November 6, 1990, Confidential, pp. 41–46, DR 2202986, Doe Run Papers. See also Craig J. Boreiko, Manager, Environmental Health, ILZRO, to Sponsors of ILZRO's Project LH-327, "Manager's Summary," January 29, 1991, Confidential, DR 11100790, Doe Run Papers.

34. Claire B. Ernhart, "Progress Report and Request for Renewal of Contract, ILZRO Project Number LH-327, Lead Level and Iron Deficiency in the Preschool Years, June 1, 1985 through May 31, 1986," [1986], p. 2, DR 5302040, Doe Run Papers.

35. ILZRO Project Summary, "LH-227-Lead Level and Iron Deficiency in the Preschool Years."

36. Rosalind Volpe, Manager, Environmental Health, ILZRO, "Manager's Summary, LH-327—Lead Level Iron Deficiency in the Preschool Years—

Ernhart—January, 1988—Progress Report," 1988, DR 2201813, Doe Run Papers.

37. Donald R. Lynam, Director, Air Conservation, Ethyl Corporation, to Jerome F. Cole, President, ILZRO, July 17, 1986, DR 5302027, Doe Run Papers. See also Dan Vornberg, Doe Run and a member of ILZRO's Environmental Health Committee, to Dick Amistadi, Doe Run, "ILZRO Environmental Health Committee and Voting," September 11, 1990, DR 2203118, Doe Run Papers: "Claire Ernhart in Cleveland is the major researcher willing to stand up and challenge the lead and mental deficiency arguments of Needleman."

38. Denworth, *Toxic Truth*, 145.

39. Ibid., 146–47.

40. Mushak, interview.

41. Denworth, *Toxic Truth*, 147.

42. D. L. Vornberg, St. Joseph Lead Company, to R. E. Peppers, "Re: LIA Environmental Health Meeting," May 4, 1983, DR 3702030, Doe Run Papers.

43. Lester Grant, Director, Environmental Criteria and Assessment Office, EPA, to Paul Mushak, March 2, 1983, Mushak Papers.

44. Expert Committee on Pediatric Neurobehavioral Evaluations, "Appendix 12-C, Independent Peer Review of Selected Studies Concerning Neurobehavioral Effects of Lead Exposures in Nominally Asymptomatic Children: Official Report of Findings and Recommendations of an Interdisciplinary Expert Review Committee," EPA-600/8-83-028A (November 14, 1983), viii, Mushak Papers.

45. Lester Grant to Herbert Needleman, November 28, 1983, Mushak Papers.

46. Mushak, interview.

47. Denworth, *Toxic Truth*, 152.

48. James D. Callaghan, Senior Vice President, Hill & Knowlton, to Ms. Sharon Begley, Science Editor, *Newsweek*, December 1, 1983, Mushak Papers.

49. Ibid. The Hill & Knowlton effort to promote the significance of the draft report, and to misrepresent it as being the "final word" from the EPA, was given legitimacy by an article that appeared in the prestigious journal *Science* the week before the public relations firm sent out its mass mailing. On November 25, 1983, a story titled "EPA Faults Classic Lead Poisoning Study" echoed the industry's position that Needleman's research had been discredited. Eliot Marshall, "EPA Faults Classic Lead Poisoning Study," *Science* 222 (November 25, 1983): 906–7.

50. Vornberg to Peppers, May 4, 1983.

51. U.S. EPA, Clean Air Scientific Advisory Committee, Science Advisory Board, "Open Meeting," April 26, 1984, p. 118.

52. Ibid.

53. Ibid., 120–21.

54. Ibid., 121.

55. Ibid., 123.

56. Ibid., 124.

57. Ibid., 125.

58. Ibid., 133.

59. Ibid., 134.

60. Ibid., 144.

61. Ibid., 145.

62. Ibid., 157.

63. Ibid., 162.

64. Ibid., 165.

65. U.S. EPA, Clean Air Scientific Advisory Committee, Science Advisory Board, "Meeting," Research Triangle Park, NC, April 27, 1984, pp. 69–70, Mushak Papers.

66. Ibid., 70.

67. Ibid., 70–71.

68. Sir Austin Bradford Hill, "The Environment and Disease: Association or Causation?" *Proceedings of the Royal Society of Medicine* 58(1965): 295–300.

69. U.S. EPA, Clean Air Scientific Advisory Committee, Science Advisory Board, "Meeting," April 27, 1984, p. 66.

70. Hugh M. Pitcher, Office of Policy Analysis, EPA, "Comments on Issues Raised in the Analysis of the Neuropsychological Effects of Low Level Lead Exposure," 1984, mimeograph, pp. 8–9, Mushak Papers.

71. U.S. EPA, Clean Air Scientific Advisory Committee, Science Advisory Board, "Meeting," April 27, 1984, pp. 83–84.

72. Denworth, *Toxic Truth*, 151.

73. U.S. EPA, Clean Air Scientific Advisory Committee, Science Advisory Board, "Meeting," April 27, 1984, pp. 83–84.

74. Henrietta K. Sachs and Donald Moel, "Leaded Gasoline Wrongly Indicted," letter to the editor, *New York Times*, April 19, 1984, A18.

75. Denworth, *Toxic Truth*, 152.

76. Jerome Cole to Paul Mushak, November 1, 1984, Mushak Papers.

77. Paul Mushak to Lester Grant, November 7, 1984, Mushak Papers.

78. D.L. Vornberg, St. Joseph Lead Company, to R.E. Peppers, "LIA Environmental Health Committee Meeting, New York City—May 12, 1982," May 13, 1982, DR 4701084, Doe Run Papers.

79. Vornberg to Peppers, May 4, 1983.

80. U.S. EPA, Clean Air Scientific Advisory Committee, Science Advisory Board, "Open Meeting," April 26, 1984, p. 13. A few years later, Schwartz turned the industry's argument on its head by showing the substantial impact on lifetime earnings of reduced IQ. See Joel Schwartz and D. Otto, "Blood Lead, Hearing Thresholds and Neurobehavioral Development in Children and Youth," *Archives of Environmental Health* (1987): 153–60.

81. "Motor Vehicles: Lead Industries Group Challenges EPA Over Cost-Benefit Analysis on Banning Lead," *Environment Reporter*, May 11, 1984, 41.

82. "Motor Vehicles: Cannon Promises EPA Proposal in July on an Early Phase-Out of Leaded Gasoline," *Environment Reporter*, June 28, 1984, 375.

83. Robert Proctor, *Golden Holocaust* (Berkeley: University of California Press, 2011).

84. U.S. EPA, "EPA Sets New Limits on Lead in Gasoline," March 4, 1985, available at www.epa.gov/history/topics/lead/01.html (accessed March 14, 2012).

85. D.L. Vornberg to G.E. Welch, "Barltrop's Steering Committee Meeting (LH-331) and Associated Conferences," February 1, 1986, DR 5300825, Doe Run Papers; Hays, "Role of Values in Science and Policy," 276.

86. John Dingell to James O. Mason, June 12, 1987, Mushak Papers. See also Mushak and Crocetti, "Methods for Reducing Lead Exposure in Young Children and Other Risk Groups," 125.

87. Agency for Toxic Substances and Disease Registry, *The Nature and Extent of Lead Poisoning in Children in the United States* (Washington, D.C.: U.S. Department of Health and Human Services, 1988).

88. Paul Mushak to Frank Mitchell, June 5, 1987, Mushak Papers.

89. Michael Weisskopf, "Authors Protest Report on Lead Poisoning: Researchers Resign, Call Changes Misleading," *Washington Post*, June 13, 1987, A14. See also Mushak to Mitchell, June 5, 1987; and Jeff Nesmith and Charles Seabrook, "After Alleged Tampering, CDC Asked for Lead Poisoning Data," *Atlanta Journal-Constitution*, June 13, 1987, 1A.

90. Weisskopf, "Authors Protest Report on Lead Poisoning." According to Mushak, "the 17 percent frequency was derived from statistical projection modeling of data in the earlier NHANES II blood-lead data sheets projected to 1984 by U.S. EPA statistician-epidemiologist, Dr. Joel Schwartz." Paul Mushak e-mail to authors, September 24, 2011. See also U.S. Department of Commerce, *1980 Census*, General Population Characteristics, U.S. Summary, Table 41, Current Population Reports, Series P-25, No. 311, available at http://www2.census.gov/prod2/decennial/documents/1980/1980censusofpopu8011u_bw.pdf (accessed March 14, 2012).

91. Weisskopf, "Authors Protest Report on Lead Poisoning."

92. Ibid., A14. Crocetti and Mushak added much detail to their reasons for resigning in a long memo to the House Subcommittee on Oversight and Investigations. In it they explained what they believed were the misrepresentations that the short summary conveyed to Congress: "The deletion of the details of the nature, range and effectiveness of abatement efforts by individual Federal and other level governmental agencies and bodies . . . shows serious problems encountered when carrying out abatement measures." Also of concern was the way the summary misled Congress into believing that the scientific community agreed about safety levels. Crocetti and Mushak worried that members of Congress would not appreciate "the relevance of recent research findings about the relationship of chronic low-level exposures and adverse health effects in children." They concluded that "if the reader does not clearly grasp that the Pb-B levels are important it is almost irrelevant to estimate the number of people at these levels." Annemarie Crocetti to Richard Frandsen and Deborah Jacobson, House Subcommittee on Oversight and Investigations, "Authors' Comments on the Third Draft (May 19, 1987) and the June 5, 1987 Draft," June 16, 1987, Mushak Papers.

93. Weisskopf, "Authors Protest Report on Lead Poisoning," A14.

94. Dingell to Mason, June 12, 1987.

95. James O. Mason to John Dingell, June 18, 1987, Mushak Papers.

96. See Barry Johnson, Associate Administrator, ATSDR, to Paul Mushak, July 14, 1987; Paul Mushak and Annemarie Crocetti, to "Scientific Peer Reviewers, ATSDR Report to Congress on Childhood Lead Poisoning," July 29, 1987; Barry Johnson to Annemarie Crocetti, August 5, 1987; and Barry Johnson to Paul Mushak, August 5, 1987, all in Mushak Papers.

97. "Draft SARAA Mandated Report Scope of Childhood Lead Poisoning 'Disturbing,'" *Inside EPA Weekly Report* 9 (April 15, 1988): 4, Mushak Papers

98. "OMB Attempt to Undermine Draft SARAA Mandated Lead Report Outrages Scientists," *Inside EPA Weekly Report* 9 (June 24, 1988): 4–5, Mushak Papers.

99. Ibid.

100. Barry Johnson, Associate Administrator, ATSDR, to Paul Mushak, July 15, 1988, Mushak Papers; "HHS Releases Lead Report to Congress Unscathed, Allaying 'Tampering' Fears," *Inside EPA Weekly Report* (July 15, 1988): 2. See also "Childhood Lead Poisoning in the United States: Report to the Congress by the Agency for Toxic Substances and Disease Registry," *Morbidity and Mortality Weekly Report* 37 (August 19, 1988): 481–85.

101. "CDC Editorial Note," in "Childhood Lead Poisoning—United States: Report to the Congress by the Agency for Toxic Substances and Disease Registry," *JAMA* 260 (September 16, 1988): 1533.

102. See various LIA documents from 1928 onward.

103. D. L. V. [Daniel L. Vornberg], "Bullet Points on Ambient Air Standard and Doe Run Strategy," May 29, 1987, DR 2301942, Doe Run Papers.

104. James Lanzafame to Walter Klinger, January 29, 1986, DR 3400322, Doe Run Papers.

105. See handwritten notes attached to James Lanzafame to Walter Klinger, January 29, 1986, DR 5901182–83, Doe Run Papers.

106. Paul W. Allen to Leslie G. McGraw, November 6, 1989, Doe Run Papers.

107. "Meeting Outline W. US EPA Re- Ambient Lead Standard," January 28, 1987, attached to John Yoder to John DePaul and Daniel Vornberg, et al., July 20, 1987, DR 6800705, Doe Run Papers.

108. Bob Carlstrom to Dan Vornberg, "Subject: Pb NAAQS Initiative," August 1, 1988, Confidential, DR 11000571, Doe Run Papers.

109. We thank Bruce Lanphear for pointing this out.

110. Kathryn R. Mahaffey, "Introduction: Advances in Lead Research: Implications for Environmental Health," *Environmental Health Perspectives* 89 (1990): 3.

111. Ellen Silbergeld, "Implications of New Data on Lead Toxicity for Managing and Preventing Exposure," *Environmental Health Perspectives* 89 (1990): 49.

112. Ibid., 52.

113. Ibid., 53.

114. R. Lansdown, W. Yule, M.A. Urbanowicz, and J. Hunter, "The Relationship between Blood-Lead Concentrations, Intelligence, Attainment and Behaviour in a School Population: The Second Study," *International Archives of Occupational and Environmental Health* 57 (1986): 225–35; M. Fulton, G. Raab, G. Thompson, D. Laxen, R. Hunter, and W. Hepburn, "Influence of Blood Lead on the Ability and Attainment of Children in Edinburgh," *Lancet* 1 (May 30, 1987): 1221–26; D.M. Fergusson, J.E. Fergusson, L.J. Horwood, and N.G. Kinzett, "A Longitudinal Study of Dentine Lead Levels, Intelligence, School Performance, and Behavior Part II: Dentine Lead and Cognitive Ability," *Journal of Child Psychology and Psychiatry* 29 (1988): 793–809; P.A. Silva, P. Hughes, S. Williams, and J.M. Faed, "Blood Lead, Intelligence, Reading Attainment, and Behaviour in Eleven Year Old Children in Dunedin, New Zealand," *Journal of Child Psychology and Psychiatry* 29 (1988): 43–52; M. Bergomi, P. Borella, G. Fantuzzi, G. Vivoli, N. Sturloni, G. Cavazzuti, A. Tampieri, and P.L. Tartoni, "Relationship between Lead Exposure Indicators and Neuropsychological Performance in Children," *Developmental Medicine and Child Neurology* 31 (1989): 181–90; O.N. Hansen, A. Trillingsgaard, I. Beese, T. Lyngbye, and P. Grandjean, "A Neuropsychological Study of Children with Elevated Dentine Lead Level: Assessment of the Effect of Lead in Different Socio-economic Groups," *Neurotoxicology and Teratology* 11 (1989): 205–13; B.A. Hawk, S.R. Schroeder, G. Robinson, D. Otto, P. Mushak, D. Kleinbaum, and G. Dawson, "Relation of Lead and Social Factors to IQ of Low-SES Children: A Partial Replication," *American Journal of Mental Deficiency* 91 (1986): 178–83; S.R. Schroeder, B. Hawk, D.A. Otto, P. Mushak, and R.E. Hicks, "Separating the Effects of Lead and Social Factors on IQ," *Environmental Research* 38 (1985): 144–54; "Report of Clean Air Advisory Committee on its Review of the National Ambient Air Quality Standards for Lead," attached to Roger O. McClellan to William K. Reilly, Administrator, EPA, January 3, 1990, Mushak Papers.

115. A major lawsuit that reached the Supreme Court was *Automobile Workers v. Johnson Controls*, where the United Automobile Workers sued the battery maker for gender discrimination, charging that a "fetal protection policy" ignored the fact that men's reproduction was compromised by lead as well. The Supreme Court ruled that under Title VII of the 1964 Civil Rights Act such gender discrimination was prohibited. For more detailed discussions of this case, see Gerald Markowitz and David Rosner, *Deceit and Denial: The Deadly Politics of Industrial Pollution* (Berkeley: University of California Press); and Warren, *Brush with Death.*

116. "Report of Clean Air Advisory Committee on its Review of the National Ambient Air Quality Standards for Lead," attached to McClellan to Reilly, January 3, 1990.

117. Ibid.

118. M. Rutter, "Raised Lead Levels and Impaired Cognitive Behavioral Functioning: A Review of the Evidence," *Developmental Medicine and Child Neurology* 22, Suppl. 1 (1980), quoted in J. Julian Chisolm Jr. and David M. O'Hara, eds., *Lead Absorption in Children: Management, Clinical, and*

Environmental Aspects (Baltimore: Urban and Schwarzenberg, 1982), 215. Bruce Lanphear explains that today "a five point IQ shift in the 'population's IQ' would result [in the population] who qualify as being mentally retarded [rising] from six million to 9.5 million." Bruce Lanphear e-mail to David Rosner, January 31, 2011.

119. Steven G. Gilbert and Bernard Weiss, "A Rationale for Lowering the Blood Lead Action Level from 10 to 2μg/dL," *NeuroToxicology* 27 (2006): 697, fig. 3.

120. David Bellinger, A. Leviton, C. Waternaux, H. Needleman, and M. Rabinowitz, "Longitudinal Analyses of Prenatal and Postnatal Lead Exposure and Early Cognitive Development," *New England Journal of Medicine* 316 (April 23, 1987): 1037–43; Kim N. Dietrich, K.M. Krafft, R.L. Bornshein, P.B. Hammond, O. Berger, P.A. Succop, and M. Bier, "Low-Level Fetal Lead Exposure Effect on Neurobehavioral Development in Early Infancy," *Pediatrics* 80 (November 1987): 721–30.

121. "Report of Clean Air Advisory Committee on its Review of the National Ambient Air Quality Standards for Lead," attached to McClellan to Reilly, January 3, 1990.

122. Jerome F. Cole to Senator Harry Reid, March 20, 1990, DR 2300347–49, Doe Run Papers. On tainted science, see Sheldon Krimsky, *Science in the Private Interest: Has the Lure of Profits Corrupted Biomedical Research?* (Lanham, MD: Rowland and Littlefield, 2003); Marcia Angell, *The Truth about Drug Companies: How they Deceive Us and What to Do about It* (New York: Random House, 2004); and David Michaels, *Doubt Is Our Product: How Industry's Assault on Science Threatens Your Health* (Oxford: Oxford University Press, 2008).

123. Jerome F. Smith, Executive Director, LIA, to Vernon N. Houk, Director, Center for Environmental Health and Injury Control, CDC, April 19, 1991, DR 2101055, Doe Run Papers.

124. Cole to Senator Reid, March 20, 1990.

125. Denworth, *Toxic Truth*, 179–205.

126. David Rosner and Gerald Markowitz, "Standing Up to the Lead Industry: An Interview with Herbert Needleman," *Public Health Reports* 120 (May–June 2005): 330–37.

127. Cole to Senator Reid, March 20, 1990. See also Krimsky, *Science in the Private Interest*; Angell, *Truth about Drug Companies*; and Michaels, *Doubt Is Our Product*.

128. J. Julian Chisolm, "Evolution of the Management and Prevention of Childhood Lead Poisoning: Dependence of Advances in Public Health on Technological Advances in the Determination of Lead and Related Biochemical Indicators of its Toxicity," *Environmental Research*, Section A, vol. 86 (2001): 120.

129. Ellen Silbergeld, quoted in Michael Weisskopf, "Persistent, Pervasive Pollutant," *Washington Post*, June 15, 1987, A4–A5.

130. Lin-Fu, untitled article in *Children Today*, 12–13.

131. Evan Charney, "Lead Poisoning in Children: The Case against Household Lead Dust," in *Lead Absorption in Children: Management, Clinical, and Environmental Aspects*, ed. J. Julian Chisolm and David M. O'Hara (Baltimore: Urban and Schwarzenberg, 1982), 86. See also Evan Charney, James Sayre, and Molly Coulter, "Increased Lead Absorption in Inner City Children: Where Does the Lead Come From?," *Pediatrics* 65 (February 1980): 226–31.

132. J. Julian Chisolm Jr., "Evaluation of the Potential Role of Chelation Therapy in Treatment of Low to Moderate Lead Exposures," *Environmental Health Perspectives* 89 (1990): 67.

133. Mushak and Crocetti, "Methods for Reducing Lead Exposure in Young Children and Other Risk Groups," 133. Some have been concerned that lead in jet fuel has largely been exempted from regulations. Marie Lynn Miranda, Rebecca Anthopolos, and Douglas Hastings, "A Geospatial Analysis of the Effects of Aviation Gasoline on Childhood Blood Lead Levels," *Environmental Health Perspectives* 119 (2011): 1513–16, suggests that lead from jet fuel is a relatively small contributor to the overall lead burden, however.

134. Interview with Ellen K. Silbergeld, March 25, 2010, Baltimore.

CHAPTER 5

Epigraph: U.S. Department of Health and Human Services, Public Health Service, Centers for Disease Control (CDC), *Strategic Plan for the Elimination of Childhood Lead Poisoning* (Atlanta: U.S. Department of Health and Human Services, Public Health Service, Centers for Disease Control, 1991), xii.

1. U.S. General Accounting Office, *Report by the Comptroller General of the United States: HUD Not Fulfilling Responsibility to Eliminate Lead-Based Paint Hazard in Federal Housing*, CED-81-31 (Washington, D.C.: U.S. GAO, December 16, 1980), 4–5.

2. Ibid., 5.

3. J. Julian Chisolm, "Evolution of the Management and Prevention of Childhood Lead Poisoning: Dependence of Advances in Public Health on Technological Advances in the Determination of Lead and Related Biochemical Indicators of Its Toxicity," *Environmental Research*, Section A, vol. 86 (2001): 119. When Dave Jacobs was sworn in by Donna Shalala as director of HUD's Office of Healthy Homes and Lead Hazard Control in 1995, he asked why in the 1970s HUD had not paid more attention to lead paint. "She told me," he recalls, "'We were told it was all gasoline and therefore there wasn't a major responsibility for HUD.' She also told me that obviously we were wrong . . . we should have done more to deal with the leaded paint problem." Interview with Dave Jacobs, December 4, 2009, Washington, D.C.

4. U.S. General Accounting Office, *Report by the Comptroller General of the United States: HUD Not Fulfilling Responsibility to Eliminate Lead-Based Paint Hazard in Federal Housing*, 11.

5. Ibid., i–ii.

6. Ibid, iii.

7. Ibid.

8. Ibid., 13–14. This was a gross underestimation, as HUD would later acknowledge in U.S. Department of Housing and Urban Development, "Comprehensive and Workable Plan for the Abatement of Lead-Based Paint in Privately Owned Housing," Report to Congress, December 7, 1990. The Report's authors identified 77 million privately owned houses of which 57 million, "or three-fourths, contain lead-based paint" (p. xvii); 3.8 million of those units were homes to young children and had "peeling paint, excessive amounts of dust containing lead, or both problems" (p. xviii).

9. Jacobs, interview.

10. Interview with Saul Kerpelman, April 12, 2011, Baltimore.

11. Evan Charney, Barry Kessler, Mark Farfel, and David Jackson, "Childhood Lead Poisoning: A Controlled Trial of the Effect of Dust-Control Measures on Blood Lead Levels," *New England Journal of Medicine* 309 (November 3, 1983): 1089–93.

12. Ibid., 1089.

13. Ibid., 1089–90.

14. Ibid., 1090.

15. Ibid., 1089.

16. Ibid., 1092.

17. Dust control for public health authorities in the 1980s and 1990s had a very particular meaning: it meant the actions that residents themselves could take to reduce the lead-containing dust in their environments. It was assumed that wet mopping, wet dusting on windowsills and other surfaces, and vacuuming, including floor mats at the entrances to homes, were necessary. Public health authorities recognized that high-efficiency particulate air (HEPA) filters needed to be used during partial or full abatement.

18. Sergio Piomelli, John Rosen, J. Julian Chisolm Jr., and John Graef, "Management of Lead Poisoning," *Journal of Pediatrics* 105 (October 1984): 529 (emphasis in original).

19. See C.S. Clark, R.L. Bornschein, P. Succop, S.S. Que Hee, P.B. Hammond, and B. Peace, "Condition and Type of Housing as an Indicator of Potential Environmental Lead Exposure and Pediatric Blood Lead Levels," *Environmental Research* 38 (1985): 46–53.

20. J.J. Chisolm Jr., E.D. Mellits, and S.A. Quaskey, "The Relationship between the Level of Lead Absorption in Children and the Age, Type, and Condition of Housing," *Environmental Research* 38 (1985): 31.

21. Ibid., 31–32.

22. "Of the 152 children discharged to old housing, 75 had 127 recurrences of PbB ≥ 50 µg/dl." Chisolm, Mellits, and Quaskey, "Relationship between the Level of Lead Absorption in Children and the Age, Type, and Condition of Housing," 31 (quotation), 39. Of the 93 children in group 1 (living in homes partially abated according to local ordinance), 13 had one recurrence; of the 12 children in group 2a (in lead-free public housing), 2 children had one recurrence and 1 child had two recurrences. Of the 15 children in group 2b (who did not visit lead-contaminated

homes), none had any recurrences. Of the 5 children in group 3 (in completely lead-abated homes), none had any recurrences. Of the 59 children in group 4 (in incompletely abated homes), 26 had one recurrence, 23 had two recurrences, 10 had three or more recurrences, and none had no recurrences.

23. Chisolm, Mellits, and Quaskey, "Relationship between the Level of Lead Absorption in Children and the Age, Type, and Condition of Housing," 40.

24. Ibid., 41 (emphasis in original).

25. Mark R. Farfel, "Reducing Lead Exposure in Children," *Annual Reviews of Public Health* 6 (1985): 334.

26. Ibid., 345. In Baltimore itself, prior to 1986, landlords were not responsible for removing lead above the four-foot level. Chisolm often critiqued these regulations, asking, "But have you ever heard of gravity?" Interview with Saul Kerpelman, April 12, 2011, Baltimore.

27. Farfel, "Reducing Lead Exposure in Children," 336.

28. Ibid., 346.

29. Ibid., 348.

30. Ibid., 349–50. See also Herbert Needleman, "Childhood Lead Poisoning: The Promise and Abandonment of Primary Prevention," *American Journal of Public Health* 88 (December 1998): 1871–77.

31. Farfel, "Reducing Lead Exposure in Children," 341.

32. Ibid., 349.

33. J. Julian Chisolm Jr., "Removal of Lead Paint from Old Housing: The Need for a New Approach," editorial, *American Journal of Public Health* 76 (March 1986): 236, 237.

34. Committee on Environmental Hazards, Committee on Accident and Poison Prevention, American Academy of Pediatrics, "Statement of Childhood Lead Poisoning," *Pediatrics* 79 (March 1987): 463.

35. Ibid. See also Yona Amitai, John W. Graef, Mary Jean Brown, Robert S. Gerstle, Nancy Kahn, and Paul E. Cochrane, "Hazards of 'Deleading' Homes of Children with Lead Poisoning," *American Journal of Diseases of Children* 141 (July 1987): 758–60; Susana Rey-Alvarez and Theresa Menke-Hargrave, "Deleading Dilemma: Pitfall in the Management of Childhood Lead Poisoning," *Pediatrics* 79 (February 1987): 214–18.

36. American Academy of Pediatrics, "Statement of Childhood Lead Poisoning," 463.

37. Ibid., 464.

38. "Current Trends Impact of the 1985 CDC Lead Statement—Savannah, Georgia," *Morbidity and Mortality Weekly Report* 36 (October 9, 1987), available at www.cdc.gov/mmwr/preview/mmwrhtml/00000982.htm (accessed January 14, 2009).

39. Claudia Ashton v. Samuel Pierce, 716 F.2d 56 (D.C. Cir. 1983), available at http://openjurist.org/716/f2d/56/ashton-v-pierce-us-hud (accessed March 16, 2010).

40. Jacobs, interview.

41. *Ashton v. Pierce*, 716 F.2d 56.

42. Jacobs, interview.

43. Ibid.

44. Ibid. See also Housing Authority Insurance Group history, available at www.housingcenter.com/HAIGroupInfo/history.aspx (accessed March 17, 2010).

45. Jacobs, interview. See also Housing Authority Insurance Group history, available at www.housingcenter.com/HAIGroupInfo/history.aspx (accessed March 17, 2010). Jacobs did a study in the late 1980s that showed that some housing authorities, specifically New Orleans's, were not safely abating lead. For a discussion of the continuing depths of the problem, see Felicia A. Rabito, Charles Shorter, and Lu Ann E. White, "Lead Levels among Children Who Live in Public Housing," *Epidemiology* 14 (May 2003): 263.

46. Jacobs, interview. In 1992 Congress passed Title X of the Housing and Community Development Act. The act "redefined what a lead paint hazard was," in Jacobs's words. In so doing, Congress rejected the previous definition of lead paint hazards as being the mere *presence* of lead paint as defined by *Ashley v. Pierce* and instead established a "new definition: . . . *deteriorated* lead paint, *contaminated* lead dust and *contaminated* bare soil." Jacobs sees this as a practical advance over the absolutist position that had produced what he characterized as policy paralysis.

47. Herbert Needleman, "The Future Challenge of Lead Toxicity," *Environmental Health Perspectives* 89 (1990): 87–88.

48. Ibid. Others, such as Dave Jacobs and Don Ryan, estimated the cost of detoxification as being much higher—at least $10,000 per house. See the discussion earlier in the chapter.

49. Needleman, "Future Challenge of Lead Toxicity," 88. HUD's own estimate, in 1990, was that the cost of testing and removing all lead paint in older housing units would be $50 billion a year for ten years. See: U.S. HUD, "Comprehensive and Workable Plan," December 7, 1990, p. 4–21.

50. Paul Mushak and Annemarie F. Crocetti, "Methods for Reducing Lead Exposure in Young Children and Other Risk Groups: An Integrated Summary of a Report to the U.S. Congress on Childhood Lead Poisoning," *Environmental Health Perspectives* 89 (1990): 132.

51. Ibid., 133.

52. As late as 2004, studies showed that the postabatement dust standard of 200 µg/dl on floors resulted in six-month-old infants, perhaps the children most vulnerable to lead's toxic neurological effects, being eleven times more likely than children more than six months old to experience an increase in blood lead concentrations of 5 µg/dl or higher. See S. Clark, J. Grote, J. Wilson, P. Succop, M. Chen, W. Galke, and P. McLaine, "Occurrence and Determinants of Increases in Blood-Lead Levels in Children Shortly after Lead Hazard Control Activities," *Environmental Research* 96 (2004): 202.

53. Denworth, *Toxic Truth*, 160. See also David Rosner and Gerald Markowitz, "Standing Up to the Lead Industry: An Interview with Herbert Needleman," *Public Health Reports* 120 (May–June 2005): 330–37.

54. Eric Felten, "Lead Scare: Leftist Politics by Other Means," *Wall Street Journal*, June 28, 1991, A12.

55. Ryan, interview.

56. CDC, *Strategic Plan for the Elimination of Childhood Lead Poisoning*, ii.

57. Ibid., xiii.

58. Ibid., xiv.

59. Ibid., 26.

60. Ryan, interview.

61. Don Ryan, "Fifteen Ingredients to Recent Progress on Childhood Lead Poisoning," mimeographed notes for talk to the Collette Chuda Foundation Jackson Hole Retreat, 1994, Don Ryan Private Papers (hereafter Ryan Papers).

62. Louis W. Sullivan, M.D., "Remarks . . . 1st Annual Conference on Childhood Lead Poisoning" (emphasis in original), in transcripts from Preventing Childhood Lead Poisoning: The First Comprehensive National Conference, Washington, D.C., October 6–8, 1991, Don Ryan Papers.

63. "Final Report," p. 3, in transcripts from Preventing Childhood Lead Poisoning: The First Comprehensive National Conference, Washington, D.C., October 6–8, 1991, Don Ryan Papers.

64. Ibid., 4.

65. See U.S. Department of Health and Human Services, Public Health Service, Centers for Disease Control, "Preventing Lead Poisoning in Young Children," October 1991, available at http://wonder.cdc.gov/wonder/prevguid/p0000029/p0000029.asp (accessed: January 24, 2012).

66. "Final Report," p. 4, in transcripts from Preventing Childhood Lead Poisoning: The First Comprehensive National Conference, Washington, D.C., October 6–8, 1991, Don Ryan Papers.

67. Ibid.

68. "Lead Hazard Reduction, Appendix C," in "Final Report," in transcripts from Preventing Childhood Lead Poisoning: The First Comprehensive National Conference, Washington, D.C., October 6–8, 1991, Don Ryan Papers.

69. Jacobs, interview.

70. Ibid.

71. Ibid.

72. William K. Reilly, Administrator, EPA, "Testimony . . . Before the Subcommittee on Toxic Substances, Environmental Oversight, Research and Development of the Committee on Environment and Public Works, United States Senate," February 21, 1991, typescript, Mushak Papers.

CHAPTER 6

Epigraph: Quoted in [Ingrid Boyum], *City Homes in Baltimore: "Minimal Rehab" to Combat Abandonment,* C16-90-1010.0 (Cambridge: Harvard Kennedy School of Government Case Program, 1990), 11.

1. Baltimore Health Department, *Lead Poisoning, Special Bulletin* (Fall 1992), Vertical File, Folder: Lead Poisoning, Enoch Pratt Library, Maryland Department.

2. Jonathan Bor and David Kohn, "Researcher Faces Outcry: Scientist Fights Claim He Put City Kids at Risk in Lead Poison Studies," *Baltimore Sun,* May 1, 2008, A1.

3. Interview with Ellen Silbergeld, March 25, 2010, Baltimore.

4. Battelle subcontract to KKI and Mark Farfel, October 30, 1990, Kennedy Krieger Institute Papers, in authors' possession (hereafter KKI Papers). See also "Affidavit of Mark Farfel, SC.D. in Support of Notice of Removal," no date, filed in Myron Higgins et al. v. Kennedy Krieger Institute Inc. et al., U.S. District Court for the District of Maryland, Northern Division, KKI Papers. We thank Suzanne Shapiro of the law firm of Saul E. Kerpelman, Baltimore, for sharing documents with us that were gathered during discovery in various lawsuits. The R&M study was organized through a contract between the EPA and Battelle, the Ohio research and development company that regularly managed government contracts in a variety of health, energy, and other technology efforts.

5. "Design of LBP Abatement, Repair, and Maintenance Study," contract between Battelle and the EPA, May 14, 1990, KKI Papers.

6. Ibid.

7. For a substantial bibliography on Maryland and Baltimore's experience, see Terry J. Harris and Lisa J. Smith, "Tort Reform Reform: Maryland's Lead Poisoning Law Needs Overhaul," *University of Baltimore Journal of Environmental Law* (Fall 2004): 27–41, available at https://litigation-essentials.lexisnexis.com/webcd/app?action=DocumentDisplay&crawlid=1&doctype=cite&docid=12+U.+Balt.+J.+Envtl.+L.+27&srctype=smi&srcid=3B15&key=f1753d13abdf9ba9b10e8e1477f7a922 (accessed March 22, 2011). For historical data from 1996 to 2002, see Maryland Department of the Environment, Lead Poisoning Prevention Program, *Childhood Blood Lead Surveillance in Maryland: 2002 Annual Report* (November 2003), available at http://textonly.mde.state.md.us/assets/document/leadcoordination/LeadAnnualReport2002.pdf (accessed March 28, 2011).

8. "Childhood Lead Poisoning in Baltimore: A Generation Imperiled as Laws Ignored," *Abell Report* 15 (September 2002): 2.

9. Kennedy Krieger Institute, "Statement of Work: Planning Activities: June 1, 1990 to August 15, 1990," KKI Papers.

10. The questions pursued in the KKI study in part grew out of the findings in Farfel's doctoral dissertation. Farfel had evaluated traditional and then-state-of-the-art methods of abatement and had found them wanting. Traditional methods actually led to an increase in exposure and a rise in blood lead levels among children returning to abated homes. See Mark Farfel, "Evaluation of Health and Environmental Effects of Two Methods for Residential Lead Paint Removal" (PhD diss., Johns Hopkins University, 1987).

11. Kennedy Krieger Institute, "Statement of Work: Planning Activities: June 1, 1990 to August 15, 1990," KKI Papers.

12. See J.J. Chisolm Jr., E.D. Mellits, and S.A. Quaskey, "The Relationship Between the Level of Lead Absorption in Children and the Age, Type, and Condition of Housing," *Environmental Research* 38 (1985): 31–41; and Mark R. Farfel, "Reducing Lead Exposure in Children," *Annual Reviews of Public Health* 6 (1985): 334–55.

13. Mark Farfel and J. Julian Chisolm Jr., "Health and Environmental Outcomes of Traditional and Modified Practices for Abatement of Residential

Lead-Based Paint," *American Journal of Public Health* 80 (October 1990): 1240–45.

14. Ibid., 1245.

15. Ibid.

16. Ibid., 1240.

17. Ibid.

18. Ibid.

19. Ibid.

20. Thomas Hendricks to Mark Farfel, "Re: Lead-Based Paint Abatement and Repair and Maintenance Study in Baltimore," May 6, 1991, KKI Papers.

21. John M. Powell, "History of Baltimore, 1870–1912," in *Baltimore: Its History and Its People*, vol. 1, ed. Clayton Coleman Hall (New York: Lewis Historical Publishing Company, 1912), 327.

22. Matthew Page Andrews, "History of Baltimore from 1850 to the Close of the Civil War," in *Baltimore: Its History and Its People*, vol. 1, ed. Clayton Coleman Hall (New York: Lewis Historical Publishing Company, 1912), 235.

23. Samuel Kelton Roberts Jr., *Infectious Fear: Politics, Disease, and the Health Effects of Segregation* (Chapel Hill: University of North Carolina Press, 2009), 11.

24. Ibid., 76.

25. Ibid., 75–76.

26. Ibid., 68–86.

27. See Joan Jacobson, "The Dismantling of Baltimore's Public Housing Program," *Abell Report* 20 (September 2007): 1–9; "Response by Housing Authority of Baltimore City, September 7, 2007," *Abell Report* 20 (September 2007): 9–19, available at www.abell.org/pubsitems/arn907.pdf (accessed January 6, 2012); "Population History of Baltimore for 1790–1990," available at http://physics.bu.edu/~redner/projects/population/cities/baltimore.html (accessed January 6, 2012).

28. [Boyum], *City Homes in Baltimore*, 1.

29. Ibid.

30. Ibid., 4.

31. Ibid., 6, 7.

32. Ibid., 9, 10.

33. Ibid., 8.

34. Ibid., 10.

35. Quoted in ibid., 11.

36. Silbergeld, interview.

37. Mark Farfel to Thomas Hendrix, "Re: Lead-Based Paint Abatement and Repair and Maintenance Study in Baltimore," June 25, 1991, KKI Papers.

38. Battelle, *Quality Assurance Project Plan for the Kennedy Krieger Institute Lead-Based Paint Abatement and Repair and Maintenance Study* (draft report to Office of Pollution Prevention and Toxics, U.S. Environmental Protection Agency, June 22, 1992).

39. Farfel to Hendrix, June 25, 1991.

40. Deposition of Mark Farfel, May 5, 1997, pp. 8–9, in Myron Higgins et al. v. Lawrence Polakoff et al., Case No. 24C95066067/CL 193461, Circuit Court for Baltimore City, KKI Papers.

41. Exhibit C, Baltimore Exhibits, pp. 449–75, in *Higgins v. Polakoff*, KKI Papers.

42. Mark Farfel to Thomas Hendrix, May 13, 1992, KKI Papers.

43. Deposition of Farfel, May 5, 1997, pp. 8–9, in *Higgins v. Polakoff*, KKI Papers.

44. Ibid., 10–11.

45. Farfel to Hendrix, June 25, 1991.

46. "Script to be Used by City Homes Personnel to Assess Interest in the Kennedy Institute Study," attached to Farfel to Hendrix, June 25, 1991. See also Battelle, *Quality Assurance Project Plan for the Kennedy Krieger Institute Lead-Based Paint Abatement and Repair and Maintenance Study*.

47. Battelle, *Quality Assurance Project Plan for the Kennedy Krieger Institute Lead-Based Paint Abatement and Repair and Maintenance Study*, chapter 1, p. 1.

48. Ibid., chapter 2, p. 2.

49. Ibid.

50. U.S. EPA, Office of Prevention, Pesticides, and Toxic Substances, "Executive Summary," in *Lead-Based Paint Abatement and Repair and Maintenance Study in Baltimore: Findings Based on Two Years of Follow-Up*, EPA 747-R-97-005 (Washington, D.C.: U.S. EPA, December 1997), vii.

51. "Attachment 1—Comparison of Elements of Repair and Maintenance Levels I–III," attached to Mark Farfel to Thomas Hendrix, "Re: Application for Renewal of RPN No. 91-05-02-01," April 17, 1992, KKI Papers. See also U.S. EPA, *Lead-Based Paint Abatement and Repair and Maintenance Study in Baltimore*, 26–27.

52. In a May 1997 deposition, Mark Farfel said, "We did try to remove deteriorated paint, but that was sometimes subject to the limitation of our resources," which was capped at $3,500. Deposition of Farfel, May 5, 1997, pp. 72–73, in *Higgins v. Polakoff*, KKI Papers.

53. "Attachment 1—Comparison of Elements of Repair and Maintenance Levels I–III," attached to Farfel to Hendrix, April 17, 1992. See also U.S. EPA, *Lead-Based Paint Abatement and Repair and Maintenance Study in Baltimore*, 26–27.

54. See note 53.

55. Battelle, *Quality Assurance Project Plan for the Kennedy Krieger Institute Lead-Based Paint Abatement and Repair and Maintenance Study*, chapter 2, p. 14.

56. Ibid.

57. Ibid., chapter 2, p. 15.

58. Ibid., chapter 2, p. 14.

59. Ericka Grimes v. Kennedy Krieger Institute Inc., No. 128, and Myron Higgins et al. v. Kennedy Krieger Institute Inc., No. 129, 366 Md. 29, 782 A.2d

807, 2001 Md. LEXIS 496 (2001); deposition of Farfel, May 5, 1997, pp. 73–74, in *Higgins* v. *Polakoff*, KKI Papers.

60. Thomas Hendrix to Mark Farfel, May 11, 1992, KKI Papers.

61. Farfel to Hendrix, May 13, 1992.

62. Mark Farfel to Thomas Hendrix, "Re: Lead Based Paint Abatement and Repair and Maintenance in Baltimore," April 25, 1993, KKI Papers.

63. "Clinical Investigation Consent Form [1991]" for the "Lead-Paint Abatement and Repair &Maintenance Study (Older Dwellings Which Have Received R&M)," Johns Hopkins Medical Institutions, attached to Farfel to Hendrix, May 13, 1992.

64. Ibid.

65. "Clinical Investigation Consent Form [1991]" Johns Hopkins Medical Institutions, attached to Farfel to Hendrix, May 13, 1992. See also Farfel to Hendrix, April 25, 1993.

66. Nancy A. Neimuth, Brandon J. Wood, Jennifer R. Holdcraft, and David A. Burgoon, *Review of Studies Addressing Lead Abatement Effectiveness: Updated Edition*, EPA 747-B-98-001 (prepared by Battelle for U.S. EPA, Office of Pollution Prevention and Toxics, December 1998), A51.

67. Farfel to Hendrix, April 25, 1993.

68. Mark Farfel to Mr. Wojtowycz, Baltimore Health Department, September 9, 1993, KKI Papers. Those standards were 200µg/ft^2 for floors, 500 µg/ft^2 for windowsills, and 800 µg/ft^2 for window wells. See *Grimes v. Kennedy Krieger Institute* and *Higgins v. Kennedy Krieger Institute*, 366 Md. 29, 782 A.2d 807, 2001 Md. LEXIS 496 at *14.

69. Farfel to Wojtowycz, September 9, 1993. Maryland required, in 1990, that there be two inspections following abatement. The first was a visual inspection to make sure that all surfaces had been attended to. The second and final inspection was done after the final cleanup at the site that collected dust samples, to make sure that their lead content was below the state's acceptable levels. Division of Lead Poisoning Prevention, Maryland Department of the Environment, "Lead Paint Hazard Fact Sheet #7, Inspections for Lead Paint Abatement," June 1990, Vertical File, Folder: Lead Poisoning, Enoch Pratt Library, Maryland Department.

70. Mark Farfel, "Renewal Request to Johns Hopkins JCCI," May 10, 1994, KKI Papers.

71. Ibid.

72. Ibid.

73. "Clinical Investigation Consent Form [1993]," for the "Lead-Paint Abatement and Repair & Maintenance Study (Older Dwellings Which Will Receive R&M)," Johns Hopkins Medical Institutions, attached to Farfel, "Renewal Request to Johns Hopkins JCCI," May 10, 1994.

74. U.S. EPA, "Executive Summary," in *Lead-Based Paint Abatement and Repair and Maintenance Study in Baltimore*, viii.

75. Ibid., xi.

76. Ibid.

77. Ibid., xiii.

78. Ibid.

79. See also Neimuth et al., *Review of Studies Addressing Lead Abatement Effectiveness: Updated Edition.*

80. U.S. EPA, "Executive Summary," in *Lead-Based Paint Abatement and Repair and Maintenance Study in Baltimore,* 63–67.

81. "Lead Paint Field Report/Spectrum Analysis for 908 N Durham, 12/1/93" and Environmental Restorations Inc. to City Homes, "Lead Paint Abatement/Construction Proposal, 908 North Durham Street . . . Scope of Work—Level II Occupied," December 29, 1993, both in KKI Papers. We thank Laura Bothwell for her detailed analysis of these two documents.

82. Jean E. Eddy, President, Environmental Restorations Inc., "Lead Paint Abatement/Construction Proposal, 1906 East Federal Street (781 Revision II) Baltimore, Maryland, Scope of Work—Level II, Vacant," April 12, 1994, attached to Clark McNutt, Environmental Restorations Inc., to Lawrence Polakoff, April 12, 1994, KKI Papers. See also Manuel Roig-Franzia and Rick Weiss, "Maryland MD Appeals Court Slams Researchers," *Washington Post,* August 21, 2001, B1.

83. Tatsha Robertson, "Subjects in Baltimore Rue Lead-Paint Study," *Boston Globe,* September 3, 2001, A1.

84. "Kathy H.," "Michael H.," "Joan M.," "Abby M.," and "Annabel M." are pseudonyms.

85. Eddy, "Lead Paint Abatement/Construction Proposal," April 12, 1994, attached to McNutt to Polakoff, April 12, 1994. See also Roig-Franzia and Weiss, "Maryland MD Appeals Court Slams Researchers."

86. "Appendix A: Abstracts of Studies Addressing Lead Abatement Effectiveness," in Neimuth et al., *Review of Studies Addressing Lead Abatement Effectiveness: Updated Edition.*

87. Neimuth et al., *Review of Studies Addressing Lead Abatement Effectiveness: Updated Edition,* x–xii.

88. "Executive Summary," in Neimuth et al., *Review of Studies Addressing Lead Abatement Effectiveness: Updated Edition.*

89. Herbert L. Needleman, "Childhood Lead Poisoning: The Promise and Abandonment of Primary Prevention," *American Journal of Public Health* 88 (December 1998): 1872.

90. Ibid., 1874.

91. Ibid., 1874–75.

92. Ibid., 1876.

93. Ibid., 1875.

94. Don Ryan, "Childhood Lead Poisoning: Ryan re Needleman," *American Journal of Public Health* 89 (July 1999): 1127.

95. David E. Jacobs, "Childhood Lead Poisoning: Jacobs re Needleman," *American Journal of Public Health* 89 (July 1999): 1128.

96. Herbert Needleman, "Childhood Lead Poisoning: Needleman Responds," *American Journal of Public Health* 89 (July 1999): 1130–31.

97. See, for example, David Rothman, "The Shame of Medical Research," *New York Review of Books*, November 30, 2000, available at www.nybooks. com/articles/archives/2000/nov/30/the-shame-of-medical-research (accessed March 16, 2012); and Marcia Angell, "The Ethics of Clinical Research in the Third World," *New England Journal of Medicine* 337 (1997): 847–49.

98. Much of the AIDS/HIV controversies over inequalities and treatment were fought over the ethics of providing research subjects with standards of care available in Western cultures. See Peter Lurie and Sidney Wolfe, "Unethical Trials of Interventions to Reduce Perinatal Transmission of the Human Immunodeficiency Virus in Developing Countries," *New England Journal of Medicine* 337 (1997): 853–56; Angell, "The Ethics of Clinical Research in the Third World," 847–49; and Rothman, "The Shame of Medical Research."

CHAPTER 7

Epigraphs: National Commission for the Protection of Human Subjects of Biomedical and Behavioral Research, *The Belmont Report: Ethical Principles and Guidelines for the Protection of Human Subjects of Research*, DHEW Publication No. (OS) 78-0012 (Washington, D.C.: GPO, 1978), 6, available at http://videocast.nih.gov/pdf/ohrp_belmont_report.pdf (accessed March 16, 2012); Ellen Silbergeld, "A Necessary Paradox: Research Has Some Risks But It Is Good for Us," *Washington Post*, September 2, 2001, B5.

1. Ruth Quinn, Outreach Coordinator, to Patricia Hughes, March 9, 1993; Ruth Quinn to Patricia Hughes, December 16, 1993; Ruth Quinn to Ms. Grines [sic], April 9, 1993; Ruth Quinn to Ms. Grines [sic], September 29, 1993, all in KKI Papers. "Enid G." is a pseudonym.

2. Ruth Quinn, Outreach Coordinator, to Ms. Grines [sic], September 15, 1993, KKI Papers.

3. Ericka Grimes v. Kennedy Krieger Institute Inc., No. 128, and Myron Higgins et al. v. Kennedy Krieger Institute Inc., No. 129, 366 Md. 29, 782 A.2d 807, 2001 Md. LEXIS 496 (2001).

4. Quinn to Grines [sic], September 15, 1993.

5. Quinn to Hughes, December 16, 1993.

6. Ruth Quinn to Patricia Hughes, December 17, 1993, KKI Papers. On May 19, 1994, Quinn wrote to the child's mother, giving the dust test results of March 9, which showed lead dust on the second floor, and advising her to "use a wet mop for these floors." Ruth Quinn to Patricia Hughes, May 19, 1994, KKI Papers.

7. Ruth Quinn to Ms. Grines [sic], March 25, 1994; Ruth Quinn to Ms. Grines [sic], March 28, 1994, both in KKI Papers.

8. "Michael H." and "Kathy H." are pseudonyms.

9. Telephone interview with Suzanne Shapiro, June 16, 2009.

10. Interview with Saul Kerpelman, April 12, 2011, Baltimore.

11. *Grimes v. Kennedy Krieger Institute* and *Higgins v. Kennedy Krieger Institute*, 366 Md. 29, 782 A.2d 807, 2001 Md. LEXIS 496 at *21–22.

12. After the cases were dismissed by the lower court, they were combined in the appeal to Maryland's highest court, its court of appeals.

13. "Memorandum of Points and Authorities in Support of Motion to Dismiss," February 22, 2000, pp. 8, 10–11 (emphasis in original), Exhibit 2 in Dontae Rico Wallace et al. v. Kennedy Krieger Institute Inc. et al., Case No. 1.07-CV-1140, U.S. District Court for the District of Maryland, Baltimore Division, in Myron Higgins et al. v. Lawrence Polakoff et al., Case No. 24C95066067/CL 193461, Circuit Court for Baltimore City, *sub nom.*, Ericka Grimes v. Kennedy Krieger Institute Inc., No. 128, and Myron Higgins et al. v. Kennedy Krieger Institute Inc., No. 129, 366 Md. 29 (2001), KKI Papers.

14. Ibid.

15. "Official Transcripts of Proceedings," April 5, 2000, in Myron Higgins et al. v. Lawrence Polakoff et al., Case No. 24C95066067/CL 193461, Circuit Court for Baltimore City, in the Court of Appeals of Maryland, KKI Papers.

16. Ibid., 29

17. "Brief of Appelle (KKI) by: Stanford Gann, Jr. and Susan Boyce in Court of Appeals of Maryland," no date, p. 24, re. *Higgins v. Polakoff*, KKI Papers.

18. Ibid.

19. Ibid., 27.

20. Ibid.

21. Ibid., 29.

22. "Lease Addendum, 1906 East Federal, 5-13-94," in *Higgins v. Polakoff*, in the Court of Appeals of Maryland, KKI Papers.

23. "Response of KKI to Co-Defendant Polakoff's Request for a Summary Judgment, March 17, 2000," in Myron Higgins et al. v. Lawrence Polakoff et al., Case No. 24C95066067/CL 193461, Circuit Court for Baltimore City, KKI Papers.

24. "Official Transcripts of Proceedings," April 5, 2000, p. 30, in *Higgins v. Polakoff*, in the Court of Appeals of Maryland, KKI Papers.

25. Ibid., 33.

26. Suzanne Shapiro of Kerpelman and Assoc., "Appeal to Court of Special Appeals of Maryland," January 17, 2001, in *Higgins v. Kennedy Krieger Institute*, No. 129, 366 Md. 29, 782 A.2d 807, 2001 Md. LEXIS 496.

27. Ibid.

28. Ibid.

29. Ibid.

30. Ibid.

31. "Motion of the National Center for Lead-Safe Housing for Leave to Participate as *Amicus Curiae* at the Maryland Court of Appeals, Higgins v. KKI," April 11, 2001, in *Higgins v. Kennedy Krieger Institute*, No. 129, 366 Md. 29, 782 A.2d 807, 2001 Md. LEXIS 496.

32. National Center for Lead-Safe Housing, "Brief of Amicus Curiae," ca. June 2001, in *Higgins v. Kennedy Krieger Institute*, No. 129, 366 Md. 29, 782 A.2d 807, 2001 Md. LEXIS 496.

33. Ibid.

34. Public Justice Center, the National Health Law Program, and the East Harbor Village Center, "Brief of Amicus Curiae," April 20, 2001, in *Higgins v. Kennedy Krieger Institute*, No. 129, 366 Md. 29, 782 A.2d 807, 2001 Md. LEXIS 496.

35. "Supplemental Brief of Appelle," ca. June 2001, in *Higgins v. Kennedy Krieger Institute*, No. 129, 366 Md. 29, 782 A.2d 807, 2001 Md. LEXIS 496 at *8.

36. Susan Reverby, *Examining Tuskegee: The Infamous Syphilis Study and Its Legacy* (Chapel Hill: University of North Carolina Press, 2009); James Jones, *Bad Blood: The Tuskegee Syphilis Experiment* (New York: Free Press, 1993).

37. "Supplemental Brief of Appelle," ca. June 2001, in *Higgins v. Kennedy Krieger Institute*, No. 129, 366 Md. 29, 782 A.2d 807, 2001 Md. LEXIS 496.

38. Suzanne Shapiro, "Supplemental Brief of the Appellants," May 24, 2001, in *Higgins v. Kennedy Krieger Institute*, No. 129, 366 Md. 29, 782 A.2d 807, 2001 Md. LEXIS 496.

39. Suzanne Shapiro, "Reply Brief of Appellants," March 19, 2001, in *Higgins v. Kennedy Krieger Institute*, No. 129, 366 Md. 29, 782 A.2d 807, 2001 Md. LEXIS 496.

40. Suzanne Shapiro, "Appellants Motion to Supplement the Record Pursuant to Maryland Rule 8-414," July 5, 2001, in *Higgins v. Kennedy Krieger Institute*, No. 129, 366 Md. 29, 782 A.2d 807, 2001 Md. LEXIS 496.

41. "Oral Arguments Taken in Reference to 'In re: Myron Higgins,'" July 10, 2001, p. 3, in *Higgins v. Kennedy Krieger Institute*, No. 129, 366 Md. 29, 782 A.2d 807, 2001 Md. LEXIS 496.

42. Ibid., 5–6.

43. Ibid., 7–8.

44. Ibid., 5–6.

45. Ibid., 10.

46. Ibid., 15–17.

47. Ibid., 18–19.

48. Ibid., 22.

49. Ibid., 23–24.

50. Ibid., 30–31.

51. Ibid., 33.

52. Ibid., 39.

53. Ibid., 47–48

54. Joe Surkiewicz, "Md. Court of Appeals Revives Lead Poisoning Suits against Kennedy Krieger Based on Study," *Baltimore Daily Record*, August 17, 2001, available at www.accessmylibrary.com/coms2/summary_0286-27347434_ITM (accessed June 22, 2009).

55. Caryn Tamber, "The Shore's Straight Shooter, Judge Dale R. Cathell Steps Down," *Baltimore Daily Record*, July 30, 2007, available at http://findarticles.com/p/articles/mi_qn4183/is_20070730/ai_n19438464/ (accessed July 1, 2009).

56. *Grimes v. Kennedy Krieger Institute* and *Higgins v. Kennedy Krieger Institute*, 366 Md. 29, 782 A.2d 807, 2001 Md. LEXIS 496 at *3.

57. Ibid. at *5–6.

58. *Grimes v. Kennedy Krieger Institute* and *Higgins v. Kennedy Krieger Institute*, 366 Md. 29, 782 A.2d 807, 2001 Md. LEXIS 496 at *7–8.

59. Ibid.

60. Ibid. at *11–13.

61. Ibid. at *14–16. The National Academy of Sciences issued a report, *Protecting Children from Housing Related Health Research*, that in part grew out of the controversies around the KKI study. It concluded that it was acceptable for vulnerable children to be involved in minimal-risk research if the benefits of the research would be used to benefit other vulnerable children. See Committee on Ethical Issues in Housing-Related Health Hazard Research Involving Children, Youth, and Families, *Ethical Considerations for Research on Housing-Related Health Hazards Involving Children*, ed. Bernard Lo and Mary Ellen O'Connell (Washington, D.C.: National Academies Press, 2005), available at www.nap.edu/openbook.php?record_id=11450&page=R1 (accessed December 15, 2011).

62. *Grimes v. Kennedy Krieger Institute* and *Higgins v. Kennedy Krieger Institute*, 366 Md. 29, 782 A.2d 807, 2001 Md. LEXIS 496 at *94.

63. Ibid. at *64.

64. Ibid.

65. Ibid. at *6.

66. Ibid. at *87.

67. Ibid. at *88–89.

68. Ibid. at *101 (emphasis in original).

69. Ibid. at *107.

70. Ibid. at *116.

71. Nicholas Wade, "Patient Dies in Trial of Gene Treatment," *New York Times*, September 29, 1999, A1, A24.

72. J. Savulescu and M. Spriggs, "The Hexamethonium Asthma Study and the Death of a Normal Volunteer in Research," *Journal of Medical Ethics* 28 (2002): 3–4.

73. Manuel Roig-Franzia and Rick Weiss, "Maryland Md. Appeals Court Slams Researchers," *Washington Post*, August 21, 2001, B1.

74. Ibid.

75. Jonathan Bor, "Kennedy Krieger Doctor Defends Lead Paint Study," *Baltimore Sun*, August 18, 2001, 1B.

76. John Biemer, "Maryland's Highest Court Scolds Researchers in Lead Paint Study," *USA Today*, August 21, 2001, available at www.usatoday.com/news/nation/2001/08/21/lead-paint.htm (accessed June 22, 2009).

77. Tamar Lewin, "U.S. Investigating Johns Hopkins Study of Lead Paint Hazard," *New York Times*, August 24, 2001, A11.

78. Manuel Roig-Franzia, "'My Kids Were Used as Guinea Pigs,'" *Washington Post*, August 25, 2001, A1.

79. Tom Scocca, "Test Case: Hopkins Arm Sued over Lead-Paint Study," *Baltimore City Paper*, August 8, 2001, available at www.citypaper.com/print-Story.asp?id=4810 (accessed June 5, 2009); Bor, "Kennedy Krieger Doctor Defends Lead Paint Study."

80. According to the *Washington Post*, the investigation "was launched before the Court's opinion was issued, although federal authorities would not say exactly when it began." Manuel Roig-Franzia, "Federal Probe Focuses on Lead Paint Research," *Washington Post*, August 23, 2001, B1.

81. David C. Bellinger and Kim Dietrich, "Ethical Challenges in Conducting Pediatric Environmental Health Research: Introduction," *Neurotoxicology and Teratology* 24 (2002): 443.

82. Gary Young, "Lead Paint Suit Breaks New Ground, Sparks Government Investigation," *National Law Journal*, August 28, 2001, available at www.law.com/jsp/article.jsp?id=900005526190&slreturn=20120901083119 (accessed October 1, 2012).

83. "Baltimore's Lawsuit Over Children Being Exposed to Lead in Johns Hopkins University Study," NPR, *All Things Considered*, August 27, 2001, available at www.highbeam.com/doc/1P1-49225418.html (accessed June 22, 2009).

84. Ellen Silbergeld, "A Necessary Paradox: Research Has Some Risks But It Is Good for Us," *Washington Post*, September 2, 2001, B5.

85. Ibid.

86. Amanda Spake, "A Study's Lasting Burden," *U.S. News and World Report*, September 3, 2001, 43.

87. Quoted in Jocelyn Kaiser, "Human Subjects: Court Rebukes Hopkins for Lead Paint Study," *Science* 293 (August 31, 2001): 1569.

88. "The Judge Went Too Far," editorial, *Washington Post*, September 29, 2001, A26. For an informative discussion of the differences between the Tuskegee research and other studies, see Amy Fairchild and Ronald Bayer, "The Uses and Abuses of Tuskegee," *Science* 284 (May 7, 1999): 919–21.

89. Scocca, "Test Case: Hopkins Arm Sued Over Lead-Paint Study."

90. Roig-Franzia, "'My Kids Were Used as Guinea Pigs.'" "Joan M." and "Annabel M." are pseudonyms.

91. Ibid.

92. Tom Pelton, "A Mother's Hope Crumbles into Despair over Lead Study Experiment," *Baltimore Sun*, August 23, 2001, 1B.

93. "KKI, JHU, UMMS, Others Ask Court of Appeals to Reconsider Lead Paint Issues," *The Gazette Online: The Newspaper of the Johns Hopkins University*, September 24, 2001, available at www.jhu.edu/~gazette/2001/24se po1/24lead.html (accessed October 1, 2012).

94. Tom Pelton, "Court Ruling Concerns Md. Researchers; Restrictions Feared after Judges' Finding in Lead Paint Case," *Baltimore Sun*, August 27, 2001, 1B.

95. Tom Pelton, "Lead Paint Rule Could Limit Research in Md.," *Baltimore Sun*, September 20, 2001, 1B.

96. Joe Surkiewicz, "Experts React to Md. Court of Appeals Ruling on Medical Research Ethics," *Baltimore Daily Record,* October 27, 2001, available at www.accessmylibrary.com/coms2/summary_0286-27348965_ITM (accessed June 5, 2007).

97. Ronald Bayer, "Beyond the Burdens of Protection: AIDS and the Ethics of Research," *Evaluation Review: A Journal of Applied Social Research* 14 (October 1990): 443–46; P. Cottin, "Is There Still Two Much Extrapolation from Data on Middle-Aged White Men?" *JAMA* 263 (1990): 1049–50. Women's groups, for example, demanded that research on AIDS drugs include HIV-infected women; they had largely been excluded from trials because of the potential harm to women who were or could become pregnant. Similarly, African Americans and Latinos were grossly unrepresented in AIDS research, leading to demands for more vigorous recruitment of these underrepresented groups. See Carol Levine, "Women and HIV/AIDS Research: The Barriers to Equity," *Journal of Applied Social Research* 14 (October 1990): 447–63. See also Gina Kolata, "N.I.H. Neglects Women, Study Says," *New York Times,* June 19, 1990, C6; and R. Steinbrook, "AIDS Trials Shortchange Minorities and Drug Users," *Los Angeles Times,* September 25, 1989, 1–19.

98. See, for example, George Annas and Michael Grodin, eds., *The Nazi Doctors and the Nuremberg Code* (New York: Oxford University Press, 1992); and David Rothman, *Strangers at the Bedside: A History of How Law and Bioethics Transformed Medical Decision Making* (New York: Basic Books, 1991). Susan Lederer's *Subjected to Science: Human Experimentation in America before the Second World War* (Baltimore: Johns Hopkins University Press, 1995) is one of the few works that explores the use of human research subjects prior to midcentury and places it in a historical trajectory.

99. See Benjamin F. Chavis Jr. and Charles Lee, *Toxic Waste and Race in the United States* (New York: Commission for Racial Justice, United Church of Christ, 1987); Robert D. Bullard, *Unequal Protection: Environmental Justice in Communities of Color* (San Francisco: Sierra Club Books, 1994); Robert D. Bullard, *Dumping in Dixie: Race, Class, and Environmental Quality* (Boulder: Westview Press, 1990); Jim Schwab, *Deeper Shades of Green: The Rise of Blue-Collar and Minority Environmentalism in America* (San Francisco: Sierra Club Books, 1994); Robert D. Bullard, *Confronting Environmental Racism: Voices from the Grass Roots* (Boston: South End Press, 1993); Phil Brown and Edwin J. Mikkelsen, *No Safe Place: Toxic Waste, Leukemia, and Community Action* (Berkeley: University of California Press, 1990); Helen E. Sheehan and Richard P. Wedeen, eds. *Toxic Circles: Environmental Hazards from the Workplace and the Community* (New Brunswick: Rutgers University Press, 1993); Committee on Environmental Justice, Health Sciences Policy Program, Institute of Medicine, *Toward Environmental Justice: Research, Education, and Health Policy Needs* (Washington, D.C.: National Academies Press, 1999); Robert Gottlieb, *Forcing the Spring: The Transformation of the*

American Environmental Movement (Washington, D.C.: Island Press, 1993); Robert Bullard, *The Quest for Environmental Justice: Human Rights and the Politics of Pollution* (San Francisco: Sierra Club Books, 2005); Ronald Sandler and Phaedra C. Pezzullo, *Environmental Justice and Environmentalism: The Social Justice Challenge to the Environmental Movement*, Urban and Industrial Environments Series (Cambridge, MA: MIT Press, 2007); Julian Agyeman, *Sustainable Communities and the Challenge of Environmental Justice* (New York: New York University Press, 2005); Kristin Shrader-Frechette, *Environmental Justice: Creating Equality, Reclaiming Democracy*, Environmental Ethics and Science Policy Series (New York: Oxford University Press, 2002); Luke Cole and Sheila Foster, *From the Ground Up: Environmental Racism and the Rise of the Environmental Justice Movement*, Critical America Series (New York: New York University Press, 2001); David Naguib Pellow and Robert J. Brulle, *Power, Justice, and the Environment: A Critical Appraisal of the Environmental Justice Movement*, Urban and Industrial Environments Series (Cambridge, MA: MIT Press, 2005); Sylvia Hood Washington, *Packing Them In: An Archaeology of Environmental Racism in Chicago, 1865–1954* (Lanham, MD: Lexington Books, 2005); Harriet Washington, *Medical Apartheid: The Dark History of Medical Experimentation on Black Americans from Colonial Times to the Present* (New York: New York : Doubleday, 2006); James Jones, *Bad Blood: The Tuskegee Syphilis Experiments* (New York: Free Press, 1981); Susan Reverby, ed., *Tuskegee's Truths: Rethinking the Tuskegee Syphilis Study* (Chapel Hill: University of North Carolina Press, 2001); Eileen Welsome, *The Plutonium Files* (New York: Dial Press, 1999); Jonathan Moreno, *Undue Risk: Secret State Experiments on Humans* (New York: W.H. Freeman and Co., 2000); and Allen M. Hornblum, *Acres of Skin: Human Experiments at Holmesburg Prison* (New York: Routledge, 1998).

100. See, for example, Adrienne Esposito, Executive Director, Citizen's Campaign for the Environment, to Michael Leavitt, EPA Administrator, "Re: Immediate Halt to Environmental Protection Agency's Children's Environmental Exposure Research Study (CHEERS) in Duval County, Florida," November 8, 2004, available at www.beyondpesticides.org/documents/Leavitt_CHEERS_04.pdf (accessed July 23, 2007).

101. David D. Kirkpatrick, "E.P.A. Halts Florida Tests on Pesticides," *New York Times*, April 9, 2005, available at www.nytimes.com/2005/04/09/politics/09pesticides.html (accessed September 28, 2011). See also David J. Rothman, "The Shame of Medical Research," *New York Review of Books*, November 30, 2000; and Barry Bloom and David Rothman, "Medical Morals: An Exchange," *New York Review of Books*, March 8, 2001.

102. Susan M. Reverby, "'Normal Exposure' and Inoculation Syphilis: A PHS 'Tuskegee' Doctor in Guatemala, 1946–1948," *Journal of Policy History* 23 (2011): 6–28.

103. These questions are explored in more detail in Amy Fairchild, Ronald Bayer, and James Colgrove, *Searching Eyes: Privacy, Disease Surveillance and*

the State in America (Berkeley: University of California Press; New York: Milbank Memorial Fund, 2008).

104. Bellinger and Dietrich, "Ethical Challenges in Conducting Pediatric Environmental Health Research: Introduction," *Neurotoxicology and Teratology* 24 (2002).

105. Paul Mushak, "Studies of Pervasive Toxic Contaminants in Children: Staying the Ethical Course," *Neurotoxicology and Teratology* 24 (2002): 463.

106. Howard Mielke, "Research Ethics in Pediatrics Environmental Health: Lessons from Lead," *Neurotoxicology and Teratology* 24 (2002): 468.

107. Don Ryan and Nick Farr, "Confronting the Ethical Challenges of environmental Health Research," *Neurotoxicology and Teratology* 24 (2002): 472.

108. Ibid., 473. See also Deborah Josephson, "Johns Hopkins Faces Further Criticism over Experiments," *British Medical Journal* 323 (September 8, 2001): 531.

109. Lynn Pinder, "Commentary on the Kennedy Krieger Institute Lead Paint Repair and Maintenance Study," *Neurotoxicology and Teratology* 24 (2002): 477.

110. Ibid., 478.

111. Ibid., 477–78.

112. Ibid., 478.

113. Herbert L. Needleman, "What Is Not Found in the Spreadsheets," *Neurotoxicology and Teratology* 24 (2002): 459–60.

114. Ibid. (emphasis in original).

115. Ibid., 460.

116. Ibid., 461.

117. Ibid. Two decades after the KKI study, the effectiveness of partial abatement strategies remains unresolved and studies continue to evaluate them. One recent study of the effectiveness of window replacement after twelve years on reducing lead dust in homes argues that "lead-safe window replacement is an important element of lead hazard control, weatherization, renovation and housing investment strategies and should be implemented broadly to protect children." Sherry L. Dickson, David E. Jacobs, Jonathan W. Wilson, Judith Y. Akoto, Rick Nevin, and C. Scott Clark, "Window Replacement and Residential Lead Paint Hazard Control 12 Years Later," *Environmental Research* 113 (2012): 14–20. Another study of children's blood lead levels in homes that were partially abated through the use of sheetrock, paint, plasterboard, paneling, and removal of friction surface on windows and doors indicated "modest success" in reducing blood lead levels, especially in children between three and six years. Jessica Leighton, Susan Klitzman, Slavenka Sedlar, Thomas Matte, and Neal Cohen, "The Effect of Lead-Based Paint Hazard Remediation on Blood Lead Levels of Lead Poisoned Children in New York City," *Environmental Research* 92 (2003): 182–90.

CHAPTER 8

Epigraph: Interview with Fidelma Fitzpatrick and John McConnell, April 8, 2011, New York City.

1. Ibid.

2. "AG Whitehouse Outlines RI Lead Paint Poison Problems, Solutions and Lawsuit for US Senate Panel," ca. 2002, available at www.riag.ri.gov/documents/reports/lead/lead.pdf (accessed September 28, 2012).

3. Originally, reformers wanted to amend the Baltimore housing code to eliminate flaking and peeling lead paint specifically but then realized that landlords could avoid liability by claiming they had not realized that the flaking paint was lead based. Hence, reformers pushed for and achieved language that was less specific but more exacting.

4. Interview with Saul Kerpelman and Suzanne Shapiro, April 12, 2011, Baltimore.

5. "Jeremy" is a pseudonym.

6. Kerpelman and Shapiro, interview.

7. Ibid.

8. Ibid.

9. Ibid. See also Thomas J. Miceli, Katherine A. Pancak, and C.F. Sirmans, "Protecting Children from Lead-Based Paint Poisoning: Should Landlords Bear the Burden?," *Boston College Environmental Affairs Law Review* 23, no. 1 (1995): 1–41.

10. See note 9.

11. Richwind Joint Ventures 4 v. Brunson, 96 Md. App. 330, 336–39, 625 A.2d 326, 327 (1993).

12. Interview with Neil Leifer, March 4, 2011, New York City. See also Paul Brodeur, *Outrageous Misconduct: The Asbestos Industry on Trial* (New York: Pantheon Books, 1985).

13. Leifer, interview.

14. Ibid.

15. Ibid.

16. See Jonathan Harr, *A Civil Action* (New York: Random House, 1995).

17. Leifer, interview.

18. Ibid.

19. Fitzpatrick and McConnell, interview.

20. Ibid.

21. See Elizabeth Blackmar, "Accountability for Public Health: Regulating the Housing Market in Nineteenth-Century New York City," in *"Hives of Sickness": Epidemics in New York City,* ed. David Rosner (New Brunswick, NJ: Rutgers University Press, 1986), 42–64.

22. Allan Brandt, *Cigarette Century: The Rise, Fall, and Deadly Persistence of the Product that Defined America* (New York: Basic Books, 2007); Robert Proctor, *Golden Holocaust: Origins of the Cigarette Eatastrophe and the Case for Abolition,* Berkeley, University of California Press, 2011; Paul Brodeur,

Outrageous Misconduct: The Asbestos Industry on Trial (New York: Pantheon Books, 1985)' Barry Castleman, *Asbestos: Medical and Legal Aspects,* 3rd ed. (Englewood Cliffs, NJ: Prentice Hall Law and Business, 1990).

23. Fitzpatrick and McConnell, interview.

24. Michael Janofsky, "Mississippi Seeks Damages from Tobacco Companies," *New York Times,* May 24, 1994, A12.

25. Fitzpatrick and McConnell, interview.

26. Janofsky, "Mississippi Seeks Damages from Tobacco Companies."

27. Ibid.

28. Fitzpatrick and McConnell, interview.

29. Ibid.

30. Ibid.

31. Ibid.

32. Ibid.

33. Ibid.

34. Ibid.

35. State of Rhode Island v. Lead Industries Association Inc., Case No. PC 99-5226, 2007 R.I. Super LEXIS 32 (2007), *rev'd,* 951 A.2d 428 (R.I. 2008). We discuss this case at length in our book *Deceit and Denial: The Deadly Politics of Industrial Pollution* (Berkeley: University of California Press; New York: Milbank Memorial Fund, 2013), esp. chapters 2 and 3.

36. Peter Lord, "Three Companies Found Liable in Lead-Paint Nuisance Suit," *Providence Journal,* February 23, 2006, A1. See also *Rhode Island v. Lead Industries Assoc.,* 2007 R.I. Super LEXIS 32 at *1.

37. Editorial, *Wall Street Journal,* February 27, 2006.

38. "Understanding Lead Pigment Litigation: What Others Are Saying, Editorials," available at www.leadlawsuits.com/index.php?s=712&item=2041 (accessed June 15, 2011).

39. "The Nuisance That May Cost Billions," *New York Times,* April 2, 2006, section 3, p. 1.

40. Quoted in Geoffrey Cowley, "Getting the Lead Out," *Newsweek,* February 17, 2003, 55.

41. *Rhode Island v. Lead Industries Assoc.,* 2007 R.I. Super LEXIS 32 at *4.

42. Abha Bhattarai, "Rhode Island Court Throws Out Jury Finding in Lead Case," *New York Times,* July 2, 2008, available at www.nytimes.com/2008/07/02/business/02paint.html?scp=1&sq=Rhode%20Island%20court%20throws%20out&st=cse (accessed June 20, 2011).

43. *Rhode Island v. Lead Industries Assoc.,* 2007 R.I. Super LEXIS 32 at *4.

44. Fitzpatrick and McConnell, interview.

45. County of Santa Clara et al. v. Superior Court of Santa Clara County, 50 Cal. 4th 35, 235 P.3d 21, 112 Cal. Rptr. 3d 697, 2010 Cal. LEXIS 7241 (2010).

46. Todd C. Frankel, "$320 Million Verdict in Lead Smelter Case Sends Clear Message," *St. Louis Post-Dispatch,* July 30, 2011, available at www.stltoday.com/news/local/metro/article_12f7e0ba-29ab-5894-8067-9a45ad255cfa.

html (accessed October 5, 2011). David Rosner appeared as an expert witness at the trial.

CHAPTER 9

Epigraph: "Children's Environmental Health: An Interview with Bruce Lanphear, MD, MPH, by Fred Lanphear," Center for Ecozoic Studies, available at www.ecozoicstudies.org/vol-4-no-4/children-s-environmental-health-an-interview-with-bruce-lanphear-md-mph (accessed July 21, 2011).

1. Herbert L. Needleman and Richard J. Jackson, "Lead Toxicity in the Twenty-First Century: Will We Still Be Treating It?" *Pediatrics* 89 (April 1992): 680.

2. See Centers for Disease Control, "National Surveillance Data (1997–2008)," available at www.cdc.gov/nceh/lead/data/national.htm (accessed September 26, 2011).

3. Needleman and Jackson, "Lead Toxicity in the Twenty-First Century."

4. Ibid.

5. Rick Nevin, "Understanding International Crime Trends: The Legacy of Preschool Lead Exposure," *Environmental Research* 104 (2007): 215. See also Jascha Hoffman, "Criminal Element," *New York Times Magazine*, October 21, 2007, available at www.nytimes.com/2007/10/21/magazine/21wwln-idealab-t.html (accessed September 26, 2011).

6. Tomás Guilarte, "Prenatal Lead Exposure and Schizophrenia: A Plausible Neurobiologic Connection," letter, *Environmental Health Perspectives* 112 (2004): A724; Tomás Guilarte, "Prenatal Lead Exposure and Schizophrenia: Further Evidence and More Neurobiological Connections," letter, *Environmental Health Perspectives* 117 (2009): A190–91.

7. Centers for Disease Control, Advisory Committee on Childhood Lead Poisoning Prevention, "Low Level Lead Exposure Harms Children: A Renewed Call for Primary Prevention," January 4, 2012, ix, available at www.cdc.gov/nceh/lead/ACCLPP/Final_Document_011212.pdf (accessed February 17, 2012).

8. See World Health Organization, *Childhood Lead Poisoning* (Geneva: WHO, 2010), available at www.who.int/ceh/publications/leadguidance.pdf (accessed February 21, 2012).

9. David Bellinger and Herbert Needleman, "Intellectual Impairment and Blood Lead Levels," *New England Journal of Medicine* 349 (2003): 500–502; L.M. Chiodo, S.W. Jacobson, and J.L. Jacobson, "Neurodevelopmental Effects of Postnatal Lead Exposure at Very Low Levels," *Neurotoxicology and Teratology* 26 (2004): 359–71; H. Hu, M.M. Téllez-Rojo, D. Bellinger, D. Smith, A.S. Ettinger, H. Lamadrid-Figueroa, J. Schwartz, L. Schnaas, A. Mercado-García, and M. Hernández-Avila, "Fetal Lead Exposure at Each Stage of Pregnancy as a Predictor of Infant Mental Development," *Environmental Health Perspectives* 114 (2006): 1730–35; K. Kordas, "Deficits in Cognitive Function and Achievement in Mexican First-Graders with Low

Blood Lead Concentrations," *Environmental Research* 100 (2006): 371–86; P.J. Surkan, A. Zhang, F. Trachtenberg, D.B. Daniel, S. McKinlay, and D.C. Bellinger, "Neuropsychological Function in Children with Blood Lead Levels < 10 microg/dL," *Neurotoxicology* 28 (2007): 1170–77.

10. For a review of this literature see Sarah Vogel, *Is It Safe?: Bisphenol A and the Struggle to Define the Risks of Chemicals* (Berkeley: University of California Press, 2012).

11. Theo Colborn, F.S. vom Saal, and A.M. Soto, "Developmental Effects of Endocrine-Disrupting Chemicals in Wildlife and Humans," *Environmental Health Perspectives* 101 (October 1993): 378–84; Theo Colburn, Diane Dumanoski, and John Peterson Myers, *Our Stolen Future: Are We Threatening Our Fertility, Intelligence, and Survival? A Scientific Detective Story* (New York: Plume, 1997); Joseph Thornton, *Pandora's Poison: Chlorine, Health and a New Environmental Strategy* (Cambridge, MA: MIT Press, 2000).

12. Interview with Ellen Silbergeld, March 25, 2010, Baltimore. For a discussion of these points, see Ana Navas-Acien, Eliseo Guallar, Ellen Silbergeld, and Stephen Rothenberg, "Lead Exposure and Cardiovascular Disease—A Systematic Review," *Environmental Health Perspectives* 115 (March 2007): 472–82. See also J.P. Wright, K.N. Dietrich, M.D. Ris, R.W. Hornung, S.D. Wessel, B.P. Lanphear, M. Ho, and M.M. Rae, "Association of Prenatal and Childhood Blood Lead Concentrations with Criminal Arrests in Early Adulthood," *PLoS Medicine* 5 (May 27, 2008): E101, doi:10.1371/journal. pmed.0050101; and R.L. Canfield, C.R. Henderson Jr., D.A. Cory-Slechta, C. Cox, T.A. Justko, and B.P. Lanphear, "Intellectual Impairment in Children with Blood Lead Concentrations below 10ug/dL," *New England Journal of Medicine* 348 (April 17, 2003): 1517–26.

13. Herbert L. Needleman, Julie A. Riess, Michael J. Tobin, Gretchen E. Biesecker, and Joel B. Greenhouse, "Bone Lead Levels and Delinquent Behavior," *JAMA* 275 (February 7, 1996): 368.

14. Bruce P. Lanphear, Richard Hornung, Jane Khoury, Kimberly Yolton, Peter Baghurst, David C. Bellinger, Richard L. Canfield, et al., "Low-Level Environmental Lead Exposure and Children's Intellectual Function: An International Pooled Analysis," *Environmental Health Perspectives* 113 (July 2005): 894.

15. Ibid., 899.

16. Joe M. Braun, Robert S. Cahn, Tanya Froelich, Peggy Auinger, and Bruce P. Lanphear, "Exposures to Environmental Toxicants and Attention Deficit Hyperactivity Disorder in U.S. Children," *Environmental Health Perspectives* 114 (December 2006): 1907.

17. Kim M. Dietrich, M. Douglas Ris, Paul A. Succop, Omer G. Berger, and Robert L. Bornshein, "Early Exposure to Lead and Juvenile Delinquency," *Neurotoxicology and Teratology* 23 (2001): 511.

18. Rick Nevin, "Understanding International Crime Trends: The Legacy of Preschool Lead Exposure," *Environmental Research* 104 (2007): 215. In another article, Nevin linked lead exposure to mental retardation rates in

the United States. See Rick Nevin, "Trends in Preschool Lead Exposure, Mental Retardation, and Scholastic Achievement: Association or Causation?," *Environmental Research* 109 (2009): 301–10.

19. Wright et al. "Association of Prenatal and Childhood Blood Lead Concentrations with Criminal Arrests in Early Adulthood." See also, D.M. Fergusson, J.M. Bowden, and L.J. Horwood, "Dentine Lead Levels in Childhood and Criminal Behavior in Late Adolescence and Early Adulthood," *Journal of Epidemiology and Community Health* 62 (2008): 1045–50, in which the authors argue that the associations between lead exposure and criminal behavior were weak. For discussion of tobacco and lead, see Tanya E. Froelich, Bruce P. Lanphear, Peggy Auinger, Richard Hornung, Jeffery N. Epstein, Joe Braun, and Robert S. Kahn, "Association of Tobacco and Lead Exposures with Attention-Deficit/Hyperactivity Disorder," *Pediatrics* 124 (December 2009): E1054–63, doi: 10.1542/peds.2009-0738.

20. M.F. Bouchard, D.C. Bellinger, J. Weuve, J. Matthews-Bellinger, S.E. Gilman, R.O. Wright, J. Schwartz, and M.G. Weisskopf, "Blood: Lead Levels and Major Depressive Disorder, Panic Disorder, and Generalized Anxiety Disorder in US Young Adults," *Archives of General Psychiatry* 66 (December 2009): 1313–19; Tomás R. Guilarte, Mark Opler, and Mikhail Pletnikov, "Is Lead Exposure in Early Life An Environmental Risk Factor for Schizophrenia? Neurobiological Connections and Testable Hypotheses" (unpublished paper, 2012), courtesy of the paper authors.

21. For example, Wieslaw Jedrychowski, Frederica P. Perera, Jeffery Jankowski, Dorota Mrozek-Budzyn, Elzbieta Mroz, Elzbieta Flak, Susan Edwards, Anita Skarupa, and Ilona Lisowska-Miszczyk, "Very Low Prenatal Exposure to Lead and Mental Development of Children in Infancy and Early Childhood," *Neuroepidemiology* 32 (February 18, 2009): 270.

22. National Toxicology Program (NTP), *NTP Monograph on Health Effects of Low-Level Lead*, prepublication copy (U.S. Department of Health and Human Services, June 13, 2012), available at http://ntp.niehs. nih.gov/?objectid=4F04B8EA-B187-9EF2-9F9413C68E76458E (accessed September 28, 2012).

23. Robin Mackar, "Panel Peer Reviews NTP Low-Level Lead Draft," *Environmental Factor* (December 2011), National Institute of Environmental Health Sciences, available at www.niehs.nih.gov/news/newsletter/2011/december/science-ntp/ (accessed January 5, 2012).

24. Federal Advisory Committee Act of 1972, 5 U.S.C. App. 2 § 5 (b)(2).

25. Silbergeld, interview. See also D. Ferber, "Critics See a Tilt in a CDC Science Panel," *Science* 297 (August 30, 2002):1456.

26. "Lead Poisoning Advisory Panel Weighed Down by Lead Industry's Friends," News from Ed Markey, U.S. Congress, Massachusetts 7th District, October 8, 2002.

27. Deposition of William Banner Jr., M.D., June 13, 2002, p. 115, in State of Rhode Island v. Lead Industries Association Inc., Case No. PC 99-5226, 2007 R.I. Super LEXIS 32 (2007), *rev'd*, 951 A.2d 428 (R.I. 2008).

28. Ibid., 136.

29. Trial testimony of William Banner Jr., M.D., July 7, 2011, in Preston Alexander et al. vs. Fluor Corporation et al., Cause No. 052-9567, Missouri Circuit Court for the Twenty-Second Judicial Circuit in the City of St. Louis.

30. *Gale Norton Nomination: Hearings Before the Senate Committee on Energy And Natural Resources*, 107th Cong. (January 18–19, 2001). Norton told the senators, for example, that "as scientific evidence became available as to problems, they [the lead companies] responded to those problems."

31. David Michaels, Eula Bingham, Les Boden, Richard Clapp, Lynn R. Goldman, Polly Hoppin, Sheldon Krimsky, et al., "Advice without Dissent," *Science* 298 (October 25, 2002): 703. Others pointed out the ways that traditional review procedures were being attacked by the secretary and the administration. See, for example, Dana Loomis, "Unpopular Opinions Need Not Apply," *Science* 298 (November 15, 2002): 1335–36.

32. The American Academy of Pediatrics summed up the state of knowledge regarding childhood lead poisoning in 2005 and reaffirmed it in 2009, acknowledging the revolution that had occurred in lead research over the preceding thirty years. There was no safe level of lead for children: "Evidence continues to accrue that commonly encountered blood lead concentrations, even those less than 10 µg/dL, may impair cognition, and there is no threshold yet identified for this effect." See "Statement of Reaffirmation," *Pediatrics* 123 (May 2009): 1421–22, available at http://pediatrics.aappublications.org/content/123/5/1421. full.pdf (accessed September 28, 2012), which provides a bibliography of supporting materials for its original statement, "Policy Statement, Lead Exposure in Children: Prevention, Detection, and Management Committee on Environmental Health," *Pediatrics* 116 (October 2005): 1036–46. See also American Academy of Pediatrics, Committee on Environmental Health, "Screening for Elevated Blood Lead Levels (RE9815), Policy Statement," *Pediatrics* 101 (June 1998): 1072–78.

33. See Jonathan Harr, *A Civil Action* (New York: Random House, 1995), for Woburn, Massachusetts, and Markowitz and Rosner, *Deceit and Denial*, for Louisiana's "Cancer Alley," the Mississippi River petrochemical corridor between Baton Rouge and New Orleans.

34. In essence, the conservative arguments against regulation rely on a view of science in general, and of epidemiology in particular, that is overwhelmingly reductionist, seeing the world in mechanistic terms that cannot account for the complexity of interactions and social relationships that determine outcomes in complex systems. Increasingly, much of mainstream epidemiology is rejecting this reductionist assumption. Scientists such as Mervyn Susser, Ezra Susser, David Ozonoff, Steve Wing, and Samuel Shapiro have developed sophisticated analyses of the role of epidemiology in uncovering environmental diseases. No single study (epidemiological or in any other discipline) is definitive, they remind us, and no discipline alone can complete the process of proving causality.

35. David Michaels, *Doubt Is Their Product: How Industry's Assault on Science Threatens Your Health* (New York: Oxford University Press, 2008);

Thomas O. McGarity and Wendy E. Wagner, *Bending Science: How Special Interests Corrupt Public Health* Research (Cambridge, MA: Harvard University Press, 2008); Naomi Oreskes and Erik Conway, *Merchants of Doubt: How a Handful of Scientists Obscured the Truth on Issues from Tobacco Smoke to Global Warming* (New York: Bloomsbury Press, 2010).

36. U.S. EPA, Office of Pollution Prevention and Toxics, "TSCA Chemical Testing Policy," 2001, available at www.epa.gov/oppt/chemtest/sct4main.html (accessed September 26, 2011).

37. U.S. EPA, "HPV Chemical Hazard Availability Study," available at www.epa.gov/hpv/pubs/general/hazchem.htm (accessed September 26, 2011)

38. "Children's Environmental Health: An Interview with Bruce Lanphear, MD, MPH, by Fred Lanphear," Center for Ecozoic Studies.

39. World Health Organization, *Childhood Lead Poisoning*, 11, 32. Hundreds of children have died and many more have been permanently injured by lead in northern Nigeria, poisoned while mining for gold as well as by the pollution produced by the mining industry. See, for example, "Lead Poisoning Continues to Plague Northern Nigeria," *Nature News Blog*, May 14, 2012, available at http://blogs.nature.com/news/2012/05/lead-poisoning-continues-to-plague-northen-nigeria.html (accessed May 15, 2012).

40. Naomi Oreskes and Erik Conway, *Merchants of Doubt: How a Handful of Scientists Obscured the Truth on Issues from Tobacco Smoke to Global Warming* (New York: Bloomsbury Press, 2010).

41. National Research Council, Committee on Environmental Epidemiology, *Environmental Epidemiology*, vol. 1, *Public Health and Hazardous Wastes* (Washington, D.C.: National Academies Press, 1991), 270.

42. J. Julian Chisolm Jr., "The Road to Primary Prevention of Lead Toxicity in Children," *Pediatrics* 107 (March 2001): 583.

43. "Executive Summary" in *Review of Studies Addressing Lead Abatement Effectiveness: Updated Edition*, by Nancy A. Neimuth, Brandon J. Wood, Jennifer R. Holdcraft, and David A. Burgoon, EPA 747-B-98-001 (prepared by Battelle for U.S. EPA, Office of Pollution Prevention and Toxics, December 1998).

Index

abatement, 132–38; CDC recommendations on, 132, 137–38, 164; conflicting meanings of, 130–31, 140; cost of, 19, 126, 133–34, 135–36, 265n48; as dilemma for public health, 27, 124–25, 164–67; Herbert Needleman on, 19–20, 135–37, 140, 141, 164–66, 216; HUD and, 125–27, 131, 133–35, 137, 146; and landlord abandonment, 2, 36, 152; limited funding for, 20, 57–58, 131, 133–34; partial, 1–2, 19–21, 27, 132, 154, 163–67, 230, 279n117 (*see also* KKI study); unsafe methods of, 126–27, 147–48, 263n17, 265n45, 267n10
ACORN, 210
acrilonitrile, 95
ACT-UP, 124
Addams, Jane, 3
ADHD, 219, 221, 228. *See also* hyperactivity
Advisory Committee on Childhood Lead Poisoning Prevention, 218, 224
African Americans, 44, 50, 149–50, 277n97; in KKI study, 1, 21, 159, 168, 178, 190, 214; lead poisoning among, 16, 30–31, 36, 48–49, 71, 92, 135, 165, 178. *See also* Tuskegee Syphilis Study
Agency for Toxic Substances and Disease Registry (ATSDR), 109–11, 145–46

AIDS, 25, 124, 145, 166–67, 192, 277n97
Alliance to End Childhood Lead Poisoning, 138–40, 164, 165, 177, 194, 210
American Academy of Pediatrics, 34, 132, 188, 285n32
American Association for the Advancement of Science, 77–78, 88
American Chemistry Council (formerly Manufacturing Chemists Association), 192
American Enterprise Institute, 228
American Journal of Public Health, 33, 35, 160, 164–66, 183
American Petroleum Institute, 228
American Public Health Association, 47–48
aminotriazole, 52
Anaconda corporation, 199
Anderson, Jack, 249n86
Angle, Carol, 99
Annual Reviews of Public Health, 130–32
Archives of Environmental Health, 40–42
Aronow, Regina, 67
arsenic poisoning, 14, 74, 94
ASARCO, 74–76
asbestos, 95, 202, 205–6, 207, 208
Ashton, Claudia, 132–33. See also *Ashton v. Pierce*